THE STORY OF
SURGERY

An historical commentary

For Stella

THE STORY OF
SURGERY

An historical commentary

Revised and expanded edition with bibliography

Robert Richardson

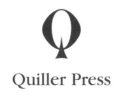

Quiller Press

First published in the UK under the title *The surgeon's tale*.
Copyright © 1958 George Allen & Unwin, Ltd

Published in the USA under the title *The story of modern surgery* (slightly revised).
Copyright © 1964 George Allen & Unwin, Ltd

Published in the USA under the title *Surgery: old and new frontiers* (revised and enlarged).
Revised text copyright © 1968 Robert G Richardson

This edition published in the UK in 2004
by Quiller Press, an imprint of Quiller Publishing Ltd
The moral right of the author has been asserted

British Library Cataloguing-in-Publication Data
    A catalogue record for this book is
    available from the British Library

ISBN 1 904057 46 2

Designed by Jo Ekin
Set in Garamond 10/13pt
Printed in England by Biddles Ltd., www.biddles.co.uk

Quiller Press

an imprint of Quiller Publishing Ltd
Wykey House, Wykey, Shrewsbury SY4 1JA, England
E-mail: info@quillerbooks.com
Website: www.swanhillbooks.com

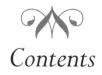

Contents

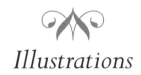

Illustrations

Horace Wells
William T.G. Morton's demonstration of ether anaesthesia
Theodor Billroth
Joseph Lister
Johannes von Mikulicz-Radecki
Theodor Kocher
An operation of the antiseptic era
Jean Zulema Amussat
Artificial anuses
Excision of the inferior part of the rectum
The intestines: from Vesalius
William Macewen
Théodore Tuffier
William Arbuthnot Lane
William Stewart Halsted
William Halsted operating
Trigeminal neuralgia – a drawing by Harvey Cushing of the surgical anatomy
Harvey Cushing

Harvey Cushing operating
Wilder Penfield
X-ray of a total hip replacement
The American Civil War: A Union Ambulance Corps
World War I: Collecting the wounded
The Carrel-Dakin treatment of wounds
World War II: A British surgical team operating in a church in Italy
X-ray of Werner Forssmann's self-catheterization of the right side of his heart
A cloth-covered Starr-Edwards mitral valve
The operating theatre at Groote Schuur Hospital, Cape Town
Christiaan Barnard, Michael De Bakey and Adrian Kantrowitz

Preface

In the pages that follow I have tried to trace in broad outline the evolution of modern surgery, including details as required or as they took my fancy. With events before, say, fifty or so years ago it was usually easy to pick out the person to whom credit should be given for suggesting and/or first performing an operation. Since then, progress has been achieved mainly by teamwork - and frequently by different teams working on the same problem - so it is often impossible to identify precisely who introduced something new, or even when. In the broadest of terms progress may be said to be occurring along two main lines: one is the refining of techniques that has allowed horizons to be broadened, and the other is set fair to transform the face of surgery in a manner that could well take its place alongside anaesthesia and asepsis in the grand order of things. I refer to minimally invasive surgery which is probably familiar to many in the shape of keyhole appendicectomy and removal of the gall-bladder; but other adventures in many other parts of the body would take your breath away. In consequence, as this book is a history and not a review of current practice, the story stops, with one or two exceptions, on the verge of what is happening in today's operating theatres - as I have said before, in the midst of events we lose perspective.

The two big differences in this new edition are, first, the addition of new material which has increased the length by about a third, and second, the inclusion of the bibliographic sources, missing from its previous manifestations. Sometimes the dates do not coincide with those given in the text; this is because, amongst other reasons, reports take time to prepare and to be published. Sometimes, too, the name of the senior author, as mentioned in the text, may not be the first to be listed - a quirk found mostly in the more modern references. I would urge those of you who would like to make most use of this book to use the indices and, particularly, the bibliography - not so much to check the source as to round out the information in the text. In the Index of Personal Names, the dates are as complete as I can make them. When they have eluded me I have simply put the date of the event with which that person was associated.

Finally, I am truly grateful to my friend Air Commodore RF Brown, FRCS, RAF (Retd) for volunteering to read and then discuss the typescript. His advice has been invaluable, particularly in regard to the surgery of warfare, and I have taken on board virtually all his many suggestions.

2004 RGR

1

By the banks of the Styx

'I saw the hand of M. Dubois held up, while his forefinger first described a straight line from top to bottom of the breast, secondly a Cross, & thirdly a Circle; intimating that the WHOLE was to be taken off....

'Yet – when the dreadful steel was plunged into the flesh – cutting through veins – arteries – flesh – nerves I needed no injunctions not to restrain my cries. I began a scream that lasted unintermittingly during the whole time of the incision – & I almost marvel that it rings not in my Ears still! so excruciating was the agony. When the wound was made, & the instrument was withdrawn, the pain seemed undiminished, for the air that suddenly rushed into those delicate parts felt like a mass of minute but sharp & forked poniards, that were tearing the edges of the wound....

'To conclude, the evil was so profound, the case so delicate, & the precautions necessary for preventing a return so numerous, that the operation, including the treatment and the dressing, lasted 20 minutes! a time, for suffering so acute, that was hardly supportable.'

When the patient was carried to her bed, she opened her eyes and 'saw my good Dr Larry [sic], pale nearly as myself, his face streaked with blood, & its expression depicting grief, apprehension, & almost horror.'

These excerpts are from no work of fiction but come from the account written by Fanny Burney, the English novelist, to her sister, Esther, some nine months after her mastectomy[1]. The operation took place on September 30, 1811, just over a year after diagnosis. The surgeon was Dominique Jean Larrey, Surgeon-in-Chief to Napoleon's Imperial Guard, who, one might have thought, would have become inured to the horrors of the appalling injuries that could be inflicted on the human body – but this was 'cold' surgery. He was assisted by

Antoine Dubois, a surgeon to the Imperial Household, and by his friend and colleague, François Ribes; two other doctors and two trainee surgeons were also present. Fanny survived to live for another twenty-nine years, dying at the age of eighty-eight.

The first half of the 19th century was a time for revolution. Following the Americans and the French, many peoples rose up to free themselves from oppression. Yet perhaps the greatest revolution of them all – certainly the greatest and the most beneficial to the entirety of mankind – took place with little more than a murmur of dissent. In 1846, anaesthesia was 'discovered' in Boston, Massachusetts. Surgeons all over the world quickly responded to their new-found freedom to operate – only to find it as illusory as the political form of freedom.

In pre-anaesthetic days a surprising variety of surgical procedures had been undertaken, though on a superficial anatomical level and mostly for trauma. Some, such as repair of hernias, cutting for stone in the bladder and couching for cataract, with some frequency and often by itinerant operators; others, such as removal of a breast for cancer, but rarely. Even more rarely a 'heroic' surgeon (with courage or foolhardiness – call it what you will) would tackle a case that would bring tears to your eyes even to think about. But when death was otherwise inevitable, any chance was worth taking – and very occasionally it would come off. Furthermore, the surgeon had at his disposal a wide selection of often beautifully crafted instruments, specially designed for given purposes. Even so, surgery was not a happy experience for either patient or surgeon; the pain was exquisite and a sensitive surgeon would sometimes be physically sick after operating. Yet despite death being more probable than life, the fact that patients would submit to the knife is testimony to the suffering they were enduring.

Although the absence of pain led to an increase in the number of operations performed, it did not have a marked effect on their scope. It was a naïve surgeon, indeed, who believed that, with the disappearance of pain during operation, all the other problems that had vexed him for centuries would miraculously disappear too. But naïve is just what most of them were. Infection could not be anaesthetized with the patient; nor could shock – the inability of the body to withstand the onslaught. And be sure it was an onslaught. Everything that happened from the moment surgery was decided upon had a deleterious effect on the patient's physiology. He himself was bound to be apprehensive at the very least and likely to be debilitated as a result of his disease. The surgeon had yet to learn the importance of delicate handling of the organs and tissues rather than the desperate pursuit of speed. And the man dripping ether or chloroform on to a gauze mask had no conception of what he was doing other than producing insensibility. There is far, far more to the art of surgery than the wielding of a scalpel on an unconscious human being, and only slowly over the ensuing generations did intensive research and experimentation bring this home.

A point that is very important to bear in mind is that, before the mid-19th century, concepts that we take as a matter of course today would have been totally incomprehensible. Doctors then would not have known what we were talking about if we tried to discuss anaesthesia, bacterial infection or virtually anything that is part and parcel of modern surgery. Entrenched ideas are always difficult to shift, but once they have been broken down and what is about to replace them has been understood and accepted, progress is rapid and perhaps explosive – until the concept of the replacement itself is challenged. Clues have usually been hovering in the wings, maybe for decades or even centuries, before a decisive discovery allows the penny to drop – and it is not always the person who makes the discovery who appreciates its significance.

Infection, often in any case already present, was the consequence of operation that mainly troubled the surgeon. Its presence was all too readily apparent, either through the formation of pus or from the patient's condition. But, within their conceptual limitations, old-time surgeons did their best and had accumulated a considerable body of understanding through careful observation – though with the ancient humoral theory of disease still being at the root of much thinking some of the conclusions were inevitably wide of the mark. As a result they had established a number of general principles: in traumatic wounds, all foreign debris (or as much as possible) had to be removed; if ligatures were inserted, they were to be left with long ends so that they could be pulled out when they had served their purpose (short ones which could not be removed were at risk of becoming foreign debris themselves); free drainage had to be established from the depths of the wound; and all shed blood had to be removed (although they weren't to know it, blood is an ideal culture medium for bacterial organisms). And they had learnt that the membranes lining the abdominal cavity (the peritoneum), the chest cavity (the pleura), and surrounding the heart (the pericardium) were highly effective barriers to infection. It was thus extremely unwise to breach their defences.

So, the difficulties that beset surgeons before the mid-19th century may be summed up in three words: pain, infection and bleeding – and, as a consequence of any one of these, shock which could be lethal. One of the effects of shock is to lower the blood pressure and this in turn lessens the force of bleeding. As an indication of human perversity and to illustrate what the early proponents of anaesthesia were up against, some people argued that it was a mistake to relieve the pain since it abolished surgical shock.

The philanthropic wave that began in the 17th century brought with it the establishment of many new hospitals and the number of surgeons increased to serve them. The benefit to surgery was not as great as might be imagined, for the standards of public health and personal hygiene were truly appalling, and owing to the almost inevitable development of postoperative infection any surgical procedure became a really hazardous undertaking. In 1651 a certain John Finch wrote to his sister from Paris:

'The Hôtel Dieu, God's House, next to the Church of Nôtre Dame, is, I believe, the best hospital in the world, either in respect of the numbers of sick persons, which is about 2000, or their accommodation, which is as good as any sick person requires, save that the multitude of the diseased makes them forced to lay six or eight in one bed, which hinder certainly the recovery of many and infects others fully that had but a little beginning of a disease in them. 'Tis to me a strange thing to see how many persons of quality come thither, their charitable dispositions making them dispense with that offensive smell which cannot but be very great where so many diseased persons infect the air…. There is scarce ever a night in the year but some die out of this place.'

Before this period infection of wounds had always been a problem, though not nearly as great, and from time to time surgeons had appeared who, by simple attention to cleanliness had shown that the production of pus was not a necessary part of wound healing. During the Middle Ages and onwards they were few and far between, since the accepted treatment of wounds was such that pus was inevitably produced and was consequently regarded as part of the natural healing process. By the 17th century, with its dirty hospitals overcrowded with even dirtier patients, no treatment then known would prevent wounds becoming infected. The concept of 'laudable pus' thus became generally accepted. The pus was termed 'laudable' because its presence indicated that the infection was due to comparatively harmless bacteria which the body could fight and, generally, ruled out infection with virulent bacteria that led to gangrene, blood poisoning and, as often as not, death – pus was therefore a good thing and to be encouraged.

As long as no one knew why infection occurred, nothing satisfactory could be done to prevent it, but in the middle of the 19th century Louis Pasteur discovered bacteria; Joseph Lister saw how this applied to surgery and with true genius introduced antisepsis. Lister realized that bacteria were in the air and could contaminate wounds, either directly or by means of the instruments that came into contact with the wound. Antisepsis implied the destruction of germs before they could reach the tissues. The use of carbolic acid was revolutionary and reduced the mortality rate from surgery, but it was only a step in the right direction, not the solution to the problem. This came in the shape of asepsis: by attention to scrupulous cleanliness the incidence of wound infection was eventually lowered to an irreducible minimum. It was indeed fortunate that anaesthetics had been discovered before Lister carried out his remarkable work, otherwise his principles might not have been so readily accepted as they lengthened the operating time and that would most certainly not have been welcomed.

If a wound becomes infected it does not heal immediately but gapes open to allow the escape of pus and finally heals by what is known as 'secondary intention'. In the absence of infection or other complicating factors the edges of a clean wound are brought together by stitching or by clips and the wound heals by primary intention. This happened in the past in the hands of a few men who unwittingly grasped the fact that it was possible for wounds to heal without suppuration. Another basic principle of wound surgery, occasionally appreciated, is that war or accident wounds will only heal by first intention if all foreign material and dead tissue are removed from the wound and the edges of the wound made clean-cut. This is the process that has come to be known as debridement, but should strictly be called wound toilet. Débridement is a French word meaning unbridling and was originally used in the surgical context to mean the relief of constriction by incision, usually the incision of a fascial layer at the bottom of a wound to relieve the build-up of tension in underlying tissues. Doubtless it owes its modern usage to an imagined derivation from debris.

Bleeding has interested mankind since earliest times and attempts to control it are just about as ancient. In the main, the story of this aspect of surgery has been one of crude and unsatisfactory methods. Styptic powders which usually provoked the formation of pus, red-hot cauteries, boiling pitch slapped on amputation stumps and other agonizing methods held pride of place for centuries. Yet even in quite early times an exceptional surgeon might employ ligation: he would tie the bleeding artery or vein or, in the case of lesser haemorrhage, he would twist the end of the vessel – a technique known as torsion. Other difficulties to be overcome, apart from the initial control of bleeding, were 'reactionary' haemorrhage and 'secondary' haemorrhage. During the operation the blood pressure fell, due to shock and loss of blood; a few hours later (with any degree of luck) recovery took place and the blood pressure began to rise with the result that any bleeding points incompletely controlled started to bleed again, and ligatures not properly applied were prone to slip off. This is reactionary haemorrhage. Secondary haemorrhage is due to infection and usually starts about ten days after operation. It was particularly common when styptics had been employed, but if death did not intervene persistence won the day. Since ligatures in those days could not be made sterile they were liable to cause infection with consequent bleeding and had to be removed – another reason why they were left with long ends. Nevertheless, in the 19th century the daring practice of cutting silk ligatures close to the knot and burying them in the wound was adopted with a fair degree of success.

Generally speaking, in those early days the surgeon's main concern was whether the patient lived or died; an operation might well be a technical success but the patient could be left a mutilated wreck. A man who had been cut for stone in the bladder might be leaking urine incontinently from the wound in his perineum. Patients could be crippled or left unable to care for themselves after amputation; satisfactory artificial limbs were unknown. The pain of disease was not infrequently exchanged for pus, blood and misery which might remain with the patient until death – sooner rather than later.

Before the beginning of the 19th century, and especially during the Middle Ages, it was almost essential that a prospective surgeon should go to the wars to obtain experience in his art and to fit himself for civil life, which for most was little else besides the treatment of injuries. The surgical staff of hospitals consisted of veterans who had seen soldiers, brave and unflinching (and probably drunk) in the face of the enemy, reduced to screaming in agony with their ministrations. Blood flowed freely, and thanks to contamination from soil and clothing and to the methods the surgeon used to staunch the bleeding and dress the wounds, pus soon followed in a riot of stench, fever and death. No wonder the average military surgeon, unable to understand the cause of all this and so unable to do anything about it, wanted a change to a quieter and more settled, though scarcely less horrific, existence. The growth of hospitals gave him the opportunity of gaining his experience at home, and so, once the challenge of infection had been met, surgery was able to progress along more ordered lines. The continuation of wars did, however, provide a stimulus to the development of surgery, and after the two World Wars remarkable advances were made by surgeons who had, on the battlefields, found that necessity was indeed the mother of invention and had returned to civilian practice to investigate and improve on the many ideas that had come to them.

Back in very early times the same inquiring spirit was already at work: the athletic contests, so much a part of Greek culture, provided a rich harvest of fractures and dislocations from which, by trial and error, the surgeon was able to devise admirable and correct methods of treatment. More bloody experience was gained from the gladiatorial bouts of the Roman Empire, which gave an excellent opportunity to those curious enough to observe the appearance, position and even workings of the internal organs.

Another essential, and this time absolute, is a sound grounding in anatomical knowledge. In the words of the 14th-century surgeon, Guy de Chauliac, 'A surgeon who does not know his anatomy is like a blind man hewing a log'. The importance of this has been appreciated since earliest times, but the acquisition of knowledge has been beset by superstition and religious prohibition. Anatomy can be learnt only by dissection of the human body, yet for various reasons such as respect or awe of the dead, the 'uncleanliness' of a dead body, and certain religions forbidding dissection, anatomical learning proceeded in fits and starts. Many incorrect assumptions, often derived from the study of animals, persisted through the ages in the writings of surgeons whose works were held to be the last word in accuracy. It was not until the early 16th century and the work of Vesalius that anatomy began to be based on accurate observations.

Throughout history there has been the occasional individual who was in advance of his time. Some of these men introduced and perfected techniques or practices which, after their death or that of their immediate pupils, faded gently into obscurity, remaining only in their writings. Their contemporaries were simply children of their time and cannot be blamed for refusing to accept these revolutionary ideas. But when the world was ready and knowledge had reached a suitable level, keen observers whose 'minds were prepared to appreciate the significance of their observations', as Pasteur expressed it, arose and incorporated the advance into the general body of learning. The man or woman who rediscovers at the right moment is hailed as the original genius, as in many ways they are, but we must not forget the pioneers who paved the way and were often scorned and hounded by their fellows.

2

A false dawn

The search for methods of relieving pain was for long periods pursued in a desultory fashion with little hope of its realization. Pain was regarded as inseparable from surgery. Nevertheless, from Ancient Egypt and on through all the major civilizations herbals – such as hebane, mandragora, indian hemp (cannabis) and the poppy (opium) – known to have a hallucinogenic effect and to dull the senses were employed. A hefty dose of alcohol was also popular. Surgeons of the ancient Hindu civilization employed wine, henbane and the fumes of cannabis, although Sushruta, an admirable recorder of the surgery of his day, recommended dashing cold water over the patient's face from time to time to ease the agony and accompanying sense of exhaustion. In Roman times, relief was attempted by pressing on the carotid artery in the neck with the aim of producing unconsciousness by depriving the brain of its blood supply. Regrettably, a satisfactory degree of unconsciousness all too often meant that the patient had reached the state where earthly troubles were of no further concern. The same difficulty was met when the ingenious Romans tried to adapt their popular method of suicide to more practical ends for, in theory, controlled bleeding from an artery in the wrist could produce unconsciousness. The correct degree of control was the problem, particularly as the operation itself added to the bleeding. A hearty blow to the head was another technique. In the 1st century AD, Dioscorides, a Greek surgeon in the Roman army, mentioned wine of mandragora for alleviating the suffering of patients being cut or cauterized, and was the first to use the word 'anaesthesia' (but remember what we said in the first chapter about grasping concepts). Besides giving the wine by mouth, he also recommended its use by instillation into the rectum, a method not reconsidered until relatively modern times.

During their period of medical supremacy, the Arabians preserved the possibility of insensibility in their translations until interest was revived in a practical manner with the emergence of the 'soporific sponge' in the 9th century. Its origin is attributed to an anonymous group of monks and for four centuries it was apparently widely used. Among those who were loud in its praise were Hugh of Lucca and his son, Theodoric of Cervia, both capable practising surgeons[1]. Recipes varied but the prime ingredient was opium followed by mandragora, hemlock, henbane, nightshade and an assortment of other herbals. The mixture was boiled with a sponge and while hot (or after heating in hot water) was applied to the nostrils as often as required. However, in the early 20th century doubt was cast on its effectiveness and, indeed, on its very existence. But whatever the truth, the English arrived at a solution which had the merit of simplicity; a bullet to bite on for ordinary seamen, rum for petty officers and junior officers, and rum and laudanum for senior officers.

The events leading up to the acceptance of ether as the first general anaesthetic were a series of disjointed fumblings that started with the isolation of nitrous oxide by Joseph Priestley in 1772[2]. Twenty-six years later, the young Humphry Davy was working as assistant to Thomas Beddoes at the latter's delightful Pneumatic Institution, a 'sanatorium' where a gullible public was allowed full rein in obtaining the benefit of recent scientific advances. The Institution specialized in the treatment of chest diseases by the inhalation of nitrous oxide and other gases, with the object of assessing their value to medicine. The inquiring mind of Davy carefully observed the effect of these gases. Being particularly impressed with the ability of nitrous oxide to render patients insensitive to pain, he carried out further experiments on himself and noted also its exhilarating effect. When he published the account of his researches, Davy mentioned that the gas might be used in surgical operations: 'As nitrous oxide in its extensive operation appears capable of destroying physical pain, it may probably be used with advantage during surgical operations in which no great effusion of blood takes place.'[3] No attention was paid to this comment and Davy himself took the matter no further.

Davy's next contact with anaesthesia came in 1824, when he was president of the Royal Society and turned down the reports of a young physician named Henry Hill Hickman who had made the first attempt to carry out scientific experiments for the relief of pain in surgery – he rendered chickens unconscious with carbon dioxide gas[4]. An anonymous writer to the *Lancet* even hoped that Hickman's letter was a hoax[5]. Hickman turned to Paris for encouragement, but the only support he got was from Baron Larrey who was unfortunately outvoted; and that was the end of that.

In a roundabout way Davy's researches had a profound effect on future progress. When he had asked his colleagues at the Beddoes Institution to inhale nitrous oxide, the exhilaration produced had been so pleasurable that they continued the practice for amusement, and the habit spread to become a popular form of entertainment. In 1818 a report, attributed to Michael Faraday but more likely written by Davy, showed that ether would produce much the same effect with the consequence that it became fashionable as an inhalant at 'ether frolics'. Wandering lecturers on chemistry had a great vogue in America at this time and helped to popularize both ether and nitrous oxide (or laughing gas as it came to be called) by demonstrating their effects to music hall audiences. As these shows were riotous affairs, it was only a matter of time before someone noticed that the revellers could hurt themselves with no recollection of having done so, and then link this observation to surgery. The credit goes to Crawford Long, a general practitioner of Georgia in the United States of America, who gave ether parties in his surgery and then, after careful consideration, decided to try the vapour for a surgical operation. On March 30, 1842, the first operation under ether anaesthesia took place, when Long removed a cystic tumour from the neck of James Venable, a student. Everything went smoothly and successfully and it might be thought that the end of the trail had been reached, but although Long continued to use the anaesthetic in his practice and made no secret about it, he did not publish an account of the operation for another seven years[6]. Consequently ether anaesthesia remained unknown to the world at large and it was not until twelve years after the event that the squabble over priority claims led to his work being widely known, and even then it was publicized by someone else.

Crawford Long was not strictly the first person to use ether for the relief of pain, since in the January three months before his operation there had been an isolated incident in Rochester, New York, of which he was unaware. On this occasion a chemistry student, William Clarke, administered ether while Elijah Pope removed a tooth from a young woman by the name of Hobbie[7]. The validity of this operation to be claimed as 'the first' seems to have gone by the board, owing to a dental extraction not being considered a surgical operation and because Dr Pope was a dentist and anyway neither of the two participants attached any significance to the event. The views of the lady involved apparently bore no weight.

However, the experiments of Long and Clarke had no effect on the course of history and are of interest value only. The events that preceded the final acceptance of ether began in 1844 when Horace Wells, another dentist, was in the audience for a demonstration of laughing gas in Hartford, Connecticut. When one of the affected gentlemen tripped over in the aisle of the theatre and obviously hurt himself, Wells noticed that he seemed unaware of the pain. Wells induced Gardner Colton, the lecturer cum music hall artist - who, incidentally, had made a close study of Davy's writings - to visit him the next day and while under the influence of nitrous oxide, had an infected tooth drawn by his assistant. Greatly impressed, he realized that the induction of insensibility was of potentially great value to surgery; wondering how to get the idea publicized, he recalled that his former partner in an unsuccessful dental practice was now a medical student at Harvard. He communicated with this man, one Thomas Green Morton, who obtained permission for Wells to demonstrate a 'painless' tooth extraction before the class of Dr John Collins Warren, senior surgeon at the Massachusetts General Hospital, Boston. By a great misfortune the patient Wells elected to use as his subject was one of those little affected by nitrous oxide (a less generous explanation is that the anaesthesia was incomplete) and at the crucial moment the patient screamed; the students hissed and Wells beat a hasty retreat. Nevertheless, he continued his researches until the death of a patient finally disheartened him.

Morton's career as a medical student was considerably interrupted by his interest in insensibility which led him to make the acquaintance of Charles Jackson, an unscrupulous chemist, who advised him to try dulling the pain of filling teeth by the local application of ether. Having tried this satisfactorily Morton then turned his attention to giving the ether by inhalation; after experiments on puppies he successfully extracted a tooth from an insensible patient on September 30, 1846. Morton next approached Warren, who must have been exceptionally long-suffering and endowed with great faith, for despite the previous failure of Wells he agreed to operate with Morton giving the ether. As Morton was not a qualified doctor, Warren must have realized that his own reputation was at stake, as well as that of the hospital which he himself had founded in 1821. But agree he did and on the morning of October 16, 1846, the steep tiers of the operating theatre were filled with the sceptical members of the hospital staff. The patient, a tuberculous printer by name Edward Gilbert Abbott, who had a 'vascular' tumour at the side of his neck, was sitting in the chair in the tiny pit feeling apprehensive and not at all sure whether he was prepared to go through with the operation. Promptly at ten o'clock all chance of escape disappeared when Warren, a tall striking figure despite his sixty-eight years, entered the theatre. Morton was missing. After waiting a few minutes, Warren, who probably never expected Morton to put in an appearance, turned to the audience and announced:

'As Dr Morton has not arrived, I presume he is otherwise engaged.'

The audience made suitably sympathetic noises and Warren picked up the knife. At this moment there was a disturbance at the door and Morton rushed in explaining that he had been delayed by having the finishing touches put to his apparatus. Completely unperturbed Warren stepped back and said:

'Well, sir, your patient is ready.'

Morton immediately applied the inhaler to the patient's mouth and after three long and anxious minutes Edward Abbott gradually lapsed into insensibility. Turning to Warren, Morton made the historic announcement:

'Dr Warren, *your* patient is ready.'

The atmosphere was tense as Warren made the incision, but when the expected howls failed to materialize, the frock-coated gathering appreciated that something unique was taking place and their scepticism gave way to respect. The operation over, Warren outwardly as calm as though he had been operating on insensible patients all his life, but with tears in his eyes, faced the audience:

'Gentlemen, this is no humbug.'

(From his use of the word 'humbug' it would seem safe to assume he was familiar with the anonymous letter in the *Lancet*[5] of some twenty years previously, disparaging Hickman's work.)

After this successful demonstration the curiosity of the medical profession was aroused, but Morton regrettably behaved in an unethical manner as, realizing the importance of ether, he tried to ensure his own financial security. He first refused to reveal the nature of the liquid and went to the extent of disguising its smell with aromatic oils. Then, calling his preparation Letheon[8], he took out a patent for his inhaler[9], hoping thereby to confuse people into believing that ether was part of the patent. The ruse failed, the inhaler became obsolete, and soon everyone knew that the liquid was ether and Morton earned the censure of the medical profession. Meanwhile, the classical mind of Oliver Wendell Holmes, to become the following year the professor of anatomy at Harvard, was distressed at the choice of name and in November 1846 wrote to Morton:

'Everybody wants to have a hand in a great discovery. All I will do is to give you a hint or two as to names.

'The state should, I think, be called "Anaesthesia".... The adjective will be "Anaesthetic". I would have a name pretty soon, and consult some accomplished scholar ...before fixing on the terms, which will be repeated by the tongues of every civilized race of mankind'[10]. The hint was taken and the word, coined by a Roman Greek, came into everyday use.

The first official account of the operation was published in the same month by Henry Jacob Bigelow, who had been present on that memorable day[11]. His paper caused an outcry that the doctors were allowing themselves to fall into the hands of quacks, but owing largely to the fact that Warren, the professor of surgery at Harvard, had performed the operation and thanks to his enthusiasm, the fame of ether for producing surgical anaesthesia spread rapidly. Before a year had passed the vapour was in widespread use in Europe as well as in America. However, the subsequent story of the first anaesthetists was far from happy. Except for Crawford Long, who was content to let others worry about his claim, they all became involved in unsavoury litigation which for most of them led to an early death. [The story of the first years of anaesthesia was well told in a book edited by Richard Henry Dana[12], the author of *Two years before the mast*, a best-selling account of his experiences working his passage round Cape Horn.

Horace Wells was an unstable character and tried to take the glory from Morton by arguing that it was he who had given Morton the idea in the days when they had collaborated over the use of nitrous oxide. Frustrated by his efforts, he became interested in chloroform anaesthesia, which had been used in 1847 in Scotland, and endeavoured to introduce this to America as superior to ether[13]. In 1848, finding himself in jail for throwing acid at two girls, he decided the time had come to put an end to his career and so committed suicide.

Morton had in the meantime petitioned the American Congress for an award in recognition of his discovery; a figure of 100 000 dollars was decided on, but he never received it as a Senator put forward Long's claim, Jackson entered one of his own and eventually the Civil War gave Congress other things to think about. Jackson, for one reason or another, seemed determined that if he himself could not get the money then Morton most certainly would not. When his own claim failed he made out that the deceased Wells was a martyr and that Wells's widow was entitled to the award; then he championed Long and finally, having ruined Morton financially and professionally, he ended his days in an insane asylum. Morton, utterly worn out by this persecution, developed nervous trouble and died a pauper on a park bench at the age of forty-nine years, unknown and forgotten.

The first time ether was used for a major operation in Great Britain was another historic occasion, and it was perhaps fitting that the surgeon should be Robert Liston, a remarkable man who had raised surgery to a degree of perfection probably unsurpassable without the aid of anaesthesia. Physically he was extremely powerful and exulted in this power, which enabled him to perform operations in a manner not available to his colleagues. Because of this he was popular with the patients, who asked nothing more than that the operation should be over quickly. Nevertheless, another school of surgeons was almost anticipating the arrival of anaesthesia and, rather than amputate, were operating to try to save limbs – much slower but, when successful, obviously gave a much better functional result. It was all the more to Liston's credit, therefore, that as soon as he heard of ether, he should decide to use the technique that would make these conservative operations an everyday occurrence.

Considering the slowness with which news travelled in those days and the little that Liston could have known about surgical anaesthesia, it was a creditable feat to undertake a major amputation within ten weeks of the first successful use of ether, but on December 21, 1846, he amputated the leg of an unconscious patient. The operation took place at University College Hospital; the patient was Frederick Churchill, a thirty-six- year-old butler who some time previously had sustained a compound fracture of his leg, in which the broken tibia had penetrated the skin. This had been set by hand but, as almost invariably happened with this sort of fracture, it became infected and when blood poisoning developed only amputation would save his life. Churchill was lifted onto the wooden table and the usual preliminary of strapping the patient down was duly performed. As he removed his coat and rolled up his sleeves Liston remarked:

'Gentlemen, we are going to try a Yankee dodge to make men insensible.'

There is some doubt over who actually administered the anaesthetic; it was either Peter Squire, a pharmacist, or his nephew William Squire, a young chemistry student (the odds would seem to favour William, since it was he who, forty-two years later, wrote an account in the *Lancet*[14]). Nevertheless, whichever one of them it was placed the sponge over Churchill's mouth and for the next few minutes the only sound was the patient's breathing. When Churchill was unconscious Liston quietly asked an onlooker to time the operation. In twenty-five seconds the leg had been removed through the thigh, done as only Liston could do it, using his right hand to cut and saw and his left to grasp the thigh pressing on the artery to stop the bleeding; an incredible performance.

As Churchill came round he asked, 'When are you going to begin?' In answer he was shown the stump, but his overwrought mind could not grasp that the operation was really ended and he broke down and wept. However, returned to his bed five minutes after he had left it, he soon recovered and became the centre of attention for many days. Back in the operating theatre, his voice shaking, Liston made the classic remark:

'This Yankee dodge, gentlemen, beats mesmerism hollow.'

Among those standing round the table was a young doctor destined to have an equally great impact on the practice of surgery. His name – Joseph Lister.

However, there is rather more to the story than simply a successful operation under ether anaesthesia. The news of Warren's operation and of the use of ether had reached Britain before mid-December in a number of letters sent by one or two writers to their friends; two included a copy of Bigelow's paper which had been reprinted verbatim in the *Boston Daily Advertiser* of November 19. But only one recipient understood the significance of the news, and that was an American, Dr Francis Boott, a friend of Bigelow's father and now living in London. Boott it was who notified Liston and Boott it was who gave the first ether anaesthetic in England and, as in America, it was for a dental extraction. But unlike the American experience there was no animosity and Boott behaved with true professionalism and did his utmost to promote the merits of ether anaesthesia.

Boott had enlisted the services of his dentist friend, James Robinson, who removed a molar tooth from a Miss Lonsdale on December 19. In his paper in the *Lancet* of January 2, 1847[15], Boott, besides recording this operation, included Liston's letter to him of December 21 describing the amputation of Churchill's leg and noting that he had also removed a great toenail of another anaesthetized patient.

Yet there was still another occurrence that was brought to the attention of the medical profession in a letter written by William Scott to the *Lancet* in 1872[16]. Scott stated that ether was exhibited on December 19, 1846, in the Dumfries and Galloway Royal Infirmary. The operation was reputed to have been the amputation of a limb. Whatever the truth of the matter, James Young Simpson, who we shall meet in a moment, was satisfied with its authenticity and included mention of it in his lectures.

Strange as it may seem now, ether anaesthesia was having a hard time in America. As the first anaesthetist of note, John Snow, wrote in the preface to his book *On chloroform*[17] 'Considerable opposition was made to the inhalation of ether in America soon after its introduction, and it seemed likely to fall into disuse when the news of its successful employment in the operations of Mr Liston, and others in London, caused the practice of etherization to revive.' This was in no small measure due to the efforts of Dr Boott.

The fickleness of history is once again demonstrated in the next phase of the story because, in Britain at all events, the name popularly associated with the discovery of anaesthesia is that of James Young Simpson. It is true he discovered the anaesthetic value of chloroform and was instrumental in getting the anaesthetic accepted, but he did not discover chloroform and his experiments with the liquid took place a year after the value of anaesthesia with ether had been demonstrated. The explanation lies in the fact that Simpson was a great man, he was already famous as an obstetrician and would have claimed a place in history had he never concerned himself with chloroform. His genius was apparent in his face, voice and manner; he completely absorbed the attention of those around him and, of particular appeal to his patients, his expression was gentle. His physical qualities also demanded attention, for though of medium build, he had broad shoulders surmounted by a large head with a flowing mane and massive brows. Added to this there is a romantic ring to the story of his career and of his experiments and later arguments over chloroform. Thus does history select her favourites.

Simpson was the seventh son of a village baker in Scotland, and thanks to the scraping and saving of his family was able to go to Edinburgh University, which he entered at the age of fourteen. The first two years he spent studying Greek and philosophy, but through a friend he became attracted to the lectures of Robert Knox, the professor of anatomy. Initially attending these lectures out of curiosity, he soon was fascinated and abandoned his classical studies to become a medical student. He received his MD in 1832 for a thesis on inflammation which attracted the attention of John Thompson, the professor of pathology, with the result that Simpson became Thompson's assistant; in his spare time he lectured on obstetrics. In 1839 the professorial chair at Edinburgh became vacant and, though Simpson was only twenty-eight, Thompson held him in such high regard that he urged him to apply for the post. In those days the appointment was in the hands of the Town Council and candidates had to campaign for votes. Simpson entered the fray with his characteristic drive and enthusiasm, lecturing and canvassing and spending nearly £300 in the process. He soon discovered that, besides the matter of age, his chief opponent, Evory Kennedy from Dublin, was married and Simpson was still single. This was likely to mean defeat, it being only right and proper for the professor of obstetrics to be a married man; so, nothing daunted, Simpson disappeared to Liverpool when his campaigning was done to return a few days later with a bride, the former Miss Jessie Grindlay, and to be elected to the Chair by a majority of one vote.

His lectures on midwifery rapidly became among the most popular in the University and his practical skill and sympathetic nature soon made him the most sought after obstetrician in Scotland. His concern for the welfare of his patients led to an interest in anaesthesia, and when he heard that his old friend, Robert Liston, had used ether for a surgical operation, he at once saw its possibilities for relieving the pains of childbirth. Accordingly, he travelled to London and what he learned from Liston so impressed him that he returned determined to give ether a try in childbirth.

The nature of childbirth, involving both mother and unborn child, and the complications to which labour was particularly prone in those days, all added to the hazards of moving into uncharted territory. Simpson was advised that by using the vapour he might cause convulsions in the mother, serious haemorrhage from the womb, the death of the baby before its birth could be completed or that it might be born an idiot. Such an array of unpleasant obstacles would be enough to make anyone think twice, which Simpson did, but as such hazards were common enough anyway, he eventually concluded that he had little to lose and much to gain. However, he was a canny Scot and waited for a suitable case in which there would be little hope for either mother or child and in which ether anaesthesia, if successful, would be life-saving. An eminently suitable patient was not long in appearing; she had a grossly deformed pelvis and in her previous pregnancy had been in labour for four days, the infant only being withdrawn after it had been mutilated in the womb to allow its extraction. On this occasion, Simpson was on hand and when she went into labour he made her unconscious with ether. With one hand in the womb and the other helping by pressure on the abdominal wall from outside, he proceeded to manipulate the child through the birth canal.

This was the first of many successes in which Simpson used ether both for performing an obstetrical operation and for easing a difficult childbirth. Yet, in spite of the success and popularity of ether, it was not long before Simpson became dissatisfied on account of the large quantities needed, its unpleasant smell and its irritating effect on the lungs which brought on coughing and, not infrequently, pneumonia. Simpson and his assistants therefore started experimenting on themselves by inhaling the vapour of almost any volatile liquid that came their way.

The experiments became social occasions and on the evening of November

4, 1847, there were gathered in the Simpson drawing-room two of his friends, Drs George Keith and James Matthews Duncan, his niece Miss Petrie, and one or two other ladies. After the men had tried the various vapours chosen for the session, all with no effect, they felt that the ladies had been deprived of their entertainment and so wracked their brains for something else to try. Simpson recalled that he had been sent a sample of chloroform but had considered the liquid too heavy and not sufficiently volatile to be of use and so had put it to one side; after a frantic search the bottle was found under a heap of papers on Simpson's desk. It was unstoppered and passed round the three men, who sniffed rather hesitatingly. The character of the party suddenly changed; the men became loquacious and indulged in a most 'intelligent' conversation to the delight of the ladies, bored by the unsatisfying scientific arguments that had been their previous fare. The sniffing continued and the voices became louder until one by one, the men fell insensible to the floor. For about five minutes the ladies fluttered round in anxious agitation, only the sound of heavy breathing reassuring them that life was not extinct. Their relief was all too evident when Simpson opened his eyes, gathered himself and looking at his still unconscious friends realized that here was an anaesthetic far more effective than ether: Matthews Duncan, lying under a chair, his mouth wide open, snoring loudly, his eyes staring at the ceiling; Keith, kicking vigorously at the upset supper table, quite oblivious to any pain. They repeated the experiment many times that same night and even induced Miss Petrie to have a sniff at the bottle. Her behaviour convulsed the others as she folded her arms across her breast murmuring, 'I'm an angel; oh, I am an angel!' The outcome of this hilarious gathering was that Simpson, within the next eleven days, used chloroform on fifty occasions for a variety of operations and before the end of the month, in the issue of November 20, had had his results published in the *Lancet*[18].

Thus the liquid, which had first been isolated independently by a French, a German and an American chemist in 1831, came to be employed as an anaesthetic agent, though its acceptance as such was not achieved without difficulty. Simpson came under fire from both the medical profession and the general public, but he was equal to fighting the onslaught from both directions and answered his attackers in terms that each could understand. The medical profession was up in arms, maintaining that anaesthesia constituted unnecessary interference and might cause convulsions or the birth of an idiot, arguments that Simpson had already considered before using ether, and which he now countered by presenting facts and figures to display incontrovertible evidence that such complications did not ensue and, in the case of operations such as amputations, that the mortality was reduced when the patient was given an anaesthetic. He used chloroform extensively in his own practice and wrote pamphlets and gave lectures that convinced scientifically minded people of its benefit to mankind. His greatest difficulty came from the church and religious bodies, for at that time a puritanical Calvinism had a hold in Scotland and the clergy raised their voices to denounce the use of chloroform in labour as unnatural and against the very teaching of the scriptures; had not God himself pronounced that women in childbirth must bear the curse of pain? The quotation illustrating their point came from Genesis 3, verse 16, 'Unto the woman he said, I will greatly multiply thy sorrow and thy conception; in sorrow thou shalt bring forth children…' Simpson contended that in this context sorrow did not mean suffering in the sense of pain, but as labour or physical exertion. In reply to the thrust that anaesthesia was unscriptural, Simpson himself quoted from the Bible: 'And the Lord God caused a deep sleep to fall upon Adam, and he slept: and he took one of his ribs, and closed up the flesh instead thereof'. Undeniably the pain of the very first operation was alleviated by unconsciousness, a point noted even by Calvin in his writings.

But still the argument continued and it was only the wisdom of Queen Victoria in allowing chloroform to be administered to her for the birth of Prince Leopold in 1853, that eventually put an end to the controversy and consolidated the place of chloroform as the most popular anaesthetic agent in Great Britain, a position it held for the next fifty years. The credit for this must really go to John Snow who gave the anaesthetic to the Queen and who did much necessary research on the use of ether, chloroform and other anaesthetic drugs[17, 19]. Although he considered ether to be the safer anaesthetic and incapable of causing death when used intelligently, the surgeons with whom he worked asked that chloroform be used in preference, despite the fact that chloroform was known sometimes to cause a sudden cardiac arrest. The extent of the surgeons' influence is seen in the fact that Snow gave chloroform nearly 4000 times in the following eleven years and ether only about a dozen times.

Amongst the upholders of ether was the doomed Morton, who took time off from his litigations to voice some well-balanced pronouncements on chloroform[20]. He had learnt that it was dangerous to give chloroform when the patient was weak from any cause, when the heart was not sound or when the patient was old or frightened; 'There is no reason for diminution of confidence in the efficacy or perfect safety of sulphuric ether; while there is an unanswerable reason why chloroform should be abandoned'. Owing to the risk of heart failure, he considered it unjustifiable to use chloroform simply because it was less disagreeable, more powerful and cheaper.

The possibility of administering ether by means other than inhalation was investigated, and a chosen method was to introduce either liquid ether or an ether and water mixture into the rectum. The first experiments were carried out on animals (three dogs and a rabbit) in 1847 in Paris[21], but at the same time

Nikolai Ivanovich Pirogoff was proceeding independently in St Petersburg. When he proposed introducing liquid ether into the rectum it was pointed out to him that this was potentially dangerous, so instead he devised a way of introducing ether vapour into the bowel and tried it on animals[22]. As this was successful he used it in eight operations including a plastic procedure on the nose which lasted three-quarters of an hour[23]. But even though the work was reported in a prestigious French journal, the idea failed to catch on and the arrival of chloroform saw the end of rectal anaesthesia for many years.

Another and more adventurous route was to inject a drug into a vein. This was first done in dogs in 1872 by Pierre Cyprien Oré using chloral[24]. He followed up these experiments two years later by treating a man of fifty-two who had contracted tetanus. After three intravenous injections of chloral at twenty-four-hourly intervals the man recovered. Inspired by this Oré removed an injured nail from a patient under intravenous chloral anaesthesia without difficulty[25]. As now seems inevitable the idea was not pursued and not until the mid-20th century and the arrival of improved techniques and more suitable drugs was it revived.

In the early days, the relationship between anaesthetist and patient cannot have been a very happy one as in most cases the anaesthetic was dripped onto a gauze-covered mask. It took some minutes for the anaesthetic to take effect, time that was largely passed subduing a struggling, half-asphyxiated, retching and sometimes vomiting patient. After the operation, vomiting was the rule and if ether had been employed the chest often became bubbly and pneumonia was a real danger. Anything that would make the anaesthetist's task easier and help to prevent post-operative complications was therefore welcome. Morphine was probably first used for this purpose in 1850, but the drug was certainly used as pre-medication by Claude Bernard in his experiments on dogs before giving them chloroform[26]. He mentioned that in 1864 a German, Neubaum, had used morphine to extend anaesthesia when he felt that the administration of chloroform had gone on for long enough. Atropine was also used in early anaesthetic times but the date when it was first used as pre-medication is uncertain; it was of the greatest value to both anaesthetist and patient, particularly when ether was used, since it reduced salivation and dried up the secretions in the lungs and air passages so lessening the chances of chest complications; it also helped to prevent the troublesome vomiting.

Without anaesthesia surgery could have progressed not at all and, though Lister might still have discovered the principles of antisepsis, his discovery could not have been exploited without the relief of pain.

3

Whitewash to carbolic

Surgeons revelled in their new-found freedom, now at last they could delve into the hidden parts of the human body sure in the knowledge that they were causing the patient no pain and could take their time to search out and eliminate disease. Operations, previously attempted only as life-saving measures, could now be undertaken as almost routine procedures; surgeons rose to the occasion and began exploring the possibilities of their art. An idea of the extent of their adventuring can be gained from the figures of the Massachusetts General Hospital, where nearly three times as many surgical operations were performed in the five years following the introduction of ether as in the previous five. Thus it might be thought that everything in the surgical garden was rosy.

Unfortunately, no. Before long surgeons discovered that although apparently free to explore where they would, the barrier of infection and sepsis raised itself in the path of their advance and made any surgical intervention a hazardous undertaking. And, with anaesthesia in such a primitive state, time was most certainly not on their side. Operations might succeed technically, only for the patient to succumb later to blood poisoning. The increasing number of operations performed, together with the ambition of the operators, made the problem of infection one of the first magnitude and one that had to be overcome before surgery could progress further. The mortality rate varied according to the surgeon, the operation performed and the hospital, so it is difficult to arrive at an accurate picture of the true state of affairs. In the period just before he introduced his antiseptic technique Lister had a mortality rate from amputations of 45 percent, and figures for other operations and other surgeons reached 80 percent. Simpson, in his well-known comment, assessed the situation rather neatly when he observed that 'a man laid on an operating-table in one of our surgical hospitals is exposed to more chances of death than the English soldier on the field of Waterloo[1]. (Nevertheless, he was somewhat wide of the mark since Digby Smith quotes a figure for *British* losses – killed, wounded and missing – of 29·9 percent of those involved and for the average losses among the entire Allied armies of 19·2 percent[2].)

The need for cleanliness had been known since very early times and practised diligently by a few, and these few, as a result, had been able to achieve healing by first intention. But, when confronted by a new idea, especially one that seems unnecessary and bothersome, it is in the nature of mankind to ask why, and if the answer is unsatisfying, to pursue the old established way with sublime indifference. So with cleanliness. No one understood the need for it. Pus was common and expected; in fact, should the wound show signs of healing naturally, the surgeon would go so far as to apply irritating dressings to provoke the desired result. However, the chance of his having to do this was remote when we consider the operating ritual. The surgeon would like as not enter the operating theatre direct from lecturing the students in the anatomy laboratory, where he had been handling the bodies; he would remove his immaculate morning coat and don his operating garb of an apron or an old morning coat liberally caked with the blood and pus of his previous endeavours. Then, without washing his hands, he would pick up the knife, admittedly sharp but soiled by many dirty fingers, and get to work on an unwashed patient lying on a wooden table that harboured a multitude of germs. The whole proceedings were closely watched by an audience breathing heavily over the point of action.

As noted in the first chapter, there are, broadly speaking, two types of bacteria that may infect a wound: those which are not particularly harmful and remain in the wound to produce masses of pus, and those which enter the blood stream giving rise to blood poisoning, erysipelas or a condition known as wound fever or hospital gangrene. This rough classification is not intended to take account of bacteria that produce specific infections such as tetanus or gas gangrene or the many other types of organism that may wreak havoc in the human body.

Strangely enough, in certain cases of plastic surgery, amputations through healthy tissue and operations on the face, most surgeons appreciated that pus formation was a bad thing, delaying healing and ruining the desired cosmetic result, but their appreciation did not extend to surgery in general. In all fairness, conditions were very much against this appreciation. Since the majority of operations were a consequence of injury, the patient was almost bound to arrive with a dirty wound or one that had already become infected, and so pus was the expected norm.

Before bacteriology appeared on the scene, attempts had been made to prevent infection, but in the absence of any scientific rationale they were all empiric and nothing more than shots in the dark, though based on accurate observation of their healing effects. Wine had been used by the ancients, for instance the Good Samaritan, to cleanse wounds, but the whole concept of infection had been utterly confused and complicated by Aristotle who had stated the theory of spontaneous generation of germ-like creatures[3]. He believed that lowly verminous creatures with no evident means of reproduction originated spontaneously from dung heaps, rubbish dumps, decaying flesh, and similar obnoxious gatherings – like unsavoury Aphrodites arising from waves of corruption. In the face of such an idea, which held its place until Pasteur discovered bacteria and showed that they had 'parents', any rational progress was impossible. Many were the fanciful speculations about the miasmata and methods of combating them; a popular weapon was the use of whitewash, which contains lime, for painting the walls of hospitals, mortuaries and other places where the danger was known to lurk, and chloride was used to disinfect dirty linen and to treat sewage. At the beginning of the 19th century France held the lead in surgery and also produced some advanced ideas for dealing with infection. The man with most influence was Antoine-Germaine Labarraque who used chloride of lime to treat infected wounds and in 1825 reported three years of uninterrupted clinical success by both physicians and surgeons[4]; he was the first to use the word disinfection in this context. At that time, the practice of washing the hands in a solution containing chlorine was recognized in Marseilles as being important in the prevention of hospital gangrene.

The next stage in the story concerns puerperal fever, an infection that attacks the womb after childbirth when its interior is nothing more nor less than a large raw wound. The fever has causes similar to those producing wound fever, although this was not realized until the 18th century. Various theories, such as the failure to produce milk, were proposed and even when Claude Pouteau in 1760[5] stated its identity with wound fever his views were not generally accepted. Shortly after, light began to dawn when there were some disastrous epidemics of the disease, particularly in Dublin. In the spring of 1787, Joseph Clarke, the Master of the Rotunda, a Dublin maternity hospital, stopped one of these epidemics by having the walls and ceilings whitewashed, the woodwork painted, and the bedding washed and exposed for days to the open air. There were to be fires by day and the windows were to be left open at night. He also advised against frequent internal examinations and manipulations. During the remainder of the year there were nine hundred and sixty deliveries and only three women were lost – one of whom had twins[6]. In 1795, Thomas Denman[7] and Alexander Gordon[8] independently published books in which they showed that puerperal fever was contagious and again established its identity with wound fever.

Epidemics continued and in Dublin the measures advocated by Clarke failed to hold them in check. Eventually in 1829 Robert Collins, a son-in-law of Clarke, decided to use the French method of fumigation. To start with, the wards were filled with chlorine gas in condensed form for forty-eight hours; the floors and all woodwork were then covered with chloride of lime mixed with water for another forty-eight hours. Next, the woodwork was painted and the walls and ceilings washed with fresh lime. Blankets and clothing were in most instances scoured and all were stoved at a temperature of 120–130° (the units were not stated but were almost certainly degrees Fahrenheit). Each ward was then treated every ten or twelve days by washing with chloride of lime and its linen was suspended in chlorine gas. The floorboards were polished. Between February 1829 and November 1833 no patient was lost. The mortality rate among 10 785 patients was 1 in 186[9]. Then, what now seems the inevitable came to pass: when Collins left the hospital his methods were abandoned, puerperal fever returned, and life (or death) settled down once again into what was then considered normality.

During the next few years more papers were written supporting the theory that puerperal fever was due to contagion, and in 1843 Oliver Wendell Holmes brought the full force of his literary talent to bear upon the subject emphasizing the practical point that puerperal fever 'is so far contagious as to be frequently carried from patient to patient by physicians and nurses.'[10] Holmes had been educated in Paris and therefore was aware of the work on disinfection proceeding in France; he had also read Alexander Gordon's book, and so in addition to his own researches he had plenty of data at his finger-tips. His paper was enthusiastically received abroad, but in America the older school of obstetricians thought Holmes was being a little too clever and attacked him vigorously. In later years Holmes got his own back by writing beautifully phrased comments on his critics: 'skilful experts, but babies, as it seemed in their capacity for reasoning and arguing'.

Nevertheless, he was not entirely deserted by his fellow countrymen. In 1846 Samuel Kneeland described most carefully and accurately the methods by which puerperal fever could spread; these included direct contact with 'fluids' from the living or the dead, the atmosphere around an already sick person and by means of clothing or bedding that had been in contact with a diseased patient[11] – and this, remember, was before bacteria, the infecting agents, had been discovered. In his second paper, he wrote: 'these two diseases [puerperal fever and erysipelas] have the same origin, one and the same contagion operating in the production of both.'[12] In Scotland, Simpson washed his hands in chlorine water after dissecting.

Thus by 1847 a system of disinfection had been developing for at least a hundred years amidst considerable opposition and difficulties; but if the scattered evidence is consolidated into a single advance it had reached a remarkably high standard. Chlorine was used for fumigation, chlorine water for washing the hands and chloride of lime for scrubbing the rooms; the identity of puerperal fever and erysipelas was known and the means by which the diseases were spread was appreciated. Yet despite the results obtained, it is a most peculiar fact that the methods were used only in one or two places, surgeons and obstetricians at large continued along their septic path. This seems so incredible that some explanation is called for; the easy answer is stubborn pig-headedness and a refusal to accept the accumulated evidence, particularly as there was no known logical reason why the methods should be effective. However, in those days knowledge of the accumulated evidence did not spread very easily as there were few medical societies where doctors could get together and argue about their discoveries, and articles in the medical press had a narrow circulation. The medical world was just not ready.

So why did the Fates smile on Semmelweis and award him such romantic epitaphs as the 'Saviour of Mothers'? The answer has to be that the controversy he stirred up and the eminent men who took sides led to a widespread awareness of disinfection, especially in Europe. Semmelweis discovered nothing new, introduced nothing new and was even incorrect in some of his beliefs; he did not consider puerperal fever to be contagious, which may seem a paradox as he knew the infection could come from dead bodies or contaminated hands or clothes. Where he went wrong was in not realizing that infection could be transmitted from one mother to another. Nevertheless, though his discoveries were not original, he arrived at the results by his own independent observations, and due to his personal zeal in promoting his methods, his name is the one popularly associated with the conquest of puerperal fever.

Semmelweis was a Hungarian, probably of German stock; he spoke both languages, the Hungarian with an accent and the German with uncertain phraseology. It is this that may have induced feelings of inferiority and accounted for his rather abnormal behaviour under stress when working in Vienna where German was the language spoken. He started his career by reading law, but soon changed to medicine and qualified at Vienna in 1844 at the age of twenty-six. An interest in obstetrics led, two years later, to his appointment at the Allgemeines Krankenhaus, the Vienna maternity hospital; before long, he noticed that the death rates in the two main wards differed markedly – a fact also well-known to the expectant mothers who would burst into tears if they found they were to be admitted to the wrong ward. Semmelweis analysed the differences between the wards and found that in the ward attended by the medical students the mortality rate was 12 percent whereas in the ward set aside for the training of midwives it was only 3 percent. Closely watching the behaviour of the students, he found that they would come from the dissecting rooms and examine the mothers internally without washing their hands. The next link was provided by the tragic death of the professor of medical jurisprudence who had cut his finger while dissecting and had developed blood poisoning. At the post-mortem examination, Semmelweis noted that the changes in the body were remarkably similar to those he was familiar with in the bodies of mothers dead from puerperal fever.

This led him to the theory that both conditions were due to some poisonous and probably living material derived from dead bodies, and that puerperal fever was transmitted to the mothers by hands contaminated in the dissecting room. Accordingly he made the students wash their hands in a solution of chloride of lime placed strategically in a bowl at the door of the ward. In the month following, the mortality rate dropped to 2 percent and in two months of the next year there were no deaths at all[13].

When his first paper appeared, Semmelweis ran into trouble with the head of the clinic, Professor Jacob Klein, who was decidedly unimpressed and attributed the favourable results to a change in whatever caused the disease. Semmelweis did not help matters by attacking Klein personally and holding him partly responsible for the shocking state of the wards. Fortunately, men eminent in other fields of medicine became interested in his work and realized its value, although the majority of obstetricians remained sceptical and were only finally convinced by the work of Pasteur and Lister.

Whether it was his future mental instability beginning to show itself or whether he believed his methods to be so obviously successful that they should be accepted on the evidence of his writings, Semmelweis did nothing further to advance the knowledge of puerperal fever. In 1850 he was given a teaching post in the Krankenhaus, but a few days after the appointment became effective he left without notice and returned to Budapest where he continued to practise midwifery, employing his method of disinfection with the same satisfactory results as in Vienna. In 1855 he was appointed professor of obstetrics at the university and began elaborating his earlier papers into book form[14]. In 1864 he showed definite signs of insanity and was admitted to a mental institution where he died the next year, ironically enough from blood poisoning from an infected finger.

During the years that Semmelweis was working in Hungary, a young French chemist was pursuing his investigations into the problem of alcoholic fermentation; at that time it was not known that yeast (the organism essential for fermentation) was a living organism and the whole process was considered to be entirely chemical. The early researches of Louis Pasteur showed Lister the way towards preventing wound infection and his later work laid the foundation of the science of bacteriology and with it an understanding of the cause of infection. As the role of bacteria in the economy of all living things is now an established fact, it is no easy matter to perceive the difficulties that Pasteur encountered in identifying something visible only under a microscope and then in showing that this microscopic organism was responsible for fermentation and disease. But Pasteur was no ordinary man of his day, content to sit back and formulate or accept theories without proof; he was a laboratory worker and experimentation was the very breath of his existence.

One of Pasteur's many achievements was to shatter the theory of spontaneous generation; this he did in a presentation to the Academy of Sciences in Paris in 1860[15] – though it took a few years longer before the pieces finally fell apart. For some time the theory had been viewed with increasing doubt, though there were still distinguished scientists who produced convincing arguments in its favour. Centuries earlier, rats and mice had been shown to reproduce quite naturally and maggots to be the larvae of flies; in the middle of the 18th century an Italian, Lazaro Spallanzani, proved to his own satisfaction that spontaneous generation from dead organic material did not occur[16]. (Unfortunately, such impact as his book might have had was rather scuppered by the notes to the French translation being written by John Needham who was convinced that micro-organisms might arise from inert organic material.)

Controversy, inevitably, continued and the next stage was the belief that 'animalcules' in the air were responsible for decomposition; in 1854 Heinrich Schröder and Theodor von Dusch designed an experiment to demonstrate this[17]. They placed some animal material in a flask and only allowed air to enter through cotton wool, thus filtering off the animalcules and preventing putrefaction. The idea was excellent but unfortunately they were not consistent in their results as their methods were faulty and, unknown to themselves, bacteria did gain entry. Far more elegant experiments were required and these were provided by Pasteur.

The experiments that initiated the science of bacteriology and that showed Lister the way to antisepsis in surgery were started quite by chance in 1854, while Pasteur was head of the newly-created faculty of science at Lille and officially engaged in the study of certain acid crystals. He was approached by a manufacturer of alcohol who was in difficulties, and out of his offer to help arose an interest in this new field which, aided by his uncanny intuition, led directly to all his future work. In Lille and later in Paris, Pasteur showed that the fermentation of both alcohol and sour milk was dependent on microscopic organisms which came from the atmosphere, and he proved his point by the exclusion of air, using a more reliable method than that of Schröder and Dusch. Moreover, he also showed the bacteria under the microscope.

Next, in 1864, the wine coming from the Jura district was being unaccountably ruined and Pasteur was called upon to investigate the crisis. He discovered that the wine was being contaminated by unwanted bacteria; these he destroyed by warming the wine to a temperature of 50–60°C for a very short period and from this simple procedure developed the practice of pasteurization. The use of heat to kill bacteria was also to find application in surgery a few years later for the sterilization of instruments and other materials.

Pasteur was also summoned to save the silk industry of France which was being crippled by disease. For five years he laboured and when eventually he discovered its cause and how to prevent it, his triumph was shattered: 'Il y a deux maladies!' Pasteur's cry of despair was echoed by the industry. After more hard, infinitely painstaking work, this second disease was also conquered.

The monumental discovery of bacteria and their effects having been made, it remained for someone to apply Pasteur's work to wound infection, and the man chosen for this was Joseph Lister, the son, curiously enough, of a prosperous wine merchant, though this had nothing to do with his interest in fermentation. The Lister family had been Quakers for a long time and so naturally Joseph was educated at Quaker schools; from quite an early age he had decided to devote his life to the alleviation of human suffering and at seventeen he entered University College, London, at that time one of the few university institutions where adherence to the Church of England was not demanded of students. He qualified eight years later and for a few years worked at experimental physiology which he considered to be essential ground-work for a good surgeon; in this belief he was ahead of his time as an understanding of the body's function is as important to a surgeon as is that of its anatomy.

When the time came for him to broaden his knowledge of practical surgery, Lister obtained a letter of introduction from his professor to James Syme, one of the most competent surgeons in the British Isles and long an advocate of conservative surgery. Syme was the professor of clinical surgery at Edinburgh and thither Lister went to study the great man's methods intending to stay only a few weeks, but so impressed was he that he accepted a post as very junior assistant. After a year, in 1854, he was appointed Syme's house surgeon and another year later he was successful in his application for the jobs of lecturer in surgery at a school outside the University of Edinburgh and of assistant surgeon to the Royal Infirmary. These vacancies arose owing to the death from cholera in the Crimea of Richard James Mackenzie, an exceptionally brilliant young surgeon for whom a great future had been predicted.

During these years Lister helped to publicize Syme's work and teachings by sending summaries of Syme's lectures to the *Lancet*; he also continued with his physiological researches, becoming particularly interested in the study of gangrene and inflammation of wounds, work that paved the way for his discovery of antisepsis. It is interesting to note that at this stage of his career he showed a scientific approach to surgery though he was not basically a scientist, as demonstrated by some of the errors and mistaken beliefs in his application of antisepsis.

In 1856 an event occurred that makes one wonder whether there may not have been something more than surgery behind his decision to stay in Edinburgh working under Syme; Lister married Agnes, Syme's eldest daughter. This must have caused him much heart-searching since Agnes belonged to the Episcopal Church of Scotland, and it was the custom for a Quaker marrying outside the Society of Friends either to resign or be compelled to do so. Lister resigned and adopted the religion of his wife, much to the regret of his family, although his father, in writing to Lister's sister showed true tolerance by remarking that one must be careful not to say anything unkind about people who may turn out to be superior to oneself. Perhaps the good man had an insight into Lister's potential and the help that Agnes was to be to him.

To ease his financial state, the remuneration from his official appointments being scarcely adequate for the upkeep of a family, Lister set himself up in private practice. Success eluded him and, to his considerable relief, in 1860 he was appointed professor of clinical surgery in Glasgow. This post enabled him to progress on his own account for, although a careful, methodical surgeon, he was without the brilliance of his father-in-law who would have continued to overshadow him had he stayed in Edinburgh; Syme acknowledging this, had encouraged him to apply for the Glasgow job.

Conditions in the surgical wards of the Glasgow Royal Infirmary were appalling; hospital gangrene was rife and the mortality from wound infection was amongst the highest in the British Isles. Lister thus had at his disposal a large number of patients to observe and on whom he could try different ideas to see if he could reach a solution to this perplexing problem. In order to devote himself wholly to the surgical care of hospital patients, he departed from the habit of his predecessors and did not engage in general practice outside his hospital duties.

For some time it had been known that infection of wounds was more likely to occur in hospital patients than in patients treated at home, in fact the incidence of wound fever was almost directly proportional to the size of the institution. Simpson called the condition 'hospitalism'[1] and speculated that it was caused by 'morbific contagious materials from the bodies of the inmates' which may seem a rather obvious remark, but was a correlation of two facts, the significance of which had not previously been grasped. However, it did not proceed beyond the stage of speculation and surgery was still waiting for someone to elucidate the real cause of infection.

Lister was soon completely immersed in the problem as he was seriously worried that patients having come successfully through their operations should still have to face a far more dangerous ordeal. Gradually over the next four or five years he accumulated the information that was to lead to the eventual solution. The first observation of importance concerned simple fractures; these would unite without wound fever intervening, whereas compound fractures in which the overlying skin was broken were almost bound to end in suppuration. Next, he noted that whenever the skin was cut by the surgeon, the wound would become inflamed and probably suppurate. He concluded that the air coming into contact with the tissues of the body through broken skin was the cause of infection, although the air alone did not always produce the infection; a link was missing in the chain of causation. Unknown to him, that link had been provided by Pasteur's discovery of bacteria. So Lister continued to puzzle over the problem until in 1865 he mentioned his perplexities to Thomas Anderson, the medically-qualified professor of chemistry. Anderson recommended a study of Pasteur's writings feeling they might be of help; little did he dream that the outcome would have such mind-blowing consequences. Lister at once saw the analogy between putrefaction and hospital gangrene. The great revelation had at last come: bacteria in the air were the cause of infection; keep them away from wounds and the surgeon's troubles would be over. This simple exposition was to undergo considerable correction with the passage of time, but it allowed surgeons to see how sepsis could be brought under control, if not eliminated.

A pleasant afternoon's walk along the banks of the Eden at Carlisle had taken Lister past the local sewage works, where he noticed that the material being discharged onto the land had been treated with carbolic acid and the usual obnoxious odour made bearable; moreover, as he subsequently discovered, the cattle that fed in the fields did not get the usual intestinal infestation. He thought that here was something worth trying in his operating theatre – although unknown to him the acid had been advocated in 1860 as a substitute for chlorine by Küchenmeister[18] and François-Jules Lemaire[19]. As with Simpson and his initial cautious use of ether in childbirth, Lister also bided his time. In March 1865 he thought he had a suitable patient with a compound fracture of the leg, but the attempt was unsuccessful. Then on August 12 of that year he treated James Greenlees, aged eleven, for a compound fracture of his left leg; with the help of carbolic dressings the wound healed in six weeks[20].

He described eleven patients, nine of whom recovered without loss of the limb, one had to have an amputation and the other died. The number of patients was certainly small, but the results were just as certainly outstanding and far and away better than any other surgeon could expect. However, the title of the paper failed to convey the fact that a new and basically important discovery had been made. Consequently, the lay press, which pounced on the paper and gave it much publicity, and the medical press, too, completely missed the point of Lister's work, believing that all he had done had been to show the value of carbolic acid as an antiseptic.

To remedy the situation, Lister described his technique in a paper read before the British Medical Association meeting in Dublin on August 9, 1867[21]. For a large wound he used 'paste composed of common whiting (carbonate of lime), mixed with a solution of one part of carbolic acid in four parts of boiled linseed oil, so as to form a firm putty' which did not excoriate the skin. The paste was covered with a sheet of blocked tin to prevent evaporation. In the nine months prior to the meeting he had not had a single case of pyaemia (pus cells in the blood), hospital gangrene or erysipelas in his wards. That was fine, but this time, as indicated by the title of the paper, 'On the antiseptic principle in the practice of surgery', he made plain for all to see the reason *why* carbolic acid (or any other suitable antiseptic) worked and *why* he used it – to create a barrier that would prevent bacteria gaining access to the wound. The antiseptic era had arrived.

Surgeons in Britain were slow to take advantage of the method, though abroad Lister's publications had a much greater impact. In France, Just Lucas-Championnière was very quick to adopt Listerism – as this accessory to surgery soon came to be known – doing so in 1868 and publishing a short book on the subject in 1876[22]. Surgeons in other Continental countries, notably Germany and Austria, were also quick to see the advantages and were thus able to bring the horror of wound infection under control. Then, as yet again seems inevitable, the widespread use of antisepsis began to uncover its dangers and complications. The most obvious of these was the fact that carbolic acid itself was unsafe. In the strengths used it was liable to cause chemical burns, and in large wounds the amount required actually caused lethal poisoning by absorption of the acid into the blood stream. This difficulty was mostly overcome by reducing the strength of the acid to a 5 percent (1 in 20) solution. Other antiseptics were used by different surgeons and there were many variations on the original 'paste' and dressings.

Another considerable danger was the complete exclusion of air from the wound, which may seem strange since this very accomplishment led to the initial success of antiseptic surgery. Lister misunderstood the situation by believing the infection to come almost entirely from the bacteria in the air – unfortunately, in the conditions with which he was dealing, this route played only a small part. He did appreciate that bacteria could infect the wound from handling and from instruments (he advised washing both hands and instruments in carbolic acid) and that they might already be present in an open injury such as a compound fracture. Although carbolic acid as employed according to the antiseptic principle kept fresh bacteria from invading a wound, Lister was ignorant of the fact that it was only partially successful in killing those already present. Thus the carbolic dressing succeeded in surgical wounds and in injuries not already infected, but was sometimes disastrous in wounds already infected; these misfortunes played a large part in the controversy that very soon surrounded him. To understand the seriousness of the failures we need to know that in order to multiply and do their damage most bacteria require oxygen, but there are others that thrive only in its absence – and amongst these are the spores of the tetanus bacterium and certain gas-gangrene organisms. If any of these happened to be present in a wound, or were introduced during operation, the outlook was bad. Lister, however, attributed these unfortunate occurrences to incomplete exclusion of air-borne bacteria at the time of operation, and so he turned his attention to overcoming this new problem – and came up with an answer that is probably the best remembered item in antiseptic surgery.

But before he arrived at this particular answer, Lister had been working on one of the hazards that faced all surgeons: the likelihood of infection and secondary haemorrhage caused by the buried ligature. He solved this by soaking catgut for lengthy periods in carbolic acid which resulted in ligatures that were not only sterile but also absorbable. As he wrote in 1869, 'The surgeon, therefore, may now tie an arterial trunk in its continuity close to a large branch, secure alike against secondary haemorrhage and deep-seated suppuration, – provided always that he has so studied the principles of the antiseptic system…'[23] So important was this to surgery that Lister chose the catgut ligature as the topic of his presidential address to the Clinical Society of London twelve years later[24].

Syme, in the meantime, had had a paralytic stroke and in 1869 Lister returned to Edinburgh to fill the post of professor of clinical surgery made vacant by his father-in-law's illness. Syme died the following year as did Simpson who, in his latter years, had been an unswerving and almost vindictive opponent of Lister, a strange lapse from the sound judgment exhibited throughout his life and the more surprising since he had shown so great an interest in the problem of hospital infection. The reason for his antagonism is usually attributed to a long-standing quarrel with Syme, the feelings underlying which spread to include Lister when he became a member of Syme's family.

After he had been back in Edinburgh a year, he produced his answer to air-borne contamination – the carbolic spray. The apparatus consisted of a pump designed to spray 2 percent carbolic acid into the atmosphere of the operating theatre; it was worked by an assistant, at first by hand, then by foot, then by an extremely bulky donkey engine and finally by a smaller steam driven contraption. The alternative was to irrigate the wound at intervals during the operation and to syringe the wound cavity after stitching. Although Lister regarded the spray as the least important aspect of antisepsis, he favoured it over irrigation as being more effective and less likely to cause carbolic poisoning; but if there was no spray available, the surgeon should still abide by the antiseptic principle[25].

While he admitted that he would joyfully give up the use of the spray if it were proved that the idea of atmospheric contamination during operation could be thrown to the winds[25], he clung to its use in his own practice for nearly twenty years. His intellectual honesty shone out when, in 1899, he wrote: 'As regards the spray, I feel ashamed that I should have ever recommended it for the purpose of destroying the microbes of the air.'[26]

Almost from the beginning quite a number of surgeons found the use of the spray unnecessary and even his closest associates felt a bit ridiculous operating under such conditions. The death knell for the spray was sounded by Viktor von Bruns in his 1880 paper 'Fort mit dem Spray!'[27] It was highly influential and came as a great relief to many.

Another technical innovation popularized by Lister was the use of rubber tubes to drain matter from cavities, such as abscesses, or in other cases where there was a danger of infection and it was necessary to allow the escape of any fluids that might accumulate. The tube had, in fact, been introduced a few years previously by a Frenchman, but in 1871 Lister had an opportunity to use it in an exceptional case and one cannot but admire him for his courage in the choice of his first patient, a lady with an abscess in her armpit. Sir William Jenner, physician to Queen Victoria, worked the carbolic spray (some unaccustomed exercise for him); much to everyone's relief the operation was completely satisfactory since the patient was the Queen herself, then in residence at Balmoral. Thus was Lister's position as premier surgeon in Scotland officially recognized – and Queen Victoria's place in the history of both anaesthesia and antisepsis confirmed.

Edinburgh became a popular centre for overseas surgeons eager to learn about the new method at first hand, and when in 1875 he went for a holiday tour to Germany, Lister was overwhelmed by the warmth of his reception and his holiday tour turned into a triumph. Not so in England. However, when Sir William Fergusson, professor of clinical surgery at King's College, London, died in 1877, Lister was invited to fill the vacancy – an invitation not appreciated by the Edinburgh students who worshipped him. But Lister knew that antiseptic surgery had made little or no impression on the London scene and so considered it his duty to spread his teachings. He accepted and arrived in London to find things even worse than expected. It is unbelievable that a method adopted on the Continent where hospital gangrene and associated troubles were nearly eliminated, should be frowned upon and criticized in London, but such was the case. Sensibly, Lister had brought with him two dedicated assistants, for otherwise he would have had difficulty finding anyone to operate his spray. One of his first operations, on October 26, 1877, was to open a knee joint and repair a fractured knee-cap with silver wire – this horrified his new colleagues who regarded opening a joint as tantamount to asking for infection and inserting wire was to make a certainty of a probability. Yet Francis Smith's knee healed well. With more results like this his methods came gradually to be respected and eventually accepted. Lister himself also faced an uphill struggle since he was a sympathetic man and a slow, careful operator who, before a difficult procedure, would stand with head bowed and say a little prayer. This did not impress his London audiences, used as they were to the flamboyant showmanship of Fergusson who had milked the spectators for all he was worth. Moreover, if students answered their examination questions from what they had learnt at his lectures, they were sure to be failed by examiners antagonistic to Listerism. In the main, students attending his lectures were those already passed in surgery and who could therefore afford to take an interest in their new professor.

Slowly, it dawned on the English that Lister had revolutionized surgery; in 1883 he was created a baronet and in 1897 he became the first medical peer. When he died in 1912 surgery had undergone another revolution; antisepsis had given way to asepsis, but through the genius and quiet persistence of Joseph, Lord Lister, antiseptic surgery had brought healing to untold thousands.

4

Stomach, gall-bladder and pancreas

S urgeons were now standing on the threshold of a great future, anaesthesia and Listerism had thrown wide the doors, light and understanding flowed in with abundance. Long was the trail still to be followed, many were the false paths and many the difficulties and disappointments ahead, but at last the way for scientific advancement was open. It would, therefore, be as well to pause for a moment and consider the state of surgery as it entered the last quarter of the 19th century, in order to appreciate to the full the remarkable strides that were to be made in a relatively short period.

Anaesthesia was still very much in its infancy, being little more than unconsciousness produced with a mask and bottle, though vaporizers, inhalers and apparatus for administering nitrous oxide and oxygen were beginning to make their appearance. The Scottish surgeon, William Macewen, in protest at the practice of introducing the anaesthetic agent through a tracheostomy (a hole made into the windpipe) for operations on the upper respiratory tract, invented a flexible brass tube which he passed into the trachea by sense of touch, a feat demanding considerable dexterity in the conscious patient whose coughs and splutterings were soon quelled by the chloroform. After preliminary experimental work on cadavers, his first clinical use of the endotracheal tube took place on July 5, 1878; the upper end was packed around with gauze to prevent blood getting into the larynx[1]. Although other surgeons intubated the larynx during the next decade, the concept of endotracheal anaesthesia was not, however, pursued for another forty years.

Surgeons did not understand the effects that anaesthesia had on the human body; they only knew that it enabled them to perform operations humanely impossible unless pain was eliminated. Speed was still important but for different reasons than before, as it was now required to minimize shock and excessive loss of blood. In the years between the discovery of anaesthesia and the acceptance of the principles underlying Listerism, the operations did not increase in scope to any great extent, only in frequency. Sepsis halted the advance that had appeared so promising. Surgeons knew that the membranes lining the body cavities were effective barriers to the spread of infection from outside and it would be a foolhardy man who intentionally opened one of these cavities unless the disease or wound had got there first. The heart and interior of the chest were highly dangerous territories; the problems of how to maintain life while operating on the heart, or to prevent the lungs collapsing when the chest was opened were not even considered.

Surgeons were, however, familiar with the inside of the abdomen, albeit relations were not friendly, as it was almost a case of slip in, cut out a length of bowel and hurriedly remove the evidence of the visit in the hope that the body would allow the insult to pass unnoticed. The peritoneum was reputed, if cut, to produce a severe and frequently lethal peritonitis, but the later arrival of asepsis taught them to look on the peritoneum as a valuable ally since, when cut it can put up a strong fight against infection and deal with any germs that gain entry by walling them off in a localized abscess. The inside of the skull was an unprofitable field and the main concern was with head injuries, as very little was known about the effect of disease on the brain. Surgeons treated scalp wounds and skull fractures, and when clots of blood or abscesses formed over the surface of the brain they relieved the pressure by opening the skull and incising the dura mater to let out the clot or pus, but not infrequently the brain itself would extrude through the opening and a lethal infection ensue.

Conditions that later became amenable to early surgery were usually watched until there was nothing left to lose. Cancers in accessible sites were removed when they had become painfully obvious, which usually meant they had spread beyond the stage when the knife could be life saving; any operation would only be palliative.

The real contribution to surgery in the anaesthetic years preceding Listerism was the accumulation of knowledge in related subjects. The strides previously made in anatomy were being continued, especially in the elucidation of the microscopic structure of tissues; physiology was progressing fast, but most important were the advances in bacteriology and pathology. Slowly the nature of disease and the processes by which diseases evolved were becoming apparent; advances were made which enabled accurate diagnoses to be made and no longer was a diagnosis just a label to an illness, it implied what was then believed to be a complete understanding of all its aspects. Progress in physics, chemistry and other branches of science helped to clarify outstanding problems and permitted the investigation of hidden parts of the body. On the technical side, instruments and materials were improved and new ones invented; experiments on animals showed that certain hitherto untried operations, for instance removal of part of the stomach, were technically possible, but too dangerous yet to be tried on human beings. Events had reached a climax, the stage was set for the next act and it had been Lister who raised the curtain.

The extensive and complicated operations made possible by anaesthesia and antisepsis, combined with the need for speed, produced a new generation of spectacular surgeons, pioneering individualists blessed with courage and resourcefulness. In uncharted spheres they often had to take split-second decisions, only rarely could they fall back on the experience of some other operator who had found the answer to the problem they were facing. Specialization had not yet divided surgery into separate compartments and surgeons had to be able to turn their hand to anything coming their way and, as is often the way with pioneers, there were many among them who were rude and rough in their methods. Although a few developed a supreme skill and dexterity and could have undertaken a modern operation with but little practice, so great were the opportunities for an individual to invent a startling new operation, that it is difficult to tell at this distance in time, whether some may not have crept into history because of their unabashed exhibitionism.

In the period between the start of antisepsis and its fulfilment as asepsis (roughly 1870–1895), the practice of surgery underwent a transformation from a risky craft to a sound, moderately safe science. During these years an amazing number of previously hazardous or impossible operations were performed successfully and many soon became routine procedures. The only serious consideration restraining abdominal surgery had been infection, and tentative steps had already been taken towards its prevention by the ovariotomists whose skill (or lack of it) lay in the removal of ovarian cysts. The first successful ovariotomy was done by an American, Ephraim McDowell, on Christmas Day, 1809[2]. The patient was Mrs Jane Todd Crawford, aged forty-seven and the operation was a success; Mrs Crawford lived to be seventy-eight. Had McDowell not been successful, a lynching awaited him from the mob howling outside his house while the operation was in progress. Ovariotomies were tried by other surgeons without success and not until 1858 were the possibilities recognized by Thomas Spencer Wells; McDowell's achievement passed unnoticed.

The two famous ovariotomists of this period, Spencer Wells and later Robert Lawson Tait, achieved remarkably good results by a technique that foreshadowed asepsis. Lawson Tait was in fact a fervent adversary of Lister's method and refused to believe in the bacterial nature of infection; he achieved his success by scrupulous cleanliness and washing out the abdominal cavity with warm boiled water when the surgery had been completed. Spencer Wells also insisted on complete cleanliness and did much to forward abdominal surgery; his most memorable contribution was the invention, reported in 1879, of artery forceps for the control of bleeding from cut blood vessels[3]. These seemingly simple

Spencer Wells forceps, first made for him in 1872 and still in use today in only slightly modified form, were of the utmost importance to surgeons who previously had had to rely on pressure, usually supplied by their assistant's fingers, to control bleeding but were now able to clamp bleeding points immediately and proceed with the operation unhampered by fists of fingers obscuring the wound. Spencer Wells was lucky to have had history smile upon him as, twelve years previously, a French surgeon, Eugène Koeberlé, had invented his haemostatic forceps; unfortunately for him he did not publish the fact until 1893[4].

The scene on the Continent was greatly different to that in Britain, where Listerism was received not at all favourably. There the methods of antisepsis were studied with great care and there many of the major advances were made. Carbolic acid was used liberally in numerous European clinics; when Richard von Volkmann took charge of the surgical clinic at Halle in 1867 sepsis almost inhibited any attempt at operation, but by meticulous attention to every detail of antisepsis he was able to rectify the situation. In addition to the carbolic spray, he had assistants walking round pouring carbolic acid from watering cans, with the avowed aim that if dirt was unavoidable at least let it be antiseptic dirt. The surgeons wore rubber boots and the floor was specially constructed to allow the acid to drain away. Due to these precautions (one might almost say in spite of them) the Halle clinic became one of the foremost in Europe and surgeons came from far afield to study and to watch Volkmann operate.

Another outstanding surgical figure and one of the great surgeons of all time was Christian Albert Theodor Billroth, head of the surgical clinic at Vienna, who collected to his credit a formidable list of successful 'first' operations, both inside and outside the abdomen. Billroth was not only a remarkable and competent surgeon, he was also an accomplished musician and a kind, gentle man who brought to all his patients a breath of humanity combined with the sure knowledge that if surgery could possibly save them, his genius would give them life.

Born on the German island of Rugen in 1829, of Swedish extraction, Billroth was only five years old when his father, an impoverished preacher, died and left him in the care of a tuberculous mother with four other children younger than Theodor to look after. The love of music which, throughout his life, vied for first place with surgery, was inherited from his maternal grandmother, a celebrated singer at the Berlin Opera, and in his early years he very much wanted to make his career in music. However, his mother and an uncle, an eminent physician, persuaded him to study medicine and in due course he was sent to Greifswald, the nearest medical school on the mainland. During his first term he took advantage of a chance to study music and rarely attended medical lectures, but in his second a doctor friend of the family managed to stimulate a real interest in medicine. From Greifswald he went to Göttingen and from there to Berlin where he finished his studies, qualifying in 1852. For the next seven years he was assistant to Bernhard Langenbeck, one of the most influential of German surgeons at this time, and became absorbed in the study of pathology which later stood him in good stead. In 1859 he was appointed professor of surgery at Zürich where his restless energy and capacity for work led him in 1863 to publish his book *Die allgemeine chirurgische Pathologie und Therapie*[5] (*General surgical pathology and therapy*). This ran into eleven editions and was translated into many languages but although a learned and brilliant work, it was not until the later editions that it showed any material advance in surgical practice. As well as this, he composed a string quartet, a piano quintet and three trios which he later burned because, as he said in one of the many letters he loved to write, 'It was awful stuff and stank dreadfully as it burned'. He was also in demand as a music critic for the local newspapers, and on two occasions was guest conductor of the Zürich music society. Then, in 1867, he came as professor of surgery to Vienna, the scene of his future life and triumphs. For some time he had been extremely concerned about wound infections and a year after his arrival he began a systematic study to see whether there was a relationship between bacteria and these infections; he quickly realized that there was and that it was one of cause and effect. He, therefore, turned to Listerism for help, but unlike others who either adopted it without question or condemned it out of hand, he understood the reasons for the technique and appreciated its faults and disadvantages. Some of his comments give a picture of antiseptic surgery at its best[6].

'In short, in every detail, to the best of my power, I carried out Lister's and Volkmann's injunctions. Unfortunately to some extent, the system is based on imperfect scientific knowledge, and thus a certain amount of faith is demanded of those who obediently carry out every detail.'

Describing his methods for dressing wounds, he recorded two cases in which he had met with severe sepsis: 'The secretion of the wound was free from odour; both patients died. For a time matters went on better, but then cases of carbolic eczema became so common, that I gave up this antiseptic, replacing it by thymol.

'Without venturing to assert that I have come to any final conclusion on the subject of antiseptic dressings over other methods of treating wounds, I think I may say that practically it is an admirable method, and I shall always recommend it as safe and reliable, until some better mode of treatment has been devised. It is especially suitable for recent wounds, and for operations on tissues that are not suppurating.

'On one point I wish particularly to insist, viz. the absolute importance of carefully watching patients treated antiseptically. I have never felt so much anxiety in any other operation cases, for if they do not go perfectly well they generally go utterly to the bad.'

The wounds that went 'utterly to the bad' were those that were not completely sterile and free of bacteria; when these were sewn up and the carbolic dressings put in place it was possible for dangerous bacteria to create havoc. Regrettably, surgeons had no way of recognizing these hazards.

Billroth's first 'first' came in 1872 with the complete removal of a larynx for cancer[7] – though Patrick Heron Watson of Edinburgh had performed a similar operation on a syphilitic larynx in 1866[8]. During the next ten years Billroth did a great deal of experimental research into intestinal surgery, removing parts of the gut and working out ways of anastomosing (joining together) the cut ends satisfactorily. The foundations of intestinal suture had been laid in 1826 by a Frenchman, Antoine Lembert who introduced the technique of sewing sero-muscular layer to sero-muscular layer[9] (the intestine has four layers; these, from outside to inside, are: serous, muscular, submucous and mucous). The careful uniting of the outer two layers made all the difference between success and failure, but before Lembert's work the significance of the different layers was not appreciated and on the rare occasions when intestinal suture had been attempted the gut was simply 'sewn together' with almost certain failure of union and consequent leakage of intestinal contents and lethal peritonitis.

Billroth is now chiefly remembered for his work on gastric surgery and is generally considered the 'Father' of this specialty, though at the time the parentage was hotly disputed, two other surgeons having preceded him in performing operations on the stomach. Jules-Emile Péan in Paris had been first on the scene on April 9, 1879, but purely by accident: on opening the abdomen he unexpectedly found a cancer of the pylorus, at the far end of the stomach; so he did what seemed to him to be the obvious thing and cut it out, sewing the remainder of the stomach to the duodenum. The operation took two-and-a-half hours and the patient died during the night of the fourteenth–fifteenth day[10]. A year-and-a-half later, on November 16, 1880, Ludwig Rydygier, a German, did the same thing but as a planned undertaking; the sixty-four-year-old man survived only twelve hours, dying from 'exhaustion'[11]. On January 29,1881, Billroth successfully operated on a forty-three-year-old woman with cancer of the stomach and pyloric stenosis (narrowing of the far end of the stomach)[12]; she died four months later due to the cancer recurring and spreading to the liver.

These three cases illustrate the difficulties with which surgeons had to contend, since patients came to them with their disease well advanced and really beyond surgical help; and when they did eventually come they were in no physical shape to withstand the onslaught of surgery. Means of making them fit in the face of serious disease were still a long way in the future. Furthermore, the operation itself was beset with dangers and although major operations were undertaken, the actual details of technique were yet to be evolved; an understanding of the effects of major surgery on the body was lacking, and the wherewithal for resuscitating the collapsed patient was non-existent.

Billroth consolidated his position as the leading abdominal surgeon by the monumental amount of research and practical work done at the Vienna clinic. The gods truly smiled on him, as the foundations of partial resection of the stomach were laid by his assistants, Alexander von Winiwarter and Carl Gussenbauer, with their experimental studies on dogs[13]. Billroth only performed the operations on living human beings after he had worked them out on cadavers and felt he could be sure of technical success. Yet in spite of this his first operation for gastric cancer was followed by two failures. The interest taken by the lay public in surgical matters and their ignorance of the nature of Billroth's studies was demonstrated by their reaction to these failures: Billroth was actually stoned in the streets of Vienna. A lesser man would probably have become utterly disheartened at this, but by 1891 he had removed, for cancer, forty-one pyloruses with sixteen operative deaths – a remarkable feat for those days in terms of both numbers of operations and low mortality rate.

The method by which Billroth dealt with his first cases was to anastomose the cut ends of the duodenum and stomach, a procedure that became known as the Billroth I operation. After a few years it was frowned on, as the anastomosis was prone to leak. On January 15, 1885, the answer came about by accident. Billroth had to operate on a man of forty-eight with cancer of the pylorus who was in a terribly debilitated state. If he were to do his usual operation the shock would probably be lethal, so he decided to make an opening in the stomach and another in the small bowel and anastomose the two, thus effectively bypassing the cancerous area – a manoeuvre known as gastroenterostomy which, as we shall see, had originally been devised by one of his assistants, Anton Wölfler, and later used for other diseases, such as peptic ulcer. Having done this and seeing that the patient was in a fair state, he went on to excise the growth and simply stitched closed the cut ends of the duodenum and of the stomach[14]. Thus, the Billroth II operation was born to hold pride of place for many years; leakage was uncommon, and by creating a gastroenterostomy the openings in the stomach and intestine could be tailor-made for an exact fit, whereas joining stomach to duodenum, as in the Billroth I, meant that the opened end of the stomach had to be partly closed to leave a hole just the same size as the duodenum – a precise estimation was needed and only a small disparity would lead to trouble from leakage. Billroth felt within his heart that the first operation was the better but practical experience told him that the second gave better results. Over the years both were modified[eg 15-17] until there was little to choose between them. Two variations are, nevertheless, worthy of special notice. With his modification, William Mayo was able to report, in 1900, on a series of over seven hundred cases with a reduced mortality rate of 14 percent[18]. Eleven years later it was superseded by the Hungarian, Jenö Pólya's variation which allowed more extensive removal of the stomach[19] and became very popular.

The first time a stomach was removed in its entirety was in Rudolf Krönlein's clinic on September 6, 1897; the surgeon was Carl Schlatter and the patient was still alive on October 11[20].

Peptic ulcer is a strange disease. In the middle years of the 20th century, it was the abdominal surgeon's pay cheque; in the opening years of the 21st century, he has to find employment elsewhere in his territory since the disease is now almost a medical one with the bacterium *Helicobacterium pylori* and smoking playing prominent roles as risk factors in its causation; surgery is infrequently required. Whether this was the situation before the 1880s or whether the disease was not recognized is a matter for debate. At all events, peptic ulcer (which means either gastric or duodenal ulcer) came into surgical prominence when Rydygier removed part of thirty-year-old Karoline Pfennig's stomach on November 21, 1881[21]. A few months after his paper had been published it was abstracted in another journal under the title, 'The first resection for stomach ulcer' the editor appending the note 'I hope it will be the last.' As with cancer, surgeons were not getting the cases early enough and the patient was often anaemic as a result of bleeding from the ulcer; the ulcer could also have perforated or become stuck to the pancreas which could make surgery technically far more difficult. Towards the end of the century, when surgeons were gaining experience in their abdominal explorations, the true frequency of peptic ulcer became apparent and, largely due to the success of Eugène Louis Doyen[22], a Parisian surgeon, gastroenterostomy came to be a popular treatment, though recurrences or fresh ulcers at the anastomotic site were not uncommon.

As the years passed, in addition to growing experience, the conditions for operating improved and the Billroth operations or the various forms of partial or subtotal gastrectomy were also used in the treatment of peptic ulcer, and remained so for gastric ulcers. However, the approach to duodenal ulcers underwent a change when, in 1943, Lester Dragstedt put into practice an idea that had been simmering in his mind since 1935[23] and so inaugurated what became known as the physiological era of ulcer surgery. He attacked the problem at its very roots by showing how nervous stimuli transmitted down the vagus nerves to the stomach led to excess secretion of hydrochloric acid. If these stimuli could be interrupted the cause of the ulcer should be removed, and so he introduced the operation of vagotomy, or cutting the vagus nerves[24]. Nevertheless, recurrences of duodenal ulcer were not entirely prevented; furthermore, the motility of the stomach was reduced, which meant that the contents tended to linger and only pass on slowly. It therefore became necessary to devise further surgical techniques to overcome these difficulties, and two main methods came into use: antrectomy, in which the hormone (gastrin)-secreting part and some of the acid-secreting part of the stomach were removed; and a drainage operation such as pyloroplasty, in which the pylorus was refashioned so as to prevent the stasis of gastric contents. Unfortunately, these were not a complete solution to the problem and arguments continued over the respective merits of the various types of operation.

One of the hazards of peptic ulceration is bleeding from the ulcer. In 1958 Owen H. Wangensteen of the University of Minnesota introduced the technique of gastric cooling as an emergency treatment for massive haemorrhage[25]. For this he passed into the stomach a tube with a balloon at the end, through which he circulated ice-cold water for prolonged periods until the haemorrhage was controlled and surgical treatment could be undertaken. Four years later he extended the idea to gastric 'freezing' as a treatment in its own right for ulcer disease – a sort of physiological gastrectomy[26]. Water and alcohol at a temperature well below freezing point were run into the balloon for about an hour, but even so actual freezing of the stomach wall seldom occurred. At first there was quite a wave of enthusiasm for the method, but before long reports started to appear showing it could be hazardous and anyway gave only temporary benefit. Accordingly it was abandoned, although the cooling technique survived for emergencies.

Statistics are, today, part and parcel of everyday life, but it was not always so, not even of medical life. Billroth was the first to introduce statistics to the surgical world and to emphasize their importance[27]. He had no wish to see surgery become a field in which only a few men excelled; he wanted to lay the foundations of sound operative methods that could be learnt and their significance appreciated, even by the average surgeon. His clinic grew into a Mecca for surgeons from all over the world, and the prestige of anyone who had watched him at work was such that men would go to great lengths to visit Vienna, and fortunate indeed were those who had been trained by him. In addition to the training itself Billroth would do all in his power to obtain leading positions for them in other European clinics.

Billroth was endowed with a noble presence, yet despite his fame he remained humble and honest with a large capacity for friendship. It is said that on one occasion Billroth was offered a post in Germany but refused as his friend Brahms was unable to leave Vienna. The composer dedicated two string quartets to the surgeon, an act, according to Billroth, that would make his name outlive his fame as a surgeon. In those days a rivalry existed between the admirers of Brahms and of Wagner to the extent that at a concert the music of one would cause the supporters of the other to leave the theatre, and many were the occasions on which the opening bars of a Wagnerian composition were the signal for Billroth to rise and march majestically down the aisle followed by other Brahmsians. When he settled in Vienna, Billroth purchased a mansion on the outskirts of the Vienna woods where he gave private concerts conducted by himself, Brahms or his other musical friend, Johann Strauss (the second).

A lover of the joys of life, he lived and entertained regally and this no doubt contributed to the corpulence and illnesses that beset him. Early in his career in Vienna he began to be troubled by the colic of gall-stones; later in life he developed stones in the kidney and for a number of years he was prone to attacks of bronchitis which culminated in a severe attack of pneumonia six years before his death and from which he never really recovered. His chest complaints affected his heart and towards his end angina pectoris and bouts of heart failure occurred with increasing frequency. His death in 1894 was deeply mourned by a wide circle of personal friends and by the whole surgical world, and though the obituary notices were glowing, many were their writers whose vision was not distant enough to perceive the lasting value of his contributions to surgery.

While Billroth was still alive, his assistants often made advances on their own account before leaving the clinic to continue their work in other major European centres. The operation of gastroenterostomy as a bypass procedure without removing part of the stomach was an unintentional invention on the part of Anton Wölfler in 1881. Because he was going away, Billroth allowed his assistant to operate on a patient with a pyloric cancer which was obstructing the passage of food; the idea was that Wölfler would simply perform a Billroth I operation. Unfortunately he met with an unexpected difficulty; the cancer had become adherent to the pancreas and could not be removed. He was about to close the abdomen and admit defeat when, according to the account given by Lord Moynihan years later, his assistant, Karl Nicoladoni, whispered to him that he had nothing to lose in attempting to bypass the obstruction[28]. Accordingly he joined the stomach to the jejunum (the first part of the small intestine after the duodenum), carrying the jejunum in front of the transverse colon[29]. Thus was the first anterior gastroenterostomy performed and by contemporary standards it was a great success as the patient lived for four months. The operation itself shortly went into permanent decline when Billroth repeated the performance a few days later and the patient died from intestinal obstruction due to kinks developing at the anastomosis.

Nevertheless, the concept had taken root in the mind of Louis Courvoisier, professor of surgery at Basel, who began experimenting on cadavers. He came to the conclusion that it was not a good thing to pull the jejunum in front of the colon, and that it would be preferable to make a hole in the membrane known as the transverse mesocolon and carry the jejunum to the stomach behind the transverse colon. The operation on October 19, 1883, on a woman of fifty-six, was a success and so well was the lady progressing, that on the eighth day after surgery the enthusiastic Courvoisier took her in a carriage to a medical meeting; alas, his zeal proved her undoing and she died five days later from an intestinal abscess, but the post-mortem examination showed perfect healing of the anastomotic line[30].

The posterior modification restored gastroenterostomy to favour of a sort; after any of these operations the surgeon was in a mental torment so dangerous were the possible complications (though, truth to tell, surgery in many instances merely postponed the inevitable; the best that could realistically be expected was an easing of the worst symptoms). Haemorrhage or leakage from the anastomosis, intestinal obstruction or shock might easily kill the patient whose tumour was often irremovable. The operative technique was slow and tedious, contributing to the shock and so many sutures were inserted (sometimes up to two hundred) that, unknown to the surgeon, the anastomosis was weakened, not strengthened. These stitches would also be liable to cut off the blood supply and cause local gangrene with resultant perforation.

To combat this, various mechanical appliances were introduced to ensure patency of the opening and yet keep the two parts of the gut in apposition without the believed need for extensive stitchery. American surgeons were largely responsible for this idea; the first on the scene was Nicholas Senn who, after experimenting with perforated discs of leather, lead and wood finally, in 1888, settled on bone plates, one of which went in the gut on either side of the anastomosis[31]. They were not entirely satisfactory and in 1892 gave way to the Murphy button which was shaped like a yo-yo, with a hollow central spindle, that could be taken in two[32], and in 1893 to the Mayo Robson bobbin, like a cotton reel made of bone[33], which enjoyed a greater popularity in Great Britain. Many other variations were tried in the attempt to reduce the rate of complications, but until the technique of suturing was perfected the Murphy button proved the most successful; it lowered the mortality rate for the operation from the 60 percent level of Billroth to about 25 percent, and held pride of place for many years.

Regurgitant vomiting was another serious complication of gastro-enterostomy, and a number of modifications were introduced for its prevention including the formation of valve-like flaps at the anastomosis to keep the gastric contents flowing in the correct direction, and various alterations to the actual technique of anastomosis; the most successful of the latter was the so-called 'no-loop' operation of William Mayo, introduced in 1905[34]. In the early years of the 20th century gastroenterostomy really went to surgeons' heads and writing in 1906 M.M. Portis of Chicago said 'One author advises that gastro-enterostomy be done for gastroptosis; another recommends it for chronic catarrh; another that it be done in hysterical vomiting; and very many advise it in the neuroses of the stomach that mask under the name of dyspepsia. Indeed, gastro-enterostomy is said to be such a panacea for all the ills that can befall the stomach, that we naturally wonder that we are not born with a gastro-enterostomy.'[35] Evidently, surgeons had not yet learnt that the operation was a success only when the disease, usually cancer or ulcer, was causing obstruction at the pylorus; if there was no obstruction the artificial orifice would tend to close and the patient would have been exposed to the hazards of the procedure for no good purpose.

A Pole who made a great impact on surgery after leaving Billroth's clinic in 1881 to become professor of surgery at Königsburg and then, in 1890, at Breslau (now Wroclaw), was Johannes von Mikulicz-Radecki (usually remembered just as

Mikulicz). He was very much at home performing and modifying most of the recently devised operations as well as introducing new techniques. For instance, on October 7, 1880, he had sewn up a perforated ulcer on the lesser curve of the stomach[36] – the man died three hours later from 'shock'. Other surgeons then attempted the operation but success did not arrive until May 19, 1892, when Ludwig Heusner closed a perforated gastric ulcer in a man of forty-one[37]; the operation was carried out in a private house in Barmen, Germany.

While still at Billroth's clinic Mikulicz developed the technique of examining the stomach with the gastroscope, a rigid angulated tube provided with mirrors[38]. At first it had been looked upon as an interesting but tricky device which, as John Bland-Sutton remarked a few years later,'requires for its successful use a surgeon with the instincts of a sword swallower and the eye of a hawk'. Mikulicz evidently possessed these attributes as he raised the status of the gastroscope to that of a valuable everyday diagnostic instrument, though it would be a long while before the instrument became thin and flexible and no longer a nightmare for the patient. After his arrival at Breslau, Mikulicz began operating in sterilized white linen gloves with a mask over his mouth in an attempt to prevent infection entering the wound from his hands and breath[39]. However, they were not received with any great enthusiasm as they interfered with the delicate sense of touch so vital to the surgeon. Rubber gloves were, however, not very far away.

The other end of the alimentary canal also commanded Mikulicz's attention and his name is enshrined in an operation for cancer of the colon – but this, and surgery of the rectum where Mikulicz's contribution was more in his skill as an operator than in making dramatic discoveries, must wait for another chapter.

Gall-stones have troubled humanity since very earliest times, and like other abdominal operations, surgery on the gall-bladder benefited from the arrival of antisepsis. But, as you might by now have come to expect, the organ had not gone unnoticed in previous days. In 1767 a Monsieur Herlin ligatured and opened the gall-bladder of a cat which recovered its normal health after the operation. He submitted the facts to an astonished Jean Louis Petit, the leading French surgeon, who was relieved of any doubt by an examination of the animal. M. l'Anglas, a colleague, then extended the operation by removing the gall-bladders from two dogs which also made good recoveries. Another colleague, M. Duchainois, also removed the gall-bladder from a dog. Herlin proposed the operation for stones in the human patient, commenting:'It seems better to try an uncertain remedy than to abandon the patient to an assured death.'[40]

John Stough Bobbs of Indiana was the first to put M. Herlin's exhortation into practice and again it was one of those occasions when the unexpected was found. In 1867 Bobbs was operating on a woman for a presumed ovarian cyst;

instead he found a distended gall-bladder full of stones. He drained and emptied the gall-bladder (cholecystotomy) and the woman made an uneventful recovery[41]. The first deliberately planned cholecystotomy was not attended by such a fortunate outcome. The surgeon was James Marion Sims of South Carolina. The patient was a forty-five-year-old woman. The operation on April 18, 1878, lasted one hour and sixteen minutes[42]. The patient died eight days later. The next planned attempt, in August 1879, was successful and the patient was in good health at the time of Lawson Tait's report in 1884[43]. By then he had operated on thirteen patients, eleven of whom were well; the other two had died. He championed cholecystotomy over cholecystectomy (removal of the gall-bladder), an operation that had been performed for the first time in July, 1882, by Carl Johann Langenbuch on a man of forty-three with success[44]. Although cholecystectomy gradually increased in favour, it did not replace cholecystotomy in appropriate cases until the early 1920s. The progress of cholecystectomy was hindered by the fact that the benefit felt by the patient after removal of the gall-bladder is roughly proportional to the degree to which it is diseased. In other words, if the gall-bladder has ceased to function properly the body will have adapted itself to this state and removal of the offending organ should relieve the symptoms; but if a normally functioning gall-bladder is removed the same happy state cannot be guaranteed. Therefore, until surgeons worked out the indications for cholecystectomy, the operation was abused and the results were not always satisfactory.

Bile from the gall-bladder is carried to the duodenum by the common duct and when stones follow the same path they frequently get stuck giving rise to biliary colic and/or jaundice. So, an important aspect of surgery for gall-stones is to make sure that the common duct is empty, and various methods have been devised for removing stones from the inaccessible lower end. In the late 1870s and early 1880s some surgeons squeezed or otherwise manoeuvred the stones on through into the duodenum while others squeezed them back into the gall-bladder. In 1884 Lawson Tait recommended crushing them with padded forceps applied outside the duct, something he had done on his fifteenth patient[45]. Theodor Kocher in 1890, however, preferred to use his fingers[46]. The duct itself was opened in 1889 and there was quite a discussion as to who had actually been the first. The credit eventually went to Robert Abbe, an American, who operated on a woman of thirty-six on April 13 of that year to remove an impacted stone; he also removed the gall-bladder and drained the hepatic duct; the patient was in perfect health four years later[47]. Charles McBurney, another American, found it easier to reach stones in the lower end of the duct if he made a vertical incision in the duodenum opposite the entrance of the duct; the first time he did this was in 1892 and with great success, although his report did not appear for another six years[48]. On June 4, 1894, Kocher adopted the same plan when he was unable to crush a stone the size of a pigeon's egg. The thirty-six-year-old man made a complete recovery[49].

Some idea of the difficulties facing the early surgeons can be gained from a look at the mortality rate for these gall-stone operations; from 18 percent in 1895, it fell to 1–2 percent in the 1950s, the reduction being due mostly to better care of the patient before and after surgery and to improved methods of draining the common duct after it has been opened.

Lying in the curve of the duodenum is the head of the pancreas, cancers of which often involve the duodenal papilla (the ampulla of Vater) through which the pancreatic duct and the common bile duct enter the duodenum. When this happens the common duct is obstructed and the patient becomes jaundiced. Surgery to relieve the condition is not something to be lightly undertaken. Yet on June 15, 1909, Walther Kausch operated on a man of forty-nine who had an ampullary cancer. He resected the head of the pancreas and upper part of the duodenum, closed off the stump of the pylorus and created a gastroenterostomy. The patient lived for another eleven months[50]. The operation lay fallow until interest was revived in America through the work of Allen Whipple who described a two-stage operation in 1935[51] and Alexander Brunschwig who, two years later reported his two-stage operation in which he removed the entire head of the pancreas and practically all of the duodenum from a man of sixty-nine. The first stage took place on January 8, 1937, and the second on February 11; the man died eighty-five days later on April 30[52].

So, returning to the 19th century, we can see that in the space of two decades, corresponding to the flourishing of Listerism, surgery within the abdominal cavity had made truly remarkable progress. The mortality rates may have been high compared to modern standards, but how very much lower they were at the end of this period than in 1874, when Sir John Eric Erichsen misguidedly declared the abdomen to be 'forever shut from the intrusion of the wise and humane surgeon'.

5

Stones in the bladder

Events destined to shape the whole future course of surgery were tumbling over themselves in their eagerness to appear before the world; some were of major importance and had an immediate impact, others, seemingly less significant, formed the solid core to logical progress. This profusion of surgical moments meant that a mass of different and sometimes unrelated subjects were developing side by side and so any strictly chronological description of events would lead to confusion. We shall, therefore, deal with the important advances at the time of their inception or, in certain cases, at the time of their acceptance, and follow them along until we come to a natural pause.

It was an ironical twist of fate that by the time a satisfactory method of dealing with stones in the urinary bladder had been evolved, the disease should decline in frequency. This was largely due to improvements in diet, hygiene and social conditions generally, and started during the mid-Victorian era; in addition, infection and various forms of obstruction within the bladder, which predispose to stone formation, were treated earlier and more satisfactorily. Stones in both the urinary bladder and the gall-bladder (which are in no way related) had troubled humanity for centuries, but as the gall-bladder lies in the upper abdomen, gall-stones had received virtually no surgical attention for that reason, and moreover the symptoms they produced were a diagnostic puzzle until the 1870s. The problem of stones in the urinary bladder was not viewed with such a jaundiced eye; the bladder was more accessible and so severely did the patients suffer that they submitted to the surgeon's knife without too great a show of reluctance. One famous patient was Samuel Pepys, who always gave thanks on the anniversary of the day (March 26, 1658) he was 'cut for stone'[1]. Trouble with passing urine, the passage of blood, intense pain, irritation of the bladder walls with inescapable infection which can spread upwards to involve the kidneys, are all possible evidence of stones. Small wonder, then, that surgery for this complaint extends back over four thousand years, since any relief the surgeon could give was welcomed even though the outcome was not always as successful as it was for Pepys.

The operation performed throughout history involved cutting into the bladder below, through the perineum (the area in front of the anus and behind the external genitalia) – perineal lithotomy. A technique whereby the bladder was approached through the lower part of the abdomen (supra-pubic lithotomy) had originally been attempted by the Hindus at the end of the pre-Christian era, but their skill was unusual and the operation lapsed until the Provençal surgeon, Pierre Franco, performed it in 1556. The patient was a child and Franco resorted to the supra-pubic route, being unable to remove the stone through the perineum. Although the child did well, Franco advised most strongly against the approach as it was attended by all the hazards peculiar to the abdominal surgery of the time[2]. Nearly two hundred years later, William Cheselden wrote a treatise on the 'high operation'[3] but as he was accused of plagiarism by another surgeon, he pursued the matter no further and turned his attention to perineal lithotomy instead. Before his day, the incision had been made in the mid-line which put the underlying structures at risk; but on March 27, 1727, Cheselden placed his incision to one side of the mid-line[4]. Thus was the lateral operation for stone brought into surgical practice, though it was, in fact, only a modification of an approach devised by the itinerant lithotomist, Frère Jacques, in 1697. The coming of anaesthesia and antisepsis ousted lateral lithotomy from favour and the supra-pubic approach became the route of choice when surgeons had to cut for stone.

The male sex supplied the majority of candidates for these operations owing to the relative inaccessibility of the male bladder and its greater liability to infection and obstruction. In the female, the urethra is short, straight and can easily be dilated, but in the male it traverses the penis, is curved and much longer. Despite this, thought was given to ways of passing an instrument into the bladder so that the stone could be crushed and the fragments passed in the urine. The crushing of stones, or lithotrity, was first performed by the Frenchman, Jean Civiale, in 1823[5]. Since the instrument he devised was poorly suited to its purpose, he continued with his experiments and by 1835 had designed a lithotrite (as these instruments are known) which had good crushing power[6]. (A lithotrite had already been designed, before Civiale's first effort, by John Elderton, a house surgeon at the Northampton General Hospital, who submitted it to Benjamin Brodie in 1817[7].)

Civiale claimed that his pre-eminence as a lithotomist was due to two simple manoeuvres: for a week before operation he passed wax dilators up the urethra to prepare the way for an easy passage of the lithotrite, and after crushing he would wash the bladder out with water. When he estimated that the stone was larger than 2cm in diameter he performed a lateral lithotomy – he knew the limitations of his instrument. The erroneous idea that the bladder was extremely sensitive to the passage of instruments originated with Civiale and retarded progress for a number of years. He believed that if trouble were to be avoided, each session should last only a few minutes, the patient returning later for the crushing of any remaining fragments. Regrettably, during the interval the patient often became ill which Civiale attributed to the instrumentation when, in reality, it was due to the sharp fragments of remaining stone resting on the floor of the bladder and setting up an inflammation that could be lethal. The post-mortem examination of some of these patients revealed the presence of fragments, and so improved methods were devised for their removal, though the actual length of the crushing part of the operation was still restricted. As the operator had to work by sense of touch alone, extreme care was needed not to crush part of the bladder wall at the same time; so fearsome and crude were the earlier instruments – straight metal catheters – that it is a wonder the bladder ever escaped injury.

In 1846 Philip Crampton invented a suction apparatus for use after the lithotrite had crushed the stones; it consisted of a glass bottle exhausted of air (to create a vacuum which supplied the suction) and connected to the catheter by means of a rubber tube with a stop-cock. This was a laborious device as the urinary bladder had to be refilled with water when the vacuum failed, but it was an idea on the right lines. The forerunner of modern apparatus was devised in 1866 by Joseph Clover, an anaesthetist with a most inventive turn of mind. Sitting at the patient's head giving chloroform through a cumbersome bag inhaler, invented by himself in 1862, he must have wondered at the inadequacy of the manoeuvres going on at the other end of the table. The tediousness of the job could be lessened and much time could be saved if the same water could be used for the washouts – so long as the chips could be prevented from returning to the bladder. Clover's answer was a rubber bulb connected to the catheter by glass tubing so arranged that it acted as a trap for the heavier particles of stone which would fall to the bottom and not be returned to the bladder.

The best known exponent of lithotrity in England was Henry Thompson; indeed his fame was such that in 1863 he was called to Brussels to see Leopold I of the Belgians. Some years previously, Civiale had unsuccessfully attempted to crush the stones in the royal bladder, but fortunately Thompson succeeded where the other had failed. Thompson did not have the patient anaesthetized although Clover had agreed to attend if it was thought necessary.

Thompson's next encounter with a royal bladder was not so happy. The Emperor Napoleon III had been plagued by stones for many years, even before the Franco-Prussian war; indeed, at the battle of Sedan in 1870 he was in such a sorry state with pain and anaemia from piles and the passage of bloody urine that he could not sit his horse or take decisions. After six months in captivity, he came to England much improved and stayed that way for eighteen months until he deteriorated to the extent that he could neither walk nor ride. He suggested that Thompson be invited to examine him; this Thompson did at Camden Place, Chislehurst, on Christmas Eve, 1872. He was not satisfied and on Boxing Day repeated the examination, this time under anaesthesia with Clover giving the anaesthetic. The operation to crush the stone, about the size of a date stone, took place on January 2; the crushing went well, but some of the fragments remained after the washout. So Thompson operated again, on the 6th, despite the Emperor's suffering from evidence of kidney failure; some more fragments were removed but not all and the next day there was another blockage which was only partially relieved by instrumentation. By now the Emperor was deteriorating rapidly and, after lapsing into a coma, he died on the morning of the 9th. The post-mortem examination showed that the bladder was grossly inflamed and that death had resulted from the almost complete destruction of the Imperial kidneys.

Thompson was a believer in crushing stones at repeated sessions limiting the time of each to two minutes; the number of sessions usually required might be anything up to ten, but it was occasionally necessary to continue for twenty-five or more. The patient might be in hospital for as long as four months. Thompson was responsible for two important modifications to the lithotrite which by this time had come to consist of two blades, one being grooved along its length (the female blade) to accommodate the other (the male blade) for ease of insertion and withdrawal. It was not uncommon for debris to get lodged in the female blade preventing complete closure with consequent damage to the urethra on withdrawal. Thompson supplied the remedy by having a hole made in the female blade, so that the debris would be squeezed out when the instrument was closed. The first satisfactory screw mechanism for opening and closing the blades had been invented by the London instrument maker, Weiss, and this Thompson improved considerably by converting the screw into a wheel screw. The unsatisfactory nature of repeated crushings was slowly being realized, for even if the small fragments were sucked out, the sharp edges of the remaining pieces of stone still irritated the bladder. The final blow to the belief that prolonged instrumentation of itself was harmful was delivered by the American, Henry Jacob Bigelow, who, it may be remembered, was present at Morton's demonstration of ether anaesthesia. He realized that an important aspect of the procedure was to remove all the stone at one sitting and that, within reason, the length of the operation was of minor significance. To this end he devised a more powerful crushing instrument and improved the evacuator, though the principle of the rubber bulb and glass bottle to trap the fragments remained the same. He also improved the actual technique by gently dilating the male urethra to a greater extent than hitherto believed possible[8]. This allowed more efficient lithotrites to be used and catheters with a larger bore to be passed, enabling larger fragments to be washed out. Before starting to crush, he filled the bladder with warm water, being careful not to overdistend the organ, and thus reduced the possibility of catching part of the bladder wall in the lithotrite.

In 1879, the year after Bigelow successfully advocated his method of lithotrity, a great advance took place that was to have far-reaching repercussions in the diagnosis of disease of the internal organs. By the use of suitably sized tubes provided with illumination and a system of lenses, it became possible to see the inside of structures such as the bladder, the oesophagus, the stomach, the rectum, and the trachea and the larger of its branches within the lungs. The scope of this form of examination was eventually to be extended so that very little of the inside of the body was hidden from view. As early as 1807 attempts had been made to see the inside of the urethra, but as only an open tube with reflected light was available, no practical purpose was served. In 1862 this primitive instrument was improved by F. August Haken who closed the business end with a glass window[9]. Five years afterwards Julius Bruck turned his attention from his usual occupation as a dentist to provide the tube with its own source of illumination in the form of an incandescent platinum loop[10]. This, however, required a complicated water-cooling arrangement. The last steps to make the apparatus of real practical value were taken in 1879 by Max Nitze and an instrument maker, Joseph Leiter, who added the lens system[11] and, in 1886, by von Dittel and Leiter who produced a carbon-filament light that required no cooling. Surgeons were now able to check the results of their labours with the lithotrite; in addition, the instrument brought tremendous benefit to the diagnosis of other conditions, such as tumours, within the bladder.

This instrument, the cystoscope, at first only allowed the operator to look, nothing more; but after much experimentation Nitze produced an operating cystoscope through which the surgeon could crush stones and perform other operations while seeing what he was doing[12]. Unfortunately, the practical application of the instrument to the surgery of bladder stones was limited, since the union of cystoscope and lithotrite meant that the strength of the lithotrite had to be reduced and so only small stones could be crushed. For the larger ones, the surgeon still had to work with his sense of touch; and if the stone was exceptionally hard, recourse had to be had to the supra-pubic approach.

6

Asepsis and sterilization

ntisepsis and asepsis were really the same thing, but achieved in different ways. Both were intended to prevent bacteria reaching the wound – antisepsis by placing a destructive barrier (carbolic acid) in their path; asepsis by ensuring that there were none anywhere near. Nevertheless, under the conditions prevailing at the time Listerism was the essential forerunner of asepsis. For surgeons who were quite happy carrying on in the same old way, something dramatic, something they could see was different, something they could fight about, was needed to grip their attention. Then, once they had grasped the underlying principle that Lister had been preaching from the start, their minds would be ready to accept the discipline of asepsis.

Even while Listerism was in full swing, many clear-thinking surgeons refused to adopt the method, maintaining that scrupulous cleanliness would prevent infection. True up to a point, but 'social' cleanliness is not 'bacterial' cleanliness and although the results obtained by these surgeons were very good, their methods were still potentially dangerous. For instance, some continued to operate in their shirtsleeves or with their frock coats on, and though their instruments might appear spotless they had not been sterilized. Other surgeons gave Listerism the benefit of the doubt and put it into practice in their operating theatres, only to become disenchanted and fall by the wayside. They failed to understand the reasons behind Listerism and used the carbolic acid in so perfunctory a manner that it would have needed miraculous powers to have had even the remotest hope of success. A number of instruments had wooden handles and the quantity of bacteria that these could harbour in the join was enormous, yet they got no more than a wiping or a quick dip in the acid. Other nasty habits, such as using the same sponge to swab the wounds of patient after patient, would scarcely have been amenable to gallons of carbolic. Another lack of understanding led some surgeons to the belief that the use of carbolic acid was the solution to all their problems and would excuse them from the niceties of surgical technique. Lister himself had emphasized that carbolic acid could not replace Nature's healing powers and was no substitute for good surgery.

Those who believed in cleanliness were not without their little lapses from grace. For instance, Lawson Tait would hold his knife between his teeth when tying ligatures and Spencer Wells held his suture needles between his lips. Thomas Annandale, a Scottish surgeon with a leaning towards urology, would blow through a catheter before introducing it to ensure that it was not blocked. William Macewen, on the other hand, was already boiling his instruments and gauze dressings round about 1880.

An astonishingly clear-sighted appreciation of where the future lay came from William Savory, a surgeon at St Bartholomew's Hospital, London, in his Address in Surgery to the 1879 meeting of the British Medical Association[1]. Listerism was, he admitted, preferable to operating in a pestilential atmosphere, but 'the surgeon's duty under ordinary circumstances is not to find the most dangerous sanitary conditions under which he dare operate, it is rather to discover the cause of the pestilence and banish them [*sic*] as far as possible from his field of action. The desiderata to be secured are a pure air, healthy conditions, and strict cleanliness generally'.

He concluded with more wise words: 'the best results have been achieved by the simplest means. Is it rash,' he asked, 'to affirm that the future practice of surgery will be most successful when it is carried on, not where antiseptics are most largely used, but under conditions least in need of antiseptics?' His audience was aghast and the *Lancet*, which reported the Address, remarked that it came as a disagreeable surprise to the advocates of the antiseptic system of surgery. No wonder that the real impetus towards aseptic surgery came from Germany where Robert Koch was securely laying the foundations of bacteriology and showing surgeons their enemy in the fight against infection.

Koch began his career as an ordinary country doctor in Wollstein, Germany (now in Poland and renamed Wolsztyn); in his spare time he investigated the blood of animals that had died of anthrax. The extent of his discoveries would have been outstanding had he been working in a well-equipped laboratory, as it was they were not far short of the miraculous. He used a microscope given him by his wife on his thirtieth birthday and, by introducing the technique of putting special oil between the slide he was examining and the lens of the microscope (oil immersion) he was able to get high enough magnifications to see the bacteria and even succeeded in taking excellent photographs. He invented solid, nutritious gelatin-like media on which to grow the bacteria, thus enabling him to study different organisms individually, uncontaminated by other types.

In 1876 he was ready to give his discoveries to the world and for once a pioneer found himself with his work recognized for its true worth. He wrote to Ferdinand Cohn, professor of botany at Breslau and an enthusiastic bacteriologist, asking permission to demonstrate his findings on the anthrax bacillus, and for three days this unknown country practitioner held a small, distinguished and highly critical audience completely spellbound. His demonstrations were flawless and from them were formulated Koch's postulates, namely, that a given bacterium must be demonstrable in every case of the disease it causes, that it must be possible to grow it in pure culture, and that when this culture is inoculated into susceptible animals it must produce the specific disease and that from these animals again must be grown a pure culture. On these postulates rests the whole structure of bacteriology.

In 1878 he published his book on wound infections, detailing the pathological effects of the different varieties of bacteria[2], and three years later he was intently studying the sterilizing action of hot air; for example, he did experiments on the sterilization of anthrax spores (10 minutes at 95°C) and of garden earth (10 minutes at 105°C). He also discovered the limitations of steam at 100°C [3]. Until his death, Koch never forgot the debt he owed to his old teacher, Jacob Henle, who had inspired in him the desire to explore under the microscope and who, in 1840, had actually laid down the conditions, very similar to the postulates, that he regarded as desiderata which would one day be achieved in practice[4]. Without doubt, this guiding hand led Koch unerringly towards his success.

The perfection of Koch's work was undoubtedly responsible for the rationalizing of asepsis, but apart from this it is difficult to say where aseptic surgery began: its component parts had been growing and developing over many years, although obviously with different ends in mind. For example, heat had been used for more than a hundred years by the experimenters on spontaneous generation and the work of Robert Collins in 1829 in Dublin has already been mentioned in connection with puerperal fever[5]. Then in 1831 William Henry was faced with the problem of how to get round the long quarantine period imposed on imported Egyptian cotton as protection against plague. In one of his experiments he showed that vaccine lymph was rendered inert by exposure to a temperature of 140°F [6]. The next year he designed and built an insulated double jacket copper steam sterilizer; with this he was able to sterilize various forms of cloth at temperatures above 200°F without the steam coming into contact with the material[7].

The origins of the autoclave (which utilizes wet steam under pressure and is familiar in the guise of the pressure cooker) are obscure but the principle was probably developed in Pasteur's laboratory. At all events a small compact autoclave for bacteriological use was manufactured by a Paris engineering firm for Charles Chamberland, a colleague of Pasteur, in about 1884[8]. The first autoclave for surgical instruments and dressings was designed by another Frenchman, P. Redard, who was decidedly disillusioned (and rightly so) with the disinfecting qualities of carbolic acid. Apart from the fact that contact with the antiseptic had to be 'very prolonged', such instruments as hollow needles, trocars, forceps and sponges could not be sterilized in this manner. Disinfection by heat was, he said, the procedure 'par excellence' and absolute disinfection could be achieved with his apparatus in 15-20 minutes with steam under pressure at a temperature of 110°C[9].

Research continued. Friedrich von Esmarch (better known for his bandage and for introducing the first field dressing during the Franco-Prussian war of 1870) showed in 1889 that the action of steam depended not so much on the temperature as on the degree of saturation of the steam. If air was present, the power of steam to destroy the microbes was very much diminished[10]. A corollary to this was that gowns, dressings and so forth had to be packed extremely carefully in autoclaves to allow the steam to penetrate every nook and cranny and drive out every last vestige of air. One obvious disadvantage of sterilization by steam is that the objects come out damp, which makes them more readily re-contaminated than if dry and, in the case of garments, very unpleasant to wear. To overcome this problem an English medical officer of health, H. Tomkins, in 1889 described an apparatus whereby a strong current of hot air could be blown through the chamber[11]; this had the double advantage of removing the last trace of moisture from the autoclaved articles and of allowing the autoclave to be used as a simple hot air sterilizer for articles that could not be submitted to steam.

The quandary in which surgeons found themselves was elegantly expressed by Charles Lockwood. Writing in 1896, he said '…the mixed method is the one which I am in the habit of using, but with an abiding faith in the efficacy of heat, and a profound scepticism as to the power of chemicals.'[12]

However, if any one place can indeed be said to have given birth to the aseptic ritual, that place was Ernst von Bergmann's clinic in Berlin in about 1886. Later, in 1892, one of von Bergmann's assistants, Kurt Schimmelbusch, described the operating ceremonial[13]. Originally, everything boilable had been boiled, but before long they changed over to the Lautenschläger sterilizer which depended on flowing steam and was preferred to autoclaving as being less complicated for ordinary use. The materials to be sterilized were placed in tin boxes perforated to allow the steam to enter: these drums were round to fit the sterilizer and right up to modern times dressing drums remained cylindrical despite the disadvantages of this shape. Tradition dies hard.

Schimmelbusch recorded how, in other parts of the ritual, leaves were taken from the bacteriologists' notebooks and their ideas put to practical use. Thus in

1875 Carl Joseph Eberth, professor of bacteriology at Zurich, had discovered that the skin harboured a multitude of bacteria and that these were also lurking in the sweat glands and hair follicles. This posed an unpleasant problem, since the bacteria would rise to the surface with the perspiration. Experiments proved that disinfecting the skin with the agents then available was far from satisfactory and so Hermann Kümmell of Hamburg introduced the practice of scrubbing up. He showed that a thorough scrubbing of the hands and forearms with ordinary soap and water was the most effective method of cleansing the skin, though not perfect. Another of von Bergmann's colleagues then drew attention to the need for paying particular attention to scrubbing under the finger nails. Nevertheless, at the time Schimmelbusch wrote his book, the ritual was not fully developed.

Despite attempts to place the credit elsewhere, there seems little doubt that the rubber gloves designed by William Stewart Halsted[14], of Johns Hopkins Hospital, Baltimore, in 1889–90 were in fact the forerunners of the modern surgical glove. As in other centres, all those involved in an operation disinfected their hands with an antiseptic after scrubbing up and not infrequently this produced a dermatitis. On one occasion the unfortunate sufferer was the theatre sister, Miss Caroline Hampton, for whom the chief surgeon, Halsted, had a warm regard. Intent that she should continue her career, he decided to protect her hands by finding some form of glove that could be rendered sterile and yet would not interfere with the job. He decided on rubber and had a pair of gloves specially made; these were so successful that before long he was persuaded by his colleague, Joseph Bloodgood, that they should become part of the aseptic ritual since they could be sterilized in a way that bare hands never could and, with the proviso that the hands were scrubbed first, the use of gloves by the surgeon himself would make surgery much safer. So that his gloves should fit as perfectly as possible, Halsted had his hands cast in bronze. Shortly after the gloves were introduced, Halsted married Miss Hampton, a sequence of events that makes one suspect that the origin of rubber gloves owed as much to a normal human emotion as it did to pure scientific zeal.

If priority should go to the surgeon who first introduced gloves specifically to protect the patient against infection, the palm should be awarded to Mikulicz even though the gloves were of linen material and compromised the surgeon's sense of touch. In the 1897 paper[15] describing his gloves he also referred to a surgical mask that was being developed in his clinic. The professor of bacteriology, Carl Flugge, had conclusively shown that bacteria-laden droplets were sprayed from the nose and mouth during speech; accordingly he persuaded Wilhelm Hubener, a surgical assistant, to devise a mask that would trap these droplets during surgery. After much experimentation Hubener eventually decided on a double layer of hydrophilic gauze stretched on a shaped wire frame, and tied behind the head.

The use of this simple and eminently satisfactory device did not have an immediate appeal and even fifteen years later it was still an optional item of equipment, though generally advised if the surgeon had a cold. The opening years of the 20th century saw surgeons arguing quite heatedly about their merits or otherwise. Infection of surgical wounds still occurred when they were used and constituted the commonest cause of death after operation. By making cultures of the air in operating theatres bacteriologists found that the number of bacteria was directly proportional to the number of spectators, and in those days it was usual for a crowd of students and visitors to come straight into the theatre with the dirt of the street on their shoes and gather closely round the surgeon asking questions, and when coughing would as likely as not turn their heads discreetly away from the patient and shower the instrument table instead. Even if they wore sterile gowns they were still a constant source of danger, and if the surgeon himself was unmasked his lecturing might help the students but was a real menace to the patient. In spite of considerations such as these, papers objecting to the use of masks appeared in the medical journals; one example of the reasons given was that the patient was frequently apprehensive when wheeled into the operating theatre (there were no separate anaesthetizing rooms) and if he saw himself surrounded by an impenetrable mass of white-clad figures with only their eyes showing, he might well be seized with ungovernable terror. Instead of the unfamiliar, he should be greeted by the kindly faces of those in whom he had put his trust.

Gloves fared no better, the chief complaint being their supposed interference with the sense of touch which, so it was said, prolonged the operation. Those who thought that way were generous enough to admit that, if a surgeon used gloves from the outset of his career, he might eventually be able to work as well as with his bare hands, but until he reached this stage he was placing his patients in considerable jeopardy. However, an American surgeon, W.P. Carr, writing in 1911, was not even prepared to go as far as this: 'It may seem a small matter, and in most operations perhaps it is, but in some cases I am sure this one thing is the determining factor of life or death for the patient. I believe firmly that more patients have died from the use of gloves than have ever been saved from infection by their use.'[16]

Except for squabbles such as these, which rumbled on for a while, asepsis and its implications had been generally accepted by the end of the first decade of the 20th century. The change from antiseptic methods begun in the 1880s took place rapidly in some centres; in others it was a gradual process occurring in stages, almost as though the surgeons were reluctant to see the end of an era and rather dubious about the efficacy of a method that ignored the use of carbolic acid. But over the years a sound technique was evolved at the right time to take advantage of the great strides that were being made in surgical pathology and physiology.

The story of sterilization continued[see 17, 18] and though our moving on for nearly half a century may seem out of place, it keeps the subject in a tidy compartment. The general approach to sterilization remained unchanged after World War I, with reliance placed firmly on the autoclave, the steam sterilizer and boiling. New ideas were not exactly plentiful, although in 1936 in America Deryl Hart found that irradiation with ultra-violet light would reduce bacterial contamination of the air in the operating theatre[19]; others experimented with the light but it was never considered worthwhile – in principle, it was not unlike Lister's spray.

World War II brought tremendous technical progress, most of which was readily convertible to peacetime uses. Surgery itself benefited directly and in an amazingly short time practically overhauled science fiction; it also benefited indirectly from materials and methods that had been developed for military purposes. Many of these new materials, most notably a wide range of plastics and a selection of useful metals, could not be sterilized by the traditional methods without destroying their properties; thus they provided a valuable stimulus to the search for other methods of sterilization.

The research also included a fresh look at the old methods and the way in which they were used, not just in the operating theatre, but throughout the entire hospital service. The fruits of this work began to appear in the middle and late 1950s and included, for instance, the vacuum assisted autoclave. This new design incorporated a vacuum pump to remove the air before the steam was admitted – a device that improved efficiency while shortening the exposure time; it transformed the sterilization of dressings. The use of dry heat, too, was attracting a good deal of attention and infra-red sterilizers (high temperature/ short time) were found to be excellent for items such as syringes and ward instruments, but to be impracticable for cutting and other instruments that had highly polished surfaces and therefore took up heat slowly. Yet another development was the substitution of disposable paper for returnable linen and of cartons for sterilizing drums; this revolutionized packaging methods.

In the 1960s, attention was directed to preventing bacteria (many of which come from the personnel in the theatre) reaching the operation site. Various means of ventilating the theatre were studied; these included the plenum system in which filtered air is introduced from above and removed at floor level while slight positive pressure is maintained inside the theatre, and systems of laminar (or uni-directional) air flow in which the air is changed three hundred or more times an hour. For operations, such as total hip replacement, where the effects of infection would be particularly tragic, plastic tent-like enclosures within the theatre were introduced; the only people inside the enclosure apart from the patient were the surgeon and his assistants who wore special suits with a vacuum system to remove the bacteria they shed[20]. Even more radical was the surgical isolater – a transparent plastic tent, distended with air and enclosing the patient's body; his or her head was outside as was the surgical team who worked entirely through glove sleeves and entry ports with air locks.

But the major problem, and the one that brought about the greatest innovations in technique, was how to sterilize the apparently unsterilizable. Heat and steam frequently damaged both the new materials and delicate new surgical equipment, and for a variety of other reasons were impracticable. The search for ways round the difficulty soon uncovered two important alternatives, each with its own range of suitability: one, gaseous sterilization, had its origins extending back into history; the other, irradiation, was a product of the atomic age.

Fumigation with chlorine gas was first practised in France at the end of the 18th century and in 1829 Robert Collins disinfected his ward linen by suspending it in the gas[5]. The power of formaldehyde to kill bacteria was discovered by Oscar Löw in 1885 and both vapour and solution are, in modern times, used for special purposes such as the sterilization of haemodialysers. Ethylene oxide, the most widely used of the gases, began its career as a disinfectant of spices and as an agent to prevent food from spoiling. Its involvement in sterilization is usually traced back to a US patent applied for in 1929 by H. Schrader and E. Bossert and granted in 1936[21]. However, in 1933, P.M. Gross and L.F. Dixon had also applied for a US patent but specifically for the use of the gas as a sterilizing agent with the backing of considerable research (which had not been the case with Schrader and Bossert); this was granted in 1937[22]. Nevertheless, ethylene oxide attracted little or no interest until 1949 when Charles Phillips and Saul Kaye demonstrated its possibilities[23]. They had been working since 1944 at the United States Army Chemical Corps Biological Laboratories at Fort Detrick on the development of gaseous sterilization and had investigated a number of gases, of which ethylene oxide seemed to have the best prospects. Its outstanding advantage was the general lack of damage it caused to many of the materials requiring sterilization, such as plastics, leather, wool, paper, electrical equipment, and delicate laboratory instruments that would be damaged by heat or moisture. Moreover, it could be used for the so-called cold or room-temperature sterilization of objects sensitive to heat, but its disadvantage in comparison with other techniques such as autoclaving was the considerably longer time required. It also suffered from the fact that bacteriological control could be difficult if the artificial (control) contaminant was carried to parts of the equipment that the gas failed to reach.

The bactericidal action of radiations was first demonstrated by Franz Minck in 1896[24], only a year after x-rays had been discovered by Wilhelm Conrad Röntgen. Having found that the rays killed colonies of bacteria on Petri dishes, Minck's train of thought moved, not to the sterilization of objects but, more ambitiously perhaps, to the treatment of internal infectious diseases, such as tuberculosis, typhus, cholera and so forth – an idea that came to nothing because of the harmful effects of radiation on the body. Fifty years then passed until the impetus given to atomic development by World War II led to vast quantities of radiations becoming available from machines – high-energy particle accelerators – and isotopes. This initiated research to find a practical use for the bactericidal effect of ionizing radiations.

Once the basic research (which had concentrated on food, drugs and pharmaceuticals) had been completed, the industrial applications were readily apparent, for here was a continuously operating sterilization process by means of which many products, including medical and surgical articles, could be sterilized in their final packaged form. Commercial development, using particle accelerators, began in the United States in the 1950s but the use of cobalt-60 as a source of gamma radiation on an industrial scale was developed by the United Kingdom Atomic Energy Authority who established a Package Irradiation Plant at the Wantage Research Laboratory. From its start in 1960, this plant dealt commercially with a wide range of surgical materials and equipment, from sutures and syringes, through catheters and cannulae, to dialysis units and prostheses, but it also accepted special items of equipment from hospitals.

Sterilization, which had stood still for the first seventy years of its existence – and even shown signs of decrepitude in the mid-1950s when reports indicated that sterilizing procedures were not always producing sterile materials (due to faults in design, installation or maintenance of autoclaves) – had finally come of age in the atomic era.

7

Appendicitis: a 'new' disease

The same year (1886) that von Bergmann introduced steam sterilization saw the emergence of an apparently new disease. In reality, it was an old disease that had simply been lurking unrecognized until Reginald Heber Fitz, professor of pathological anatomy at Harvard, gave a clear description of inflammation of the appendix, named the condition 'appendicitis' and thus rescued a common disease from the welter of confusion then surrounding intra-abdominal pathology[1]. Before 1886 no one knew the origin of an illness in which pus collected in the right side of the abdomen and which not infrequently ended in death. No surgeon would have been insane enough to operate early in a bout of abdominal pain, and when the patient died and came to post-mortem the inflammation, suppuration and other changes (possibly the result of previous attacks) had so distorted the normal appearance that it was impossible to say where the disease had started. However, once surgery within the abdomen became a fact of life it was only a matter of time before the situation was clarified. Diagnosis remained difficult, and even when surgeons had gained experience they still had to agree on the indications for operation which, in the main, meant the ability to recognize the disease in its early stages, and the courage to operate then and not wait until an abscess had formed or the appendix had burst and peritonitis was killing the patient.

It seems reasonable to assume that appendicitis has afflicted mankind from earliest times since study of ancient Egyptian mummies shows that these people suffered, and died, from appendicitis though there is no evidence that their contemporaries had the remotest idea what ailed them. The first reasonable account of what may have been a case of acute appendicitis which perforated and led to peritonitis was given in 1567 by Jean Fernel in his record of the post mortem of a seven-year-old girl[2]. There is, however, doubt as to the precise anatomical structure he was describing, since the same word was used at that time for both the appendix and the caecum. Ignorance continued to surround the appendix and the diagnoses that probably covered most instances of appendicitis were 'typhlitis', and 'perityphlitis', though doubtless the disease also accounted for some cases of colic and 'iliac passion' (which just meant pain in the iliac region or lower side of the abdomen). Typhlitis is the old word for inflammation of the caecum or blind-gut, and derives from the Greek *typhlos* meaning blind. Treatment was in keeping with the times and consisted of purging, bleeding, enemas and the popular practice of tobacco-smoke enemas; this last was also used in cases of irreducible hernias. From the 18th century onwards a few accounts of appendicitis appeared, but in nearly all the fact that the appendix was to blame was only found at the post-mortem examination and it would appear that the discovery occasioned no little surprise. With one or two exceptions the accounts were solely case histories with no mention made of surgery or even of its possibilities.

These descriptions failed to attract attention, chiefly because nothing could be done, even had an early diagnosis been made, and pain in the abdomen continued without an accurate diagnosis; the condition either cleared up or the patient died, usually of peritonitis. However, on December 6, 1735, there occurred a most remarkable case in which the appendix was removed by a surgeon when operating for a completely different condition. Claudius Amyand, a surgeon at St George's Hospital, London, had a boy of eleven brought to him with a hernia in the groin that had been present for a number of years and the swelling had extended into the scrotum. Associated with the hernia was a faecal fistula, or leakage of faeces through an abnormal opening produced by disease. Amyand decided that the only way to cure this leakage was to cure the hernia. When he opened the swelling in the scrotum he found the appendix in this unusual position and, moreover, that the appendix was perforated by a pin. He removed the appendix with some difficulty and then dealt with the hernia and the fistula, taking about half an hour to complete the operation. The wound healed well and uneventfully[3]. Pause for a moment to imagine what that boy must have gone through.

The appendix not uncommonly became the centre of an abscess and this accounted for most cases of 'perityphlitic abscess'. In 1759, at the St André Hospital, Bordeaux, M. Mestivier made an incision through the abdominal wall of a man of forty-five to release a pint of foul-smelling pus. When the man died, the surgeon carried out the post mortem and found a large encrusted pin in the appendix[4]. (Unfortunately, neither Amyand nor Mestivier recorded how the pins came to be swallowed, but as pins are commonly held between the lips, the two cases are probably not quite so much of a coincidence as it might seem.) In 1827, another Frenchman, François Mêlier, reported on a few cases of acute appendicitis and showed that the inflammation could cause the appendix to perforate and lead to abscess formation[5]. He suggested the possibility of operating if the diagnosis could be made with certainty, but with surgery as it then was, no one was prepared to put the suggestion into practice. Furthermore, inflammation in the right lower part of the abdomen was still believed to arise in the caecum rather than in the appendix – surgeons had difficulty in accepting the fact that inflammation of such a small and useless structure could be responsible for the death of a fit and hitherto healthy patient.

Willard Parker of New York took the next step forward when he operated successfully on more than one patient and set out what he regarded as the indications for surgery. His first patient was a fellow doctor from Brooklyn with an appendiceal abscess which he incised in 1843 (before the arrival of anaesthesia). Dr T. recovered in a short time and was in good health at the time of the report in 1867. Parker had three more successes in 1865–6[6]. However, his recommendations of the course to adopt fell short of the desirable, possibly because the risks of surgery were too great or because he believed he had found the answer to the problem. Having made the diagnosis of acute appendicitis, instead of operating at once he advised waiting till the fifth to twelfth day by which time an abscess would have formed [or the inflammation would have settled and surgery not be required – one can see his point], then incising the abscess to allow the pus to drain off. Parker's intervention was early compared to that of other surgeons who would wait for longer until gas had started to collect in the abscess. This operation of surgical drainage (without removing the appendix) was performed in a few isolated cases in the years that followed but failed to gain any degree of popularity.

Henry Hancock, an English surgeon, had beaten Parker into print with the account of his opening of the abdomen of a thirty-year-old woman, on April 17, 1848, to evacuate a quantity of excessively offensive turbid serum; she survived[7]. Although his paper failed to create a stir, Hancock deserves credit for recognizing the abscess as being of appendicular origin and operating at once before gas had begun to collect.

It was Lawson Tait, the bold, unconventional and progressive surgeon, famed as an ovariotomist, who on September 17, 1880, first operated on an appendiceal abscess and removed a diseased appendix from its normal position. The abscess had already been present for a few months when Tait opened the abdomen; expecting to find peritonitis, he found only a large abscess in the middle of which was a gangrenous appendix – 'I therefore snipped it off'. All went well and the girl of seventeen made a complete recovery[8]. On March 4, 1886, he diagnosed another case of appendicitis at an early stage before perforation had occurred and took the courageous step of removing the organ, again with a perfectly satisfactory result[8].

In the first half of the 1880s Mikulicz, in Germany, had been devoting much attention to the general problem of any form of perforation within the abdomen and we have already seen how, in 1880, he had been the first surgeon to sew up a perforated gastric ulcer. Three or four years later he recommended that all patients with acute appendicitis should have the appendix removed and, to demonstrate his faith in his belief, on December 19, 1883, he operated on a man of forty-nine with a perforated appendix, intending to remove the organ. Unfortunately, he was unable to find the appendix and the man died five days afterwards[9]. Two months later, on February 14, 1884, Rudolf Ulrich Krönlein of Zürich opened the abdomen of a seventeen-year-old patient with acute appendicitis, removed the diseased organ and washed out the peritoneal cavity with antiseptic solution – as a good follower of Lister would do – but the patient died after two days[10]. On July 26, 1885, he again made a diagnosis of acute appendicitis and operated; but like Mikulicz before him he could not find the appendix despite a prolonged search which was brought to an end by a deterioration in the man's condition. Krönlein washed out the peritoneal cavity, inserted a drain and closed the incision; much to everyone's surprise, the eighteen-year-old patient lived[10]. (As if to justify his actions he referred to both Mikulicz and Lawson Tait throughout his paper.) One way or another Krönlein is credited with the first *planned* attempt to operate on a patient with acute appendicitis with the intention of removing the offending organ.

The prevailing state of surgical opinion was still retarding progress and surgeons seemed unable to abandon the past in spite of general agreement that the appendix was to blame and not the caecum. This hesitancy was no doubt fortified by the fear, not yet dispelled, of unnecessarily cutting the peritoneum. What to do about appendicitis remained uncertain until Fitz's brilliant exposition.

Fitz graduated at Harvard, obtaining his MD in 1868, and then, like so many other American doctors of his generation, he came to Europe for two years. There he was extremely fortunate in being able to study under two of the most influential pathologists of the day, Carl Rokitansky, a Czech, at Vienna and Rudolf Virchow, at Berlin. Rokitansky believed a sound knowledge of pathology to be essential to the practice of clinical medicine and surgery and this view had a considerable influence on Fitz's future work. When he returned to Harvard, Fitz devoted himself to the study of pathology, being appointed professor at the university in 1879, and seven years later giving to the world the results of his research into appendicitis. The occasion was the first meeting of the American Association of Physicians, and here he read his paper entitled 'Perforating inflammation of the vermiform appendix; with special reference to its early diagnosis and treatment'[11]. This gave for the first time a lucid description of the disease and correlated the clinical picture with the findings in the body after death; in all, he analysed four hundred and sixty-six cases, in two hundred and fifty-seven of which the diagnosis was unquestionable, having been made post mortem, and in the remaining two hundred and nine the diagnosis had been made clinically as either typhlitis, perityphlitis or perityphlitic abscess. Fitz showed that the vast majority of these latter cases were in fact due to inflammation of the appendix and he therefore proposed naming the disease 'appendicitis'.

His paper drew the attention of the medical profession in no uncertain manner to disease of the appendix, and surgeons were soon able to recognize appendicitis as a distinct entity, though at first they continued to operate only when abscess formation and perforation had occurred. In 1887, Thomas George Morton of Philadelphia was presented within a man of twenty-six who had had attacks of acute abdominal pain for three or four years; the present illness had lasted ten days. Leeches were first applied before, on April 27, Morton went in through an eight-inch incision to be met by a free flow of pus when he opened the peritoneum. He found the appendix to contain a faecalith (a 'stone' formed from compacted faecal material) like a cherry stone at the site of a large perforation near the origin of the appendix at the caecum. He tied one silk ligature close to the caecum and another at the end of the appendix, and then removed the intervening section together with a large piece of omentum lying in the abscess cavity which he washed out with warm water. Finally he drained the wound; the patient made a good recovery. At the meeting of the Philadelphia College of Physicians where his work was presented, Morton remarked, '...an incision should be made as soon as the symptoms indicate the possible or probable formation of abscess or perforation. Now that the abdominal cavity can be sectioned there should be no delay in promptly making at least an exploratory incision. The delay in such cases constitutes one of the chief sources of the well recognised great mortality.'[11] This recommendation was not only influential but also indicated considerable progress in attitudes towards abdominal surgery.

At the end of the year, on December 30, Henry Sands of New York made a diagnosis of perforated appendicitis. At operation he found one faecalith in the peritoneal cavity and another escaping from a hole at the base of the appendix. The margins of the hole were not gangrenous, so 'these were very slightly trimmed with scissors, and then brought together with three interrupted silk sutures'. The boy recovered[12]. That Sands's devotion to the useless organ was short-lived was indicated by Charles McBurney who recorded the next year that he had assisted Dr Sands in a number of successful appendicectomies at an early stage of the disease[13].

In England the idea of early operation with sacrifice of the appendix did not meet with immediate approval and even Lawson Tait, despite his two previous successes, believed that removal of the appendix was a risky undertaking. For instance, on August 20, 1889, he operated on a man of twenty-seven who had had recurrent attacks of appendicitis and found the swollen appendix surrounded by inflamed tissues. He proceeded to slit open the organ and, with a small celluloid catheter, pushed a faecalith back into the caecum. The catheter was left lying in the lumen of the appendix with its other end outside the abdomen and was removed three days later. The patient went on to make a good recovery[14]. Tait then announced that he would continue to drain the appendix in this manner until he found a good reason to revert to his old method of removal. Frederick Treves provided another example of the lengths to which surgeons would go in order to preserve an appendix. He was a great believer in operating between acute attacks and on February 16, 1887, he found a thirty-four-year-old man's appendix to be kinked. So he straightened it and bared its convex side hoping that new adhesions would hold it straight. He did have the courage to admit, 'In the majority of cases it would probably be wiser to remove the appendix.'[15] [What, unfortunately, I have been unable to discover is how many of these patients who kept their appendices subsequently developed recurrent attacks and perhaps had to have the organ removed.]

Charles McBurney, a colleague, as we said, of Sands was in charge of the surgical division of the Roosevelt Hospital in New York. He had carefully observed many cases of appendicitis and as a result in 1889 was able to describe what has since become known as McBurney's point. He laid great stress on the fact that a useful diagnostic sign of acute appendicitis was the finding of a certain tender point and he was most exact in its localization: 'And I believe that in every case the seat of greatest pain, *determined by the pressure of one finger*, has been very exactly between an inch and a half and two inches from the anterior spinous process of the ilium on a straight line drawn from that process to the umbilicus.'[13] The symptoms now recognized as those of the usual type of appendicitis were first recorded in 1889 by the Chicago surgeon, John Murphy[16]. The patient initially complains of fairly generalized pain in the abdomen, most often intense around the umbilicus, and accompanied by nausea, which proceeds to actual vomiting, and finally the pain changes in character and settles in the lower right side of the abdomen. This order of symptoms and McBurney's point of maximum tenderness put Fitz's original description of abdominal pain and tenderness into good clinical perspective.

Attention was now directed towards discovering the best technique for performing the operation itself. The surgeon could not simply pick up his scalpel and cut straight down to the appendix; he had to consider the arrangement of the muscles of the abdominal wall and how to get through them, so that after operation their function would be unimpaired. Important nerves had to be avoided, and if the appendix was not found in its usual place, the incision had to be such that it could be extended to enable the surgeon to explore further afield. McBurney gave much thought to the problem, eventually devising a method of approach that he first used on December 18, 1893[17], and which, with few modifications, is still popular today. Besides being named after its originator, it is also known by the more descriptive titles of 'muscle-splitting' and 'grid iron' and is performed by making an incision about three inches long over McBurney's point or directly over the appendix, if this can be felt when the patient is anaesthetized. The incision classically slopes from above downwards and in an inward direction, though some surgeons prefer to make it more horizontal thereby cutting along the line of the skin creases. The underlying muscles are not cut but are carefully split, hence the origin of one name; the grid iron part comes about because the muscles of the various layers run in different directions. The only cutting required is to open the sheaths of the muscles as these are reached, then when the all the muscles have been drawn back and a good view obtained the peritoneum is incised and the intestines exposed.

In 1895 another famous incision was introduced by William Henry Battle of London, not a spectacular surgeon, but always reliable, neat and quick. Since he started his career in pre-aseptic days he was accustomed to operating in white cotton gloves and took some time to adjust to rubber gloves. His incision, known not unexpectedly as Battle's incision, was a vertical one and nearer to the mid-line than McBurney's[18]; it was supposed to have the advantage of being suitable for further exploration in obscure cases, but in reality it could be dangerous to nerves and blood vessels and, if it had to be extended, there was a risk that the scar would bulge. The incision was heavily criticized at the time. Nevertheless, it is strange that an unsatisfactory incision should have the names of other surgeons, from different parts of the world, attached to it – Adolphe Jalaguier[19] (French) in 1897; Frederic Kammerer[20] (American) also in 1897; and Karl Gustav Lennander[21] (Swedish) in 1898 – whereas McBurney's incision is associated with his name only. Strange again because he was not the first to describe the grid iron incision; that honour goes to Lewis Linn McArthur of Chicago. [But see pp. 88-89.] Presentation and publication of McArthur's paper was delayed by the summer recess: 'During that time Dr. Chas. McBurney in the *Annals of Surgery* for July has advocated the same procedure. This will therefore be a recommendation in itself for the suggestion.' McArthur had been using the incision for over two years and had demonstrated it before his colleagues to their complete satisfaction; his results in fifty-nine patients were excellent[22]. When McBurney learnt of this, he acknowledged McArthur's priority to the grid iron incision[23].

Like quite a number of other diseases, appendicitis soon had a terrific vogue which in England was touched off by Edward VII, who caused a dramatic postponement of his coronation by developing the complaint in 1902 and was successfully operated on by Frederick Treves. As might be expected, the operation was a drainage of an abscess without removal of the appendix. So fashionable did appendicitis become that almost any 'tummy ache' was suspect and surgeons were guilty of excess in their enthusiasm to operate. The subsequent reaction was due to the belief that many of the deaths were really the result of injudicious surgery, and it took the shape of non-operative management, devised in America by Albert Ochsner[24] and in England by James Sherren[25]. The Ochsner-Sherren regimen consisted in nothing being taken by mouth, nutrient fluids instead being given into the rectum while the patient was very closely watched in bed. It was carried out whenever the patient was first seen more than thirty-six hours after onset, except in children. When the treatment was successful, the appendix was removed a few weeks later at a time chosen by the surgeon and not dictated by the disease. Ochsner lowered his mortality rate by more than three-quarters by adopting the regimen. Nevertheless, there were many objections to the acceptance of the routine which was impractical except in hospital where operation could be undertaken immediately should it prove necessary. Sherren, in fact, did always operate if he was in any doubt at all.

Largely owing to the work of American surgeons, appendicitis emerged from virtual obscurity to become a commonly recognized disease and one eminently suitable for cure by the surgeon's knife.

8

Abdominal wounds and early colostomies

Many past surgical struggles with disease of the large bowel were influenced by attempts to save the anal sphincter and so preserve faecal continence. Unfortunately, these were sometimes detrimental to the patient because, though they may have spared him the inconvenience (or worse) of a colostomy or ileostomy, they also spared the disease. Contrariwise, many other struggles were concerned more with the disease than the patient. Whichever course his surgeon chose, the patient's lot was not a happy one. Only with modern technical progress have surgeons been able to give their whole-hearted attention to both disease and quality of life.

As so often happened with other parts of the body, surgical attitudes to the bowels were moulded by Nature's response to trauma and disease – and from antiquity until as recently as the 19th century, her response was generally agreed to be bad. Hippocrates's aphorism on the subject was widely interpreted as referring to all penetrating wounds of the abdomen, yet he had in fact been more specific: 'A severe wound of the bladder, of the brain, of the heart, of the diaphragm, of the small intestines, of the stomach, and of the liver, is deadly.'[1] Thus, by implication, wounds of the large intestine were not so disastrous, and from time to time a casualty evidently survived, since Galen, in his commentary on the aphorism, said that wounds of the bowels were not necessarily 'very dangerous' – which was what he believed Hippocrates meant by 'deadly'.

Celsus had been of like mind, for he wrote, 'sometimes the abdomen is penetrated by a stab of some sort, and it follows that intestines roll out. When this happens we must first examine whether they are uninjured, and then whether their proper colour persists. If the small intestine has been penetrated, no good can be done. The larger intestine can be sutured, not with any certain assurance, but because a doubtful hope is preferable to certain despair; for occasionally it heals up.'[2] Yet despite this encouragement, abdominal surgery slid, along with everything else, into the gloom of the Dark Ages. Certain despair was, with reason, natural.

Matters remained unchanged until the 18th century, although surgeons and, in particular, itinerant herniotomists had long been familiar with the occasional spontaneous breakdown of a gangrenous strangulated hernia to form a life-saving enterostomy (a hole in the intestine through which faeces are discharged to the surface); with the abdominal wound, the wound itself became an unnatural anus. Admittedly these were uncommon, but by way of compensation they were usually dramatic.

One of the first to give Nature a helping hand was William Cheselden: Margaret White had had an umbilical hernia since she was fifty. All went well until 'her seventy-third year, when, after a fit of the cholic, it mortified, and she being presently taken with a vomiting, it burst. I went to her, and found her in this condition, with about six and twenty inches and an half of the gut hanging out, mortified. I took away what was mortified, and left the end of the sound gut hanging out at the navel, to which it afterwards adhered; she recovered, and lived many years after, voiding the excrements through the intestine at the navel; and though the ulcer was so large, after the mortification separated, that the breadth of two guts was seen; yet, they never at any time protruded out at the wound, tho' she was taken out of her bed, and sat up every day.'[3]

Two of Cheselden's contemporaries, one French and the other German, followed their respective armies – which, so far as any modern concept of treating the wounded is concerned, was just about all they were allowed to do. Their experience did, however, give them an insight into wounds of the bowel (and elsewhere) denied to surgeons in civilian life.

The Frenchman, Henri François Le Dran, a much under-rated surgeon, had noticed that it was quite common for poor people with incarcerated ruptures to mistake the painful, inflamed swelling for an abscess and to incise it themselves. When these patients at last came to him in severe pain with faeces discharging from a suppurating wound, he usually found that nothing more than daily cleaning and dressing were required. At the most he would dilate the incision to allow free drainage of pus and faeces. Many patients recovered 'more by Nature than by Art', the wound either healing or remaining open to form a new 'anus' in the groin. Le Dran made full use of the lesson when dealing with wounded gut; moreover he was fully alert to the dangers of peritonitis:

'If the loss [of intestinal substance] be considerable, two or three threads must be passed through in the nature of a loop, to keep it fixed at the most depending part of the wound; to the end, that if any chyle, or matter, should issue from it, they may not be discharged into the belly.'[4]

Gangrenous intestine left within the abdomen could only have lethal results. 'To prevent this inconvenience,' Le Dran wrote, 'we must anticipate the operation of nature, by cutting off the part that is mortified, and then fix the open intestine, by one or more stitches of the looped suture, at the lower part of the wound, as we before advised when speaking of a wound of the intestine attended by loss of substance.'[5] He twisted the sutures, rather than tying them, so that they could easily be withdrawn since it was his hope that the enterostomy would close of its own accord – Nature always prefers to send faeces along the natural route when this is still available.

From 1707 to 1709, the German, Lorenz Heister, attached himself to the Dutch camp in Flanders where the war with France gave him many practical opportunities as well as the chance to study the methods of English, Dutch, and other German surgeons. His writings have much in common with those of Le Dran and he sometimes refers to the practice of the younger man. The principles on which these two managed wounded bowel marked the transition from the old to the new.

Until then, penetrating wounds of the intestine – when the casualty survived to reach a surgeon, and when the surgeon dared to intervene at all – were closed with the continuous glover's suture and the gut returned to the abdomen. The stitches were close together and the ends of the final knot hung for a foot outside the abdomen so that the silk thread could be withdrawn when the intestine was healed. As this technique was only very rarely successful, Heister instead fastened the hole in the intestine to the internal aspect of the wound in the abdominal wall with waxed thread. The thread was then firmly fixed with sticking plaster so that the gut could not slip back inside and no faeces could enter the peritoneal cavity. It is not entirely clear from his description whether he had the same hope as Le Dran of spontaneous closure or whether he fashioned only permanent enterostomies. Although he failed to comment on the fate of the distal length of gut, he certainly created permanent stomas for he wrote: 'there have been Instances where the wounded Intestine has been so far healed, that the Faeces which used to be voided per Anum have been voided by the Wound in the Abdomen: Which, from the Necessity of wearing a Tin or Silver Pipe, or keeping Cloths constantly upon the Part to receive the Excrement, may seem to be very troublesome: But it is surely far better to part with one of the Conveniences of Life, than to part with Life itself. Besides, the Excrements that are voided by this Passage, are not altogether so offensive, as those that are voided per Anum.'[6]

This excerpt contains one of the rare descriptions of how stomas were managed in those early days. But, apart from his obvious concern with the patient's welfare, Heister's great contribution was his appreciation of how eagerly the wounded gut would adhere to other structures: the surgeon's job was to give this proclivity time to work and to make sure that it did so to the patient's advantage.

Yet, despite the encouraging approach of Heister and Le Dran, enterostomies were still rarities and objects of surprise in the second half of the 18th century. Pierre Joseph Desault, the great teacher of clinical surgery at the Hôtel Dieu in Paris, for instance, could report only two cases of unnatural anus, one the result of a wound, the other of a strangulated scrotal hernia[7].

Then, as if born to mitigate the horrors of the Napoleonic battlefields there appeared a surgeon who behaved with all the confidence and insight that were still being learnt more than a hundred years later. Dominique Jean Larrey genuinely cared for the wounded man; not only did he bring him first aid – and often definitive surgery – where he lay, he also organized a complete system of casualty evacuation; and, to complement these talents, he had an uncanny appreciation of a surgical situation. At the assault on Cairo in 1799, a soldier was wounded in the abdomen by a ball that divided the ileum. Larrey described the subsequent course of events:

'Being on the field of battle, I attended to him immediately and found the two ends of intestine to be separated and swollen. The upper end was turned back on itself, like the prepuce in paraphimosis, and had strangulated the intestinal canal. Although I almost despaired of the man's recovery, I endeavoured to apply a remedy to his singular case.

'I divided the neck of the strangulation with four small incisions made with curved scissors. I then passed a ligature through the mesentery of the two ends, which I brought up to the edge of the abdominal wound. I took care to dilate this wound. After applying dressings, I awaited the result. The first days were unpromising; then the symptoms abated – those connected with the alimentary evacuations improved daily. After two months' attention the two ends of the ileum were in apposition and ready to adhere. I assisted Nature. I had the patient dressed with a tampon (according to Desault's ingenious plan) which was continued on and off for two more months. This soldier left hospital completely cured.'[8]

For gun shot wounds, Larrey mostly followed Le Dran's technique, stitching the injured intestine to the abdominal wound which was kept dilated until the injury was ready for healing; this took place from intestine outwards. 'After many battles I have had occasion to treat a great number of soldiers with wounds of this kind, and they have generally been cured in this way.'[9] Incised or punctured wounds were a different matter (because the disturbance, and consequently the formation of adhesions, was less). In these cases Larrey considered creating a colostomy based on that suggested by Littre in 1710 but he discarded the idea:

'Littre's technique in wounds of the intestine, whatever their nature, is undoubtedly the least calculated to aggravate the irritation of the injured parts; but it also has the inconvenience of prolonging the disease and creating an artificial anus for some time.' He feared, too, the risks of the colostomy slipping back inside the abdomen and of its prolapse and strangulation. For these reasons he preferred the suture, providing it could be done immediately after the accident.

'In suturing wounds of the intestines, it is necessary to keep in view the following points:

'*First*. To preserve the lips in exact contact.

'*Second*. To include within the points of the suture only the least possible portion of the intestinal tube, lest we so diminish its diameter as to obstruct the passage of faecal matter.

'*Third*. That this is the most suitable method of suture; for, whatever may be asserted to the contrary by other authors the reunion of wounds of the intestines is effected, as in other parts of the body, by their own vessels; and the adhesions will be prompt and easy in proportion as the divided parts are brought into exact contact, and preserved in this state by the suture indicated.'[9]

Thus, by a quarter of a century, did Larrey anticipate the Lembert suture[10] on which hangs the success or failure of intestinal anastomosis (see p. 38).

But unfortunately, despite the evidence from twenty-five years of almost continual bloody warfare, Larrey's experience was soon forgotten. Until World War I wounds of the abdomen carried a high mortality rate and there was considerable doubt whether to operate or not. The general opinion, however, was that to interfere was to make a certainty of a probability. By the time of World War II, surgery and its supportive techniques had entered a new era; nevertheless surgeons were fearful of returning sutured colon into the peritoneal cavity in case the adjacent bowel might have been devitalized by the injury. 'A step which I have repeatedly advocated since the outbreak of war, the exteriorization of colon injuries, is, perhaps the greatest single factor in the improved results we are able to record,' wrote William Heneage Ogilvie. 'The principle that all damaged parts of the large intestine must be excluded till the process of repair is complete applies to all parts of the large bowel, particularly the extraperitoneal portion of the rectum.'[11] The wound in the bowel thus became the stoma. However, on occasion when the surgeon did suture the wounded colon and returned it into the peritoneal cavity, a defunctioning colostomy was routinely created.

From what we know of 18th century military surgery, it is scarcely surprising that contemporary civilian surgeons were singularly reluctant to fashion colostomies ab initio, even in cases of dire need. Their operating repertoire was sorely limited and, besides, they had their reputations to consider. Surgery was slowly emerging into respectability and shaking itself free of the aura of barbers, charlatans and mountebanks; so, during the transformation period certain despair was much to be preferred to a hope so doubtful that the majority of surgeons had neither the faith nor the courage to chance their scalpel. Only a fool would venture into a body cavity and, whatever else they may have been, these men were not fools. They knew their limitations and were content to leave most of the chancy stuff to the quacks who, not being fools either, were itinerant. Broadly speaking, the mentality of the 18th-century surgeon was such that, when he did intervene, it was only to use his art to aid Nature – not to do something she was incapable of doing for herself.

Nevertheless, the evidence of spontaneous and traumatic enterostomies did make one or two surgeons wonder about the possibility of imitating Nature in cases of intestinal obstruction. The first person to make the suggestion publicly was Alexis Littre in an observation to the Royal Academy of Sciences in Paris in 1710. In carrying out a post-mortem on a six-day-old baby he had found the rectum to be in two parts joined only by a few threads of tissue about an inch long; the upper pouch was full of meconium (the first faeces of a newborn baby), the lower was empty. Littre put forward two plans for dealing with similar situations, 'if the diagnosis could be made'. The first was to open the two closed ends and stitch them together; the second was to bring the upper end out onto the abdominal wall where it would function as an anus – this became known as the Littre operation.[12] 'It is often sufficient just to know that we have a choice, to keep us from despair at the first sight,' he said, paraphrasing Celsus.

But his remark about diagnosis was much more to the point and draws attention to one of the big difficulties holding back progress – surgeons had very little idea of what they were dealing with. An imperforate anus was obvious, but if a stab with a knife failed to open a passage for meconium they, and the patient, were lost. Congenital abnormalities of the rectum were more of a diagnostic problem and as a result the babies were simply left to die. Acquired obstruction, often due to cancer, was, diagnostically speaking, almost a closed book – 'iliac passion' covered a multitude of sins both inflammatory and obstructive. Laxatives, purges, enemas and blood-letting were about the sum total of the general treatment, and the swallowing of metallic mercury (to force a passage through the obstruction by its weight alone) constituted the specific therapy in those cases where the obstruction was too high to be reached by a wicked variety of instruments and chemical cauteries designed to force or erode a passage. No one attempted to emulate the performance of Praxagoras who, in about 330 BC practised 'audacious surgery' on a patient in 'acute torment' – a diagnosis on a par with iliac passion, although between them they conjure up a pretty picture of serious low abdominal pathology. Praxagoras opened his patient's belly and extracted a mass (faecal?) causing the blockage. The patient apparently survived[13].

No one, either, risked putting Littre's suggestion of a colostomy to the test until the end of the 18th century and the first attempt, by Dubois, was a failure – but at least he had tried. Antoine Dubois, later to become a surgeon-consultant to Napoleon's imperial household and accoucheur to Marie Louise, operated on a three-day-old child with imperforate anus in 1783. The baby died ten days afterwards[14].

Meantime, though, a provincial surgeon in Rouen had already performed the first planned enterostomy with complete technical, if not lasting, success. This operation by Pillore is somewhat of a historical misfit since it was first reported, after a lapse of twenty-two years, to the Medical Society of Lyons by Martin the younger. In 1798, having spoken of Duret's recent Littre operation (see below), Martin said that 'Pillore, a Rouen surgeon, had also done it with success; but his incision was made in the right iliac fossa and utilized the caecum.'[15]

This news aroused the interest of the handful of colostomy enthusiasts of the day, and of the Geneva surgeon, Pierre Fine, in particular. Fine wrote to Pillore and, after the old man's death, to his son (also a surgeon) asking for details, but was unable to rekindle the enthusiasm. Dupuytren tried in his turn, and he, too, failed. Not until the late 1830s did Pillore fils part with his father's records, and the man who winkled them out was Amussat, at that time preparing his own memoir on a form of colostomy which was to push the abdominal variety into the shade for about fifty years. Nevertheless, both the concept and the execution of Pillore's operation were magnificent.

M. Morel, a country wine merchant, had been referred to a physician in Rouen because of increasing difficulty in getting his bowels open. Laxatives helped for a while until the obstruction became complete, whereupon the physician fed M. Morel two pounds of mercury. A month later, as no mercury had appeared, Pillore was called in. He examined the rectum thinking to find a mass of impacted faeces, but instead discovered a large, fixed, obstructing rectal cancer. For several days he tried to force a passage with sounds of many shapes and sizes, all to no avail.

'I therefore proposed that I should make him an artificial anus. He agreed and even drew my attention to the case of a man in his village who for several years had had an artificial anus provided by Nature when his hernia strangulated. I did in fact know of this case and also of another similar one in a woman.

'I was now determined to carry out the operation, but as the case was extremely delicate, I first asked five or six of my colleagues to see the patient with me. Not one of them agreed with my opinion. But the patient, a sensible man, asked my colleagues if they knew of any other means by which he might be saved. They knew of none. "Very well," he answered, "in that case operation is essential since my illness is mortal and you know of no other way to save me."

'Encouraged by the force of his argument, I operated in the presence of my colleagues and of six students. I chose the caecum on account of its position and because it would act as a reservoir. Before operation my patient and I had discussed the matter and together we had devised a small plate with, attached to it, a sponge in the shape of a large button. Held in place with an elastic bandage, this served instead of a sphincter and allowed the patient to remove it whenever he felt the need. Also, by means of a small enema, he could from time to time cleanse the reservoir.'

Pillore made his incision a little above the right groin and found the caecum without difficulty. He opened it transversely and stitched the opening firmly to the two lips of the wound. Faecal matter ran out freely and abundantly for several days, but of the mercury there was no sight despite M. Morel's adopting a variety of postures to encourage it to appear. For a fortnight his condition steadily improved and the wound healed well, but then he began to complain of abdominal pain; on the twentieth day his belly became swollen and on the twenty-eighth he died. Post-mortem revealed a loop of gangrenous jejunum weighed down into the pelvis by two pounds of mercury[16].

The operation next in order after Dubois's was the first entirely successful colostomy and was performed in the left inguinal region in a baby with an imperforate anus. But, as did Pillore, its author suffered in the early priority stakes from delaying publication. C. Duret, the surgeon in question, was a professor at the Military and Naval Hospital in Brest. In October 1793 a day-old boy (who also had a genital malformation) was brought to him on account of the imperforation. After making an examination, Duret called a meeting of physicians and surgeons from the Brest hospitals to discuss the case. Predictably, they all agreed that the perineum should be cut at the site of the missing anus and the rectum sought for. Duret did this, but could find no trace of the lower end of the large bowel. He went home that evening convinced the child would be dead by morning. He was wrong, and it was this inborn determination to survive that decided him. He called a second meeting of his colleagues and told them that he proposed to fashion an artificial anus.

'To give me confidence in this unusual task, I practised first on the dead body of a 15-day-old child taken from the poorhouse. I made a two-inch incision on the left side between the bottom rib and the iliac crest. I exposed the kidney and part of the colon; I opened the latter. Then I injected some water into the anus – part came out through the opening; part escaped into the belly. I next opened the belly and discovered that, in the baby, this area of colon is not extraperitoneal, as it is in the adult, but has a mesocolon which renders it free and floating. This finding made me abandon the idea of operating in this manner for fear that it would cause meconium to escape into the belly.'

Duret had thus had the idea of reaching the descending colon from behind without entering the peritoneal cavity. Unfortunately he believed the anatomy of the newborn to be against him; but if only it could be followed, how much safer this route appeared as it avoided the seemingly inevitable hazard of those days – peritonitis.

In spite of this setback, Duret was determined to attempt surgery. 'I opened the belly of the little patient in the left iliac region, close to the place where the sigmoid colon was forming a visible bulge and where the meconium had already given a slightly darker colour to the skin. Through an incision about an inch and a half long I crooked my index finger round the sigmoid colon and lifted it out. To prevent it slipping back inside, I passed two waxed threads through the mesocolon; I then opened the gut longitudinally.' No other sutures were inserted.

The child steadily improved, though on the fourth day when the stools decreased in quantity Duret again used his initiative and ordered a washout with plain water to which was added two drops of syrup of rhubarb. This had the desired result. The waxed threads were removed on the fifth day as their task seemed to have been achieved. On the sixth day one of the curses that was to plague enterostomies for many a long year made its unwelcome appearance – the mucosal layer of the bowel prolapsed. 'I tried to reduce the prolapse by passing a lead cannula into the stoma; this instrument would also obstruct any further prolapse and keep the passage open for faeces, but the child's cries made me desist. The instrument has, however, since been perfected by Citizen Morier, a skilled cutler.' On the seventh day, 'the child was so well, both at the site of the operation and in the exercise of his functions, that I judged him no longer in need of professional care or supervision.'[17]

Duret had ploughed more furrows than he realized – quite apart from the fact that his patient lived well into adult life and died at the age of forty-five.

The first case to be published – and this, after all, is important when tracing the development of an operation – was Desault's failure in 1794 with a Littre colostomy in a two-day-old baby with an imperforate anus. He used no sutures; instead he packed a dressing into the bowel with the two-fold intention of keeping the passage open and encouraging the intestine to adhere to the edges of the wound. The child died four days later[18].

The outlook seemed bleak, until a man whose voice had the ring of authority swung into action. Charles Louis Dumas was professor of medicine at Montpellier, a prestigious appointment. In 1797, safe behind his defence of being a physician, he took a side-swipe at a surgical colleague when reporting, to the Medical Society of Paris, a case of imperforate anus that had been in his care in 1790. The surgeon, by name Estor, had already made several unsuccessful attempts to find the large bowel through the perineum when Dumas suggested he might establish an artificial anus in the left iliac region. To this, Estor is reputed (by Dumas) to have replied, 'I agree, but I haven't the courage to put it into practice. The parents are opposed to the idea and I shall undoubtedly compromise my reputation by attempting so serious an operation when success is so uncertain.' The baby died and at the post-mortem Dumas seized the opportunity to demonstrate the technical feasibility of his plan. He also urged that iliac passion due to obstruction in the rectum could be relieved in like manner; furthermore he believed that an incision in the line of the muscle fibres would have a sphincteric effect and prevent both prolapse and retraction[19].

Where Dumas obtained his inspiration is open to doubt. He simply said that the surgeon should follow the guidance of Nature in creating an artificial anus. He made no reference to Littre and gave no indication of having heard of Duret's work; but his integrity on these two points has been challenged and if we ask why he should have waited seven years before announcing his suggestion, the inescapable answer is that he had heard rumour of Duret's operation. Yet no matter; he brought colostomy out of the shadows, stimulated discussion, and was indirectly responsible for Duret publishing his case.

A short while after Dumas had presented his paper, Pierre Fine in Geneva operated on Madame Helliger whose rectal cancer had caused a complete obstruction for the previous fortnight. Fine had long wanted to perform an enterostomy in these cases but had never been able to get permission. On this occasion he succeeded and, though aware of previous operations, he planned to imitate Nature's behaviour in strangulated hernia as precisely as he could by using ileum for the artificial anus.

On October 12, 1797, he made his incision just below the umbilicus, withdrew a loop of bowel, passed a holding suture through the mesentery, opened the gut, and stitched it to the abdominal wall. The sixty-three-year-old patient lived for another three-and-a-half months, and only at the post-mortem did Fine discover that the artificial anus was transverse colon and not ileum as he had fondly imagined[20].

Dumas' report had another indirect effect: it drew attention to a hitherto little-known textbook of surgery by a Dane, Hendrik Callisen[21]. In the section on imperforate anus Callisen described an approach to the colon through the left lumbar region. The incision was vertical and placed at the border of the quadratus lumborum muscle. Thus it was essentially the same operation as that practised by Duret on the dead baby, except for the incision being more posterior and vertical instead of (presumably) horizontal (Duret's description was not precise).

However, when Callisen's book was brought into the daylight by Allan, Duret had still not published, and Callisen's was the name that became attached to the operation. Allan, the recorder for the Medical Society of Paris, in 1797 concluded his report on the Dumas paper with the words: 'We think that Callisen's procedure merits consideration, and, if it could be made safe and easy, the results would be infinitely less disagreeable and incommoding for those whose lives would be saved.'[22]

At the time few agreed with this assessment and, in 1810, Raphael Bienvenu Sabatier wrote rather sarcastically: 'Instead of making an incision above the groin, Mr. Callisen, a surgeon who enjoys a distinguished reputation in Copenhagen, has suggested a search for the descending colon in the left lumbar region, where he supposes that it lies partially outside the general peritoneal cavity. The end result would be the same, but the artificial anus would be less disagreeable because the patient would be able to make himself more comfortable and because his disability would be further from his sexual organs. Callisen attempted the operation on the body of an infant dead with imperforate anus. He failed to observe the landmarks carefully and in consequence opened the peritoneal cavity. Having made a second incision more posteriorly he discovered the colon, as he had intended. However, he did not deny that his fingers, which he introduced through the first incision to help him secure the bowel, were most useful in performing the posterior operation. The procedure is commendable but the difficulties of execution are not worth the slight benefits that would result.'[23] Callisen had found the same trouble as had Duret, and the raison d'être of the lumbar approach disappeared if damage to the peritoneum could not be avoided.

Indeed the only time a Callisen type of operation was attempted before the end of the 1830s was in 1818 when Guillaume Dupuytren of the Hôtel Dieu in Paris failed in a baby with an imperforate anus. His operation differed, however, in that he went in through the right flank to the caecum; unfortunately, although he did not penetrate the peritoneal cavity, the baby died of peritonitis[24]. (Amussat – see p. 82 – was worried about this operation: the account had not been published until after Dupuytren's death; the caecum seemed a strange place in view of the diagnosis; there were technical difficulties; and, he wondered, had Dupuytren been deliberately trying to avoid the peritoneum or not. In fact, he all but queried the truth of the report[25].)

While the theoretical arguments were being mulled over in Paris, Duret's patient lived on, a constant, if localized, reminder that Man as well as Nature could form a functioning artificial anus. In consequence, while it would be an exaggeration to say that Brest became a Mecca for imperforate anuses, the surgeons there had the opportunity of creating about twelve more iliac colostomies in the next twenty or thirty years. Duret's second patient died after four days, but three operated on by Miriel all survived and were recorded in his son's thesis sustained at the Faculty of Medicine of Paris in 1835[26].

Although the French dominated the colostomy scene and continued to do so for the first half of the 19th century, three Englishmen entered the fray at this period, the first appropriately enough in the year of Waterloo. More significantly though, two of them were as concerned with the aftercare as with the operation itself.

In 1815, George Freer of Birmingham created a left iliac colostomy for a newborn baby with an imperforate anus. The colostomy functioned well and the edges united, but sadly the baby died of marasmus after three weeks. Freer's next patient was a farmer, aged about forty-seven, with rectal obstruction. On February 5, 1818, he fashioned a left iliac sigmoidostomy which, apart from prolapsing, behaved itself admirably until the fourteenth when the patient died, seemingly due to an excess of therapeutic zeal (in the shape of daily purgation and numerous enemas through the artificial anus) which ruptured the caecum[27].

The second British surgeon was Daniel Pring of Bath who had a sixty-four-year-old patient with complete obstruction of the rectum from cancer. As the patient, Mrs White, was 'desirous of living on any terms', Pring, on July 7, 1820, brought the sigmoid colon to the surface in the left inguinal region. The contents were under considerable pressure (patients sometimes died from rupture of the gut behind an obstruction), so when he incised the bowel, Pring had to retreat smartly from an eruption of faecal material. The course for the first four or five weeks after the operation was very stormy, the faeces irritated the skin and the wound sloughed extensively. But the patient slowly began to pick up until six months later she was in good health and could walk about the house.

Mrs White usually had two evacuations a day: 'she does not, upon the whole, experience so much inconvenience from the manner of evacuation as might have been expected.' The bowel did, however, prolapse easily, an annoyance that Pring attributed to the sloughing of the wound, and one that he attempted to control: 'She has a truss, somewhat similar to that for exomphalos, constructed with a circular spring, and a large pad containing a weak spiral spring, which is preserved in its place by means of straps: this contrivance has not, however, yet answered so well as a compress, confined by a band, pinched tightly around her.'

Pring concluded his paper with these words: 'the inconveniences of an anus in this situation are not such as to have caused her any regret for having submitted to the operation: on the contrary, so far from her having any reason to lament this circumstance, I believe myself that it has afforded her a moral, as well as a physical advantage; for she is now at no loss for an interest, and is provided with something to think of for the rest of her life.'[28] Everything is for the best in this best of all possible worlds.

Richard Martland of Blackburn, the last of this British trio, operated on Henry Baron, a forty-four-year-old bookkeeper, on July 24, 1824, having explained that the only hope of overcoming the cancerous obstruction lay with an artificial anus but that it was not without danger. He used a left iliac incision, then fixed the colon to each end of the wound with a suture and made a one-and-a-half-inch incision in the bowel. The wound healed in a month. On September 9 a truss 'was procured for him on the plan of the self-adjusting one, with this difference, that, in the centre of the pad, a tin box was placed for catching the feces. This box could be taken out and replaced at pleasure. On the 12th he left Blackburn to resume his employment. I was informed on the 21st of October, that the truss had not answered our expectations. When he used it, the invagination was very great, and sometimes the feces escaped from the edges of the pad. The best contrivance yet discovered is a piece of soft sponge, and about the size of a hen's egg, and common bandages. This, he says, permits the passage of wind, and obstructs the feces until he has an opportunity to relieve himself.'[29]

But by August 1825, Baron, an intelligent man, had modified this arrangement. First, he applied a small piece of cotton, then a piece of waste paper and on top of this further folds of cotton, all of which he bound on by a firm six-inch cotton bandage. Finally, he applied the truss, though in place of the tin box he put a piece of box-wood two-and-a-half inches in diameter. Baron lived for another five years.

Even in those early days thought was given to closing colostomies when faeces were being passed per anum – these cases were mostly traumatic. As the natural passage took over, so the unnatural opening tended to close, sometimes completely, sometimes leaving a persistent and troublesome fistula. Failure to close was nearly always due to the development of a spur. (A spur, quite simply, is formed by the contiguous walls of the two barrels of a colostomy adhering to each other. This is a good thing and is encouraged when the colostomy is functioning, as it helps to prevent faeces entering the distal barrel. It is a bad thing when one wants to restore intestinal continuity as it is then an obstruction to reunion.) Accordingly, various methods were devised to overcome the spur when it became a hindrance. Among the first were sponges, tents, balloons, and the 'ingenious plan' of Desault using a tampon which Larrey employed successfully in 1799. However, as these were rather hit-or-miss measures, Dupuytren decided to ligate the base of the spur; when the spur sloughed off, he completed the separation of the two barrels with scissors but regrettably opened the peritoneum and the patient died of peritonitis. He then suggested that the spur should be crushed with an enterotome – a technique that has survived to the present day. (The problems associated with closing lumbar colostomies were somewhat different – see p. 87.)

9

Later colostomies

J ean Zuléma Amussat was saddened by the general attitude of leaving the obstructed patient to die either through ignorance of what surgery might offer or through fear of compromising oneself. He referred to Dupuytren who, in 1829, had written, 'If the rectum, for instance, is obstructed and all medicines and all manoeuvres fail to re-establish continuity, would it not be legitimate to incise the abdominal wall towards the left flank, to draw out a part of the descending colon, and to open an artificial anus? The establishing of this would check the fatal outcome and prolong the life of the subject.'[1]

But far from praising this attitude, Amussat was building up for a scathing criticism of the late doyen of French surgery: 'Dupuytren himself had undoubtedly had several opportunities for practising this operation, notably on Talma [a celebrated tragedien]. However, he did not dare to attempt it.' Amussat had not overlooked Dupuytren's possible operation in 1818, but this had been for imperforate anus and the subject under discussion was obstruction in the adult. Nevertheless a more generous man would have been less harsh in his judgment, since one very real reason why colostomies were rare was the frequent difficulty of establishing during life just where the obstruction was situated. The surgeon's grasp of what he was dealing with was still extremely weak. Furthermore, the operation was dangerous, but not quite so hazardous as popular surgical imagination would have it. So Amussat set out to draw a picture of the true situation.

He gathered all the cases he could trace between Pillore's operation in 1776 and 1839 when he wrote his first memoir[2]. In those sixty-three years twenty-seven colostomies were known to have been performed, twenty-one for imperforate anus (one a recto-vaginal fistula, one a recto-urethral fistula) and six for obstruction in adults. Four of the infants were long-term survivors (another lived for three years, and another for twenty-seven months). Two of the adults (Pring's and Martland's patients) had made worthwhile recoveries, and some of the others had been technical successes; not bad, one might think, considering the patients were in very poor clinical shape. Yet Amussat was dissatisfied. He attributed all the deaths to peritonitis resulting from damage to the peritoneum – like everyone else he had a deep mistrust of the peritoneal cavity – and so he determined to make Callisen's lumbar approach safe and reliable. The final stimulus to his resolve was standing helplessly by while his patient and colleague François Joseph Victor Broussais died slowly and unpleasantly from an obstructing rectal cancer.

Amussat took himself off to the dissecting room where he found that the posterior surfaces of both ascending and descending colon were (in most cases) bare of peritoneum. For the descending colon, he emphasized the fact by distending the bowel with air pumped in by tube and bellows. The anatomy of the region had been badly neglected and the Callisen lumbar operation, suitably modified in the light of his dissections and trials on living animals, seemed a distinct possibility despite the disapproving noises made by other surgeons past and present. The significant modification was a horizontal incision taken well posteriorly to the border of the quadratus lumborum muscle.

On June 2, 1839, in the presence of a number of colleagues, including a British visitor, John Erichsen, Amussat operated on a forty-eight-year-old woman with cancer of the lower end of the sigmoid colon. She had been completely obstructed for twenty-six days. Having made the incision and resected most of the excessive fat, 'I recognized the intestine perfectly; it was very distended, ballooned and devoid of peritoneum.' The bowel was held by three torsion forceps, opened, and the edges fixed to the skin at the anterior end of the wound with four interrupted sutures 'turning back the mucous membrane' (note this seemingly insignificant detail). The posterior end of the wound was closed with a single suture. Everything went satisfactorily and by the beginning of July, Madame D. was walking about her room, eating with pleasure, and having four or five regular motions a day. She wore a compress and bandage and was well content until her death five months later from malignant peritonitis.

With his second case, Amussat showed great clinical courage, since the tumour in the patient's upper rectum was causing only partial obstruction. He was most reluctant to operate, but was eventually persuaded to do so when the patient began to go rapidly downhill. Operation was successful and the sixty-two-year-old man was still alive two years later.

By 1841, Amussat had performed two more lumbar colostomies, but on the right side, in the ascending colon, since in both patients the precise site of obstruction was in doubt. The second of these failed, in the sense that the patient died of advanced cancer ten days after operation. Doubt also surrounded the diagnosis of a third case; the obstruction was thought perhaps to be in the neighbourhood of the ileo-caecal junction and for this reason Amussat departed from his usual practice and created a right iliac caecostomy (a Littre procedure). However, the cause of the obstruction was an intussusception and the patient died twenty-four hours later[3].

Amussat's operation was good news and the bearer of this news to England was John Eric Erichsen. He was most enthusiastic, praising the advantages that Amussat himself had emphasized. Pride of place went to the absence of peritonitis, but there was also the point that the colon was more firmly fixed than in the Littre operation and consequently prolapse was less likely. Erichsen was delighted at the inconspicuousness of the spur as this made closure, should it become possible, so much easier – surgeons were still unaware of the problems of overflow of faeces into the distal bowel, though Amussat must have had an inkling since he considered the possibility of creating a spur but decided it was too dangerous in the relatively immobile lengths of colon.

Among the indications Erichsen gave for lumbar colostomy were 'Scirrhous affections of the rectum, as soon as there is much difficulty in defecation. The establishment of an artificial anus is, in these cases, the only means of retarding the progress of the disease.'[4] The influence of Amussat's second case is evident in this brave step towards the earlier treatment of rectal cancer.

Nevertheless we must not run away with the idea that colostomies were now done at the drop of a hat. Far from it. They were still occasional enough for each to merit an individual write-up. One particularly successful case, and one of the first done under anaesthesia (chloroform), was that of John Wilson Croker Pennell, an English surgeon working in Rio de Janiero, in 1849. His patient was a fifty-year-old merchant whose troubles had begun with a fistula-in-ano. Treatment of one sort and another had led to rectal stricture and the opening of a false passage into the bladder and urethra. The man passed faeces through his urethra in exquisite agony. Croker Pennell created a left lumbar colostomy through an oblique incision that corresponded with the outer margin of the quadratus lumborum muscle[5]. The result was admirable and a much relieved merchant was able to return to his business and to mix freely in society. He died fifteen years later of an unrelated disease. Yet, despite this example, surgeons continued to use the ancient excruciatingly painful methods of treating fistulae.

After Amussat the surgical initiative slipped out of French hands, but for a number of years was not firmly grasped again by any one country in particular, though British surgeons had most influence in sorting out the problems peculiar to colostomies themselves as opposed to those of the diseases for which they were employed. The period was the most momentous in the whole of surgical history and surgeons were bewitched by the possibilities opening before them as first anaesthesia, then antisepsis, and later asepsis drew back the barriers of centuries. They were also not a little confused. Amussat's operation was designed in an era when the peritoneum was feared; when that fear was overcome its raison d'être ceased to exist and its one-time advantages became disadvantages.

Representative of the old school were William Allingham of St Thomas's Hospital, and Thomas Bryant of Guy's Hospital. Allingham firmly believed that, for the adult, Amussat's operation was the first choice and it was his opinion that when mistakes were made it was because the surgeon did not look for the colon in the correct place. In more than fifty post-mortem dissections he had located it accurately every time and had never opened the peritoneum at operation (eleven cases by 1871). His patients were usually able to get up at the end of four weeks when 'they should wear a well-fitting india-rubber pad to prevent the escape of wind and motion. I now have the pad made with a little hollow and fill the concavity with cotton wool, which will absorb any slight moisture and keep the part dry. Some of my patients preferred merely a pad of wool and a napkin over it, to any mechanical appliance.'[6] When his patients survived for several months, a degree of prolapse always appeared but it was of little concern as it could easily be replaced by passing a softened bougie. (Indicative perhaps of Allingham's character is his remark about Amussat: 'It is by no means certain, however, that he ever performed the operation.')

By 1876 Bryant had performed twenty-seven lumbar colostomies through an oblique incision which, he said, seemed to lessen the possibility of prolapse; he never regretted operating though in many instances he fervently wished he could have done so earlier. At operation he oiled the margins of the wound to prevent irritation by faeces, and in the immediate postoperative days he used as the dressing a piece of oiled lint covered with oakum and kept in place with a soft towel. After healing was complete he found that a pad covered by a folded napkin and fastened on with a lumbar binder was best[7]. He had no time at all for the ivory balls or plugs which some surgeons advocated as these could neither be kept in place nor prevent prolapse.

That all was not well with the Amussat operation is evidenced by the suggestions made for overcoming the difficulties. Edward Lund of Manchester, for instance, took a leaf out of the originator's book and proposed the routine use of an air syringe and rectal tube to make the bowel more obvious. He had other ideas too: 'I also employ vaseline and eucalyptus (one-tenth) as the permanent dressing, for I have found it to decrease in a marked degree, if not entirely destroy, the unpleasant odour of the feculent discharges.'[8]

John Neville Colley Davies-Colley, in 1885, reported three instances of left lumbar colostomy in which he had brought the bowel to the surface but delayed opening it for between one and six days in order to give the bowel time to adhere to the wound edges, thus lessening the risk of infection and abscess formation and preventing soiling by faeces should the peritoneum be damaged. He furthermore suggested that a general plan might be adopted for growths of the colon: namely, a two-stage procedure in which the loop bearing the growth was first exteriorized through an abdominal incision, and then later amputated by cautery or knife[9].

Charles Bent Ball of Dublin had no liking for this scheme as he reckoned it produced symptoms of intestinal strangulation due to the need to hold the bowel up in the wound. Instead he devised special clamps for preventing peritoneal soiling and relied on the belief that once the patient had settled down after operation he usually had one motion in twenty-four hours with sufficient warning to prepare for it and so be able to avoid contamination of the wound. In his textbook of 1887[10] he wrote that the Amussat operation with the oblique incision recommended by Bryant (but not mentioning its use by Croker Pennell) was the one then generally used in adults, though for babies with imperforate anus Littre's operation was preferred.

But the days of the lumbar colostomy were numbered – even though as late as 1912, Frank Paul felt that it had a use in the temporary relief of obstructions distal to the caecum, and had the advantage of not interfering with any subsequent abdominal operation; it was particularly valuable, he thought, in the old or exhausted patient.

We shall never know the complete and true picture of colostomies in Victorian times since records were bad and many patients were operated on in their homes with no record kept at all. Yet judged by such evidence as we possess and by the reluctance to operate even when the bowel had been totally obstructed for months, it must have been pretty gloomy. The patient who could return to work, horseback, and an active social life did exist, but he was the lucky one.

The operation of lumbar colostomy itself could be a disaster. The stoma could easily be established below the obstruction and it was not unknown for the ileum to be opened by mistake and with rapidly fatal results – boding ill for the future by prejudicing the surgical mind against ileostomies. Whether or not the patient achieved any degree of control was in the lap of the gods who usually looked the other way: laudanum was then favoured as a constipating medicine. Stenosis, probably due to chronic, low-grade infection of the wound, was fairly common and demanded regular dilatation. Prolapse in moderation was welcomed by most surgeons as it helped prevent the spill-over of faeces into the distal end of bowel. And it was this spill-over that caused a good deal of trouble.

Out of sheer cussedness an unreasonable quantity of faeces seemed to get into the distal end where it would accumulate and set up antiperistaltic movements to the great discomfort of the patient; sometimes, too, it would be responsible for perforation. The problem was usually attacked simply by washouts, but some surgeons attempted to create a spur when the bowel was sufficiently mobile – their success was inconspicuous. Another surgical solution, proposed by Albert Schinzinger of Freiburg in 1881[11] and by Otto Wilhelm Madelung in 1883[12], was to divide the bowel completely (rather than just incise it), make the upper end a terminal colostomy, and close the distal end before dropping it back. This carried the danger of leaving an undrained closed loop of bowel in the abdomen. (The question of closed loops was already bothering surgeons who practised inguinal colostomies at this period; we will return to it in the chapter on rectal cancer.) And, finally, should the obstruction later be overcome, closure of the colostomy could be more hazardous than its creation, since it was frequently necessary to excise the portion of bowel that had formed the stoma (thus entering the peritoneal cavity) and anastomose the fresh ends (an unperfected art in those days). These dangers erected a formidable barrier to the performance of lumbar colostomy for potentially curable conditions.

Nevertheless, while lumbar colostomies were in the ascendant, the inguinal variety had not been entirely ignored and towards the end of the 1870s when abdominal surgeons spread their wings it began a slow but steady comeback. No one person was responsible; the movement simply gathered momentum. With the peritoneal cavity no longer forbidden territory, it was permissible to go in through the abdomen and bring a loop of mobile colon to the surface in such a manner that a good spur was formed from the outset.

Henry Albert Reeves of the Hospital for Women, London, had been promoting iliac colostomy since about 1880 and emphasizing the merits of simplicity. 'The simplification of operative measures should, in the interests of patients, be the aim of the surgeon,' he wrote, 'and experience abundantly proves that the simpler an operation is the better are its results.'[13] His technique was to bring a loop of colon to the surface and pass a vulcanite rod through its mesentery to hold it above skin level and create a sort of spur before the bowel was incised. The longer the rod was left the better the spur, but Reeves usually opened the intestine between three and six days later[14]. He frankly admitted that he could not understand the modifications of other surgeons such as Maydl of Vienna, but this seems to have been affectation in the pursuit of simplicity since Maydl's principles differed little, if at all, from his own.

Karl Maydl, whose first modified operation took place on February 4, 1884, drew out the sigmoid until he could see its mesocolon, through which he then pushed a rigid rod. If the operation had to be completed at once, he sutured the bowel to the edges of the wound and incised it transversely. Otherwise he waited for four or six days before opening the bowel with a thermocautery. On the fourteenth day after surgery he cut away all superfluous bowel above the rod and sutured the edges of the mucous membrane to the skin[15].

In the United States Charles B. Kelsey of New York used a hare-lip pin passed successively through skin, parietal peritoneum, mesentery close to bowel, parietal peritoneum, and out through skin to hold the loop firmly in position and to form a satisfactory 'spur'[16].

Among the enthusiasts of inguinal colostomy, and one of the first to state his preference in print (in 1887[17] – on the strength of six operations) was the son of William Allingham, Herbert William Allingham. He, too, emphasized the importance of getting a good spur which he achieved by bringing the sigmoid well out of the wound and passing sutures through the mesocolon. He also delayed opening the bowel for two or three days (though sooner if the patient's condition deteriorated rapidly) and cut away the edges of his incision in the gut so that the two openings were as near as possible at skin level.

The name of Frank Thomas Paul of Liverpool is perhaps the best remembered from this period as his work and that of Mikulicz of Breslau marked a significant step forward in the surgery of the large bowel. The major troubles with a colostomy were the perennial ones of faecal soiling of peritoneum and skin and the spill-over into the distal loop. To deal with the latter, Paul emulated Madelung by closing the distal opening and returning it inside the abdomen. To prevent soiling, he devised a glass tube (flanged so that it could be held more securely in the proximal opening) with a rubber extension for carrying the faeces away. He first used this tube on March 3, 1890, in a man of forty-six with cancer of the rectum. The rectum was removed at a second operation on March 24, and the patient survived for about a year with a satisfactorily functioning artificial anus.

In his report[18], Paul proposed that a similar plan might be adopted for the ileum as a means of averting death in a patient in extremis from internal strangulation. The ileostomy could, in Paul's eyes, be only temporary and he was emphatic about the need for a subsequent operation to restore intestinal continuity. This suggestion attracted no comment, but Allingham junior carped about the colostomy technique[19]. He was troubled by the idea of closing a loop since the intestine might be twisted when it was brought out and the wrong end closed; also the faeces already in the distal loop had to be removed for fear of ulceration – not an easy task – and finally he believed that faeces could still escape while the bowel was being sewn to skin. Time, however, proved that in a well-ordered house Allingham's fears and those of surgeons who shared his views were groundless.

The extent of surgical inventive genius in its first flowering at the end of the 19th century is well shown by the ideas that were tried in an attempt to give the patient some sort of control over his colostomy. Skin flaps were toyed with, but were no use. The emerging bowel was subjected to external pressure in a variety of ways such as passing it subcutaneously over the iliac crest and bringing it to the surface two inches below; leading it through a V-shaped groove gouged out of the symphysis pubis; carrying it subcutaneously down the anterior surface of the thigh; and using clips held in place by tubular skin grafts. All these ran the risk of prejudicing the blood supply of the gut. Maydl brought his colostomies out through a muscle-splitting incision (this was McBurney's grid-iron

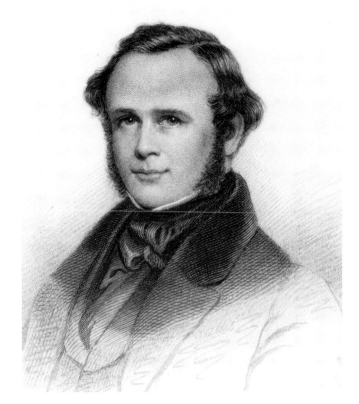

Horace Wells. (By courtesy of the Harvard Medical Library in the Frances A. Countway Library of Medicine.)

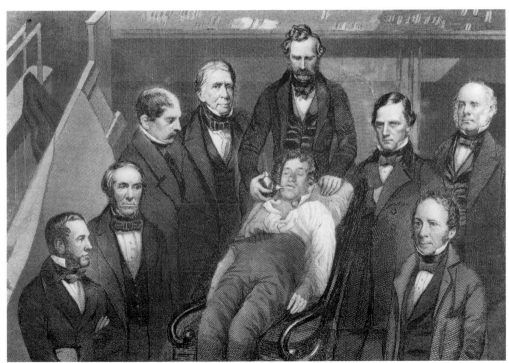

William T.G. Morton's demonstration of ether anaesthesia in 1846. (By courtesy of the National Library of Medicine, Bethesda, Maryland.)

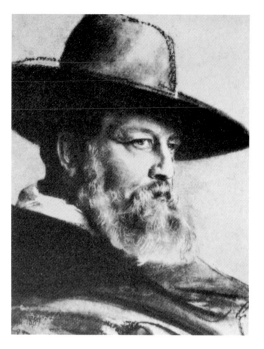

Theodor Billroth. (By courtesy of the Wellcome Library, London.)

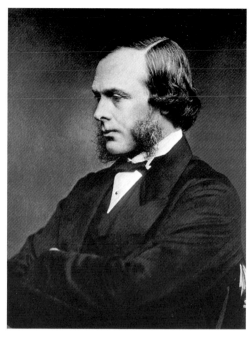

Joseph Lister. (Photo: T. and R. Annan and Sons Ltd. By courtesy of the Wellcome Library, London.)

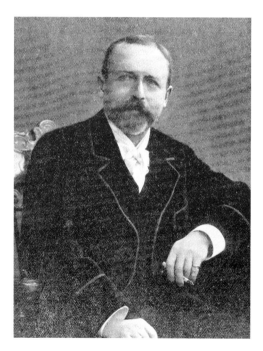

Johannes von Mikulicz-Radecki. (By courtesy of the Wellcome Library, London.)

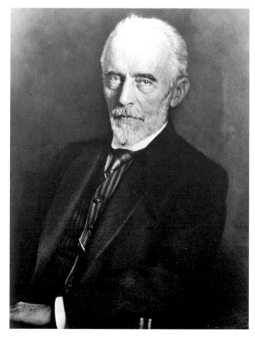

Theodor Kocher. (By courtesy of the Wellcome Library, London.)

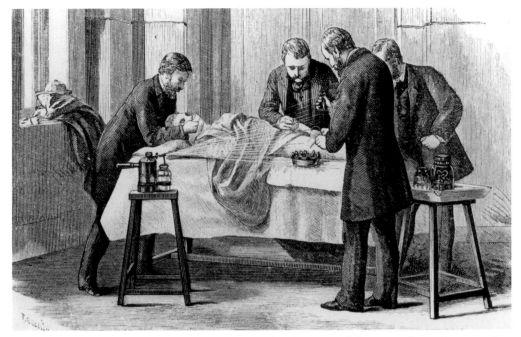

An operation of the antiseptic era. Shown are the distance of the spray from the wound, the arrangement of the wet towels, the position of the trough containing the instruments, the position of the house surgeon (facing) so that he continually has his hands in the cloud of carbolic spray and the action of the dresser (right) who hands the instruments through the spray to the surgeon. Intriguingly, the original caption described this as 'an operation performed with complete aseptic precautions'. (From Cheyne WW. (1882). *Antiseptic surgery*. London; Smith, Elder.)

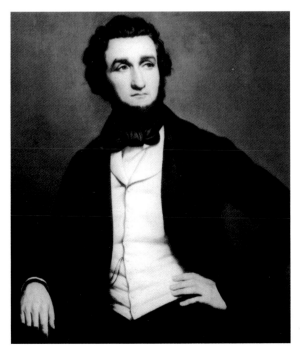

Jean Zulema Amussat. (By courtesy of the Wellcome Library, London.)

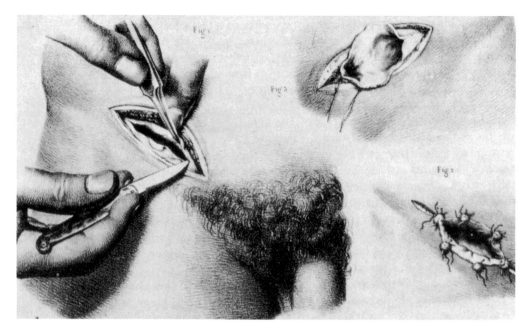

Artificial anuses. Figs 1 and 2 depict the creation of a caecal 'anus' – Pillore's procedure.
Fig 1 shows the caecum being opened through an oblique abdominal incision. In Fig 2,
the wound has been closed with six twisted waxed sutures. Two threads passed through
each angle of the intestine and tied to a musculo-cutaneous suture prevent faecal matter
from entering the abdominal cavity. Fig 3 shows the appearance, at the end of the operation, of an artificial iliac anus – Littre's procedure. The mouth of the proximal loop (right)
has a funnel-like shape. A thread passed behind the distal opening (left) keeps the
intestine in place. (From: Bourgery (1840). *Traite complet de l'anatomie de l'homme
comprenant la medecine operatoire*. Atlas, vol 7. Paris; Delaunay. By courtesy of the
Wellcome Library, London.)

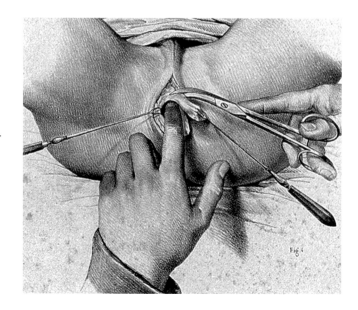

Excision of the inferior part
of the rectum – Lisfranc's
operation. The anal end
of the rectum has been
mobilized through two semi-
eliptical lateral incisions.
The rectum, steadied by the
surgeon's left index finger,
is excised above the cancer
with long-bladed curved
scissors. (From: Bourgery
(1840). See above. By
courtesy of the Wellcome
Library, London.)

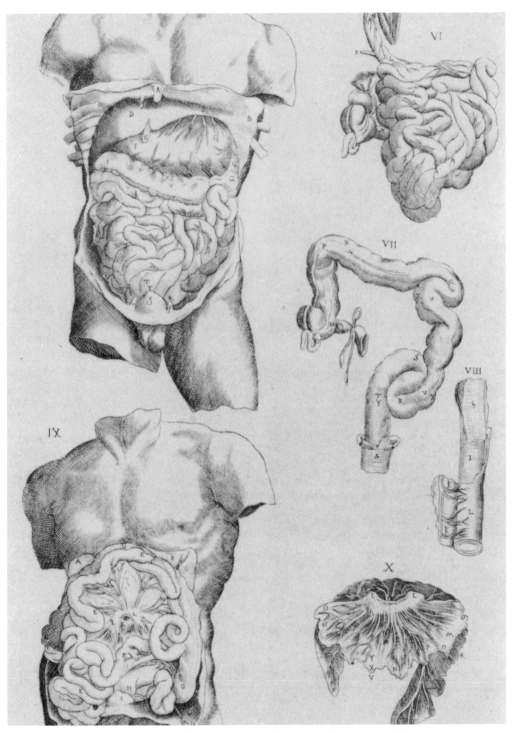

The intestines from: Vesalius (1642). *Librorum de humanis corporis fabrica epitome,*
cum annotationibus Nicolai Fontam. Amstelodami; Janssonium. (First edition, 1543.)
Andreas Vesalius broke with the past and by the descriptions of his dissections he
unshackled anatomy from the chains of Galenism. As is evident from this illustration he
was well served by his artist, Jan Stephan van Calcar (1499–1546), a pupil of Titian.

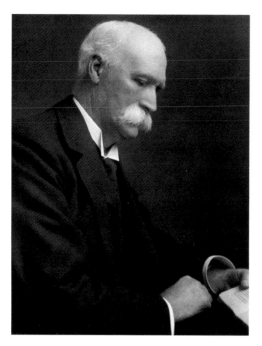

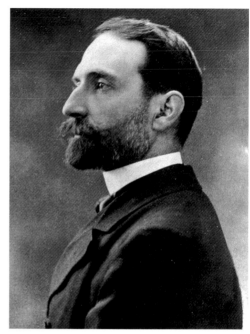

William Macewen. (Photo: T. and R. Annan and Sons Ltd. By courtesy of the Wellcome Library, London.)

Théodore Tuffier. (From an original photograph lent by Dr E.A. Underwood. By courtesy of the Wellcome Library, London.)

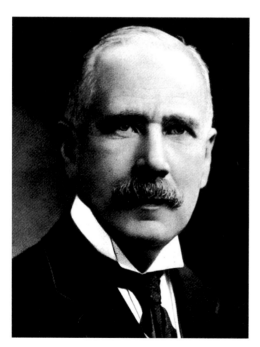

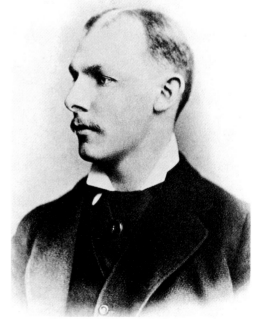

William Arbuthnot Lane. (By courtesy of the Wellcome Library, London.)

William Stewart Halsted. (From: The *Surgical papers of William Stewart Halsted*. By courtesy of the Wellcome Library, London.)

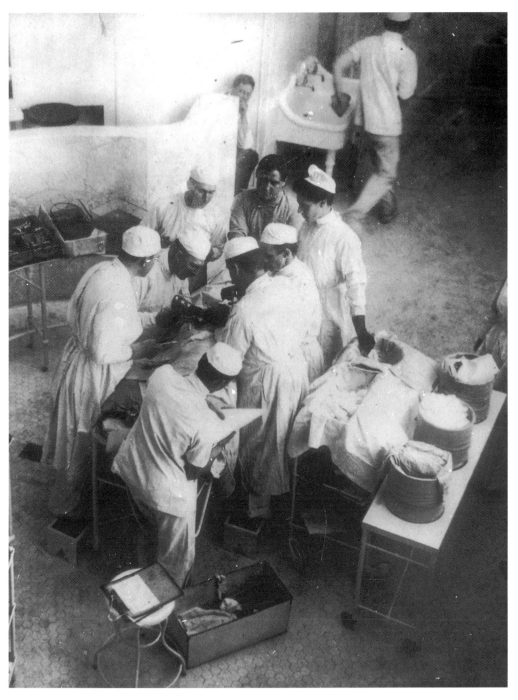

William Halsted (*left centre*) performing the first operation when the new surgical amphitheatre of Johns Hopkins was opened in 1904. Harvey Cushing was his second assistant and Miss Caroline Hampton, his theatre sister. Note the use of gloves, gowns and drapes, but the casual use of caps and the absence of masks. (From: MacCallum WG. (1930). *William Stewart Halsted. Surgeon.* Baltimore; Johns Hopkins Press. London; Oxford University Press. By courtesy of Yale Medical Library, the Clements C. Fry Collection.)

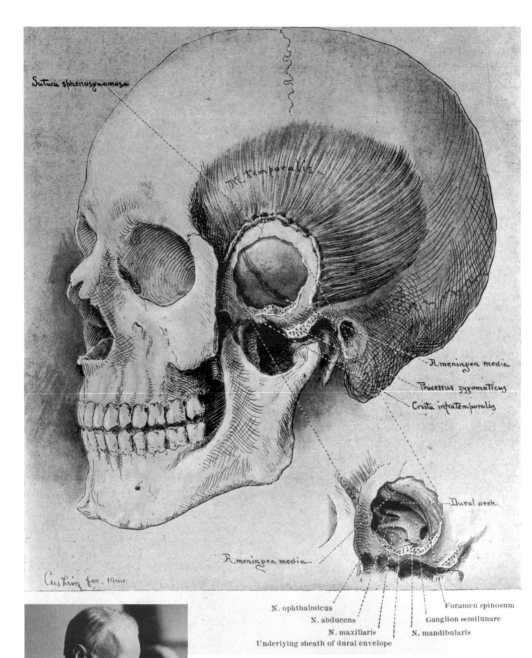

Sutura sphenosquamosa

M. temporalis

A. meningea media

Processus zygomaticus

Crista infratemporalis

Dural arch.

A. meningea media

Cushing fec. 1900.

N. ophthalmicus

N. abducens

N. maxillaris

Underlying sheath of dural envelope

N. mandibularis

Ganglion semilunare

Foramen spinosum

A drawing by Harvey Cushing to demonstrate the anatomical relations encountered during surgery to remove the Gasserian ganglion (ganglion semilunare) in the treatment of trigeminal neuralgia. It shows the relations of the middle meningeal artery to the operative foramen before and after elevation of the dura and exposure of the ganglion.

Harvey Cushing. (By courtesy of the Wellcome Library, London.)

appendicectomy incision which he described in 1894, six years after Maydl's paper and 100 years after Dumas had suggested this way into the abdomen). The object of Maydl's incision was to provide a sphincter of a sort; other surgeons used the rectus abdominis muscle; others passed the bowel behind the sartorius muscle in the thigh; and yet others simply twisted the gut. In the mid-1950s, in chosen cases, the Australian surgeon Edward Stuart Reginald Hughes, passed a long loop of sigmoid colon (with its marginal artery) through an incision in the left iliac fossa and then carried it beneath the skin to the midline below the umbilicus where he brought it to the surface[20]. The idea was that the passage of faeces along the subcutaneous part would create a definite sensation and so warn the patient of an impending bowel action.

All these techniques may have seemed fine in theory but none worked consistently in practice; the anal sphincter was not to be mimicked. Appliances were non-existent, so the patient arrived home to find he had to work out his own salvation – the surgeon had done his job and subsequent management was none of his concern. This attitude was particularly unfortunate as the inguinal region was a bad site; every time the patient moved the colostomy was liable to leak. The change to a better site nearer the centre of the abdomen began only at the end of the second decade of the 20th century. At this time, too, surgeons finally overcame their reluctance to create colostomies other than with the sigmoid colon; hitherto many had feared that increasing the length of bowel distal to the stoma was asking for trouble.

At the start of its career a colostomy was neither more nor less than a means of relieving obstruction at the far end of the large bowel, regardless of the cause of that obstruction. But in the last quarter of the 19th century a subtle change in attitude became noticeable as surgeons began to attack diseases in their own right: a colostomy became part of the management of the disease, not an end in itself. Evidence of this adjustment can be seen in the gradual dropping of the word colotomy from about 1892 onwards and its replacement by colostomy; the emphasis had shifted from cutting into bowel to the formation of a stoma.

10

Cancer of the rectum and colon

C ancer, the commonest cause of chronic intestinal obstruction in the adult (though often in the past optimistically mistaken for faecal impaction), was the first of the diseases of the large bowel to be hived off from the general run and treated as other than a straightforward blockage.

The story customarily begins with the operation of the Parisian, Jean F. Faget, for bilateral ischiorectal abscesses ('customarily', because for a long time it was erroneously believed that the patient had had cancer). The patient, a man of twenty-three, had had the abscesses opened elsewhere and when Faget saw him, the integrity of the rectum was virtually destroyed. So, on June 9, 1739, Faget resected the last part of the rectum and restored continuity; the bowels subsequently functioned satisfactorily[1].

The first successful excision of the rectum for cancer was by Jacques Lisfranc on February 13, 1826. His report dealt with nine patients all of whom had had cancer below the level of peritoneal reflection and six of whom survived operation to leave hospital, though some were obliged to wear a packing of lint in the rectum to prevent leakage of faeces[2]. However, the idea of such radical surgery was not at all attractive and nothing more was heard of it until almost half a century later when surgeons were able to explore more freely, but even so conditions around the rectum were unpleasantly restricted. Then in 1873 Aristide Verneuil published his paper on resection of the coccyx in the surgery of imperforate rectum; this recorded his first success in 1864 with a four-year-old boy who had normal bowel function afterwards[3]. Amussat had, in fact, been the originator of this scheme for giving the surgeon more room and had used it once in 1842[4]. However, Verneuil gave no acknowledgement to his predecessor for the idea – could he have been unaware of Amussat's third memoire? But whatever the truth, Verneuil reintroduced the operation at the right time, although it was not to make its mark in neonatal surgery.

The idea was quickly seized upon by that impeccable operator in Berne, Theodor Kocher, who used it to improve the exposure when operating for cancer[5]. The excision, however, remained below and outside the peritoneum and also remained a thoroughly inadequate cancer operation. The mortality rate did drop from about 80 percent to about 60 percent, but this was largely owing to an increasing awareness of antisepsis.

The next step (and on the surface an apparently logical one) was to add excision of part of the sacrum – again an original Amussat suggestion[4]. This was first done by the German, Paul Kraske, who on May 11, 1885, removed the lateral part of the lower end of the sacrum in a man of forty-eight. Kraske freely opened the peritoneal cavity and mobilized the pelvic colon which he brought down[6]. Where possible he saved the perianal skin and external sphincter, but if end-to-end anastomosis was impracticable he established a sacral anus. This reduced the mortality rate to about 20 percent and since Kraske wielded considerable influence, the technique rapidly became the most popular in Germany and Austria where a variety of modifications were introduced. More and more of the sacrum was removed; muscle attachments and blood supply were damaged in the process and the pelvic floor sagged ominously. The German enthusiasts were obsessed with preserving the anal sphincter at all costs and only rarely did they create a preliminary defunctioning colostomy.

In Great Britain, France and the United States, the Kraske operation never became popular, though when it was performed a preliminary colostomy was favoured. The reasons for the dislike are not difficult to find: the anastomosis was prone to break down and produce an intractable sacral fistula; the recurrence rate was still in the region of 70–80 percent; prolapse was a frequent complication; and a sacral anus was uncontrollable – even when the sphincters were saved their function was often impaired. This last failing may have been due to damaged nerve supply since the experience of William Harrison Cripps at St Bartholomew's Hospital, London, with straightforward excision was just the opposite. In his view, destruction of the internal sphincter and even a fair amount of damage to the external sphincter did not always result in incontinence. Out of thirty-six patients (not all his own cases), twenty-three defaecated normally, six were satisfactory provided the motions were not too fluid, and only seven were incontinent. He reckoned that it was useless to attempt to stitch the cut end to the anus, as it quickly formed attachments to the sides of the cavity and during cicatrization (scar formation) was drawn downwards. Cripps avoided the tendency to stenosis by not removing the whole circumference of bowel; he left intact a strip of wall extending down to the anal margin[7].

Frank Paul of Liverpool, however, brought down the bowel and sutured it to the anus when this had been left behind or to the posterior angle of the wound when it had been excised. By 1895 he had operated on fourteen patients with twelve recoveries; the first, a man of forty-seven, operated on in 1881, was still alive ten years later when Paul lost sight of him[8]. In his paper, Paul challenged British surgeons with not being adventurous enough; three inches was the usual upper limit of excision. He also disagreed with those Germans who thought that a new sphincter developed or that defaecation could become normal again after the lower end of the rectum had been excised. To help control postoperative prolapse (and, to a lesser extent, incontinence also) he designed a special truss equipped with a rectal pad and knob.

In general, though, the fate of a patient with a sacral anus or with a 'saved' sphincter was pretty miserable. 'It was sentiment and not sense', said Charles Horace Mayo, 'that dictated an uncontrollable outlet in the anal region'. One also wonders whether Victorian sensibility may not have been equally responsible.

The first enterostomy done as a preliminary to removal of a carcinoma was not in fact a colostomy but an ileostomy. In 1878 Wilhelm Georg Baum of Danzig daringly fashioned an inguinal ileostomy in a man of thirty-four with intestinal obstruction of uncertain site. Seven days later the abdomen was no longer swollen and a tumour could be felt in the ascending colon. Baum therefore opened the abdomen and removed the growth together with a wedge-shaped piece of mesocolon containing an enlarged lymph node. The bowel was reunited by end-to-end anastomosis. Throughout, the operation was conducted under the protection of an antiseptic spray[9]. Unfortunately, the anastomotic line was insecure and three days after operation faeculent fluid exuded from the wound; the ileal anus discharged less and less and on the ninth day the patient died.

Maurice Pollosson of Lyons originated the idea of establishing a colostomy with closure of its distal end as a routine preliminary to excision of the rectum[10]. This would avoid irritation of the growth by faeces, improve the patient's condition before radical surgery, and lessen the serious risk of wound infection, the cause of death of most of these patients. Like Madelung, Pollosson was using lumbar colostomies and he became most incensed if anyone confused the principle underlying his preliminary colostomy with that of Madelung which was simply to prevent faecal over-spill[11]. (Madelung reported his suggestion to a congress in Berlin on April 13, 1883, and Pollosson had his idea in the June of that year, though it did not appear in print until 1884 – for some reason Schinzinger seems to have been completely ignored by these two contestants.)

In Germany credit for the concept of preliminary colostomy goes to Max Schede of Bonn who published his work in 1877[12]. Despite the other claims to priority his stake is good as his colostomy was abdominal and placed in the descending colon (rather than the usual sigmoid) so that it would be out of the way when he came to excise the rectum. Unlike the others, his colostomy was double barrelled and designed to be closed subsequently.

The opening moves towards the Paul-Mikulicz technique came from Germany and Denmark – and, to demonstrate yet again the fickleness of fame, both depended on the same principle of exteriorization as the Paul-Mikulicz. In his textbook of 1886, Walther Hermann Heineke described a three-stage procedure for resection of the colon[13]. At the first, he exteriorized the bowel and excised the affected loop (with its mesentery); he then sutured the two cut ends together side by side to form the spur before anchoring them to the abdominal wall. The second stage was crushing the spur, and the third was closure of the colostomy.

In 1892, Oskar Bloch of Copenhagen reported on one hundred and eighty-six cases (eighty growths were in the sigmoid, twenty-four in the caecum, and the remainder in other parts of the colon – at last we have a reasonably sized series). His first stage consisted in exteriorizing the cancer-bearing loop and inserting a tube to drain the bowel above the growth. A few days later, when the loop was firmly stuck to the abdominal wall, the offending bowel was excised. Then finally the spur was crushed and the colostomy closed[14].

And so we come to Paul's first successful case on February 15, 1894. The patient was a thirty-six-year-old woman with a malignant stricture of the ascending colon, and the operation was virtually a carbon copy of Heineke's except that Paul inserted one of his glass tubes into each barrel of the colostomy[15]. The tubes usually remained in situ for seven to ten days before long dressing forceps were introduced to crush the spur. The colostomy was 'closed by separating the mucous membrane and turning it in with Lembert sutures, and then bringing together the skin edges above it,' Paul wrote in 1900[16]. In one case though he wondered whether he should have brought the muscles together as well, since the outer wall of the colon tended to herniate and had to be supported with a belt and pad.

Mikulicz followed more the Bloch pattern, as he excised the growth forty-eight hours after exteriorizing the bowel. His report appeared in 1903[17]. Before long, a staged excision of colon in the style of either Paul or Mikulicz became known as a Paul-Mikulicz operation. It dramatically reduced the operative mortality rate from about 43 percent to about 12 percent, but it had its disadvantages as it was unsuitable for the extreme ends of the colon and incomplete crushing of the spur could lead to a stricture. But infinitely more important than either of these was the fact that it was a poor cancer operation since it ignored the lymphatic drainage. However, it was safe and that was a prime consideration in the early part of the 20th century. When all our modern resources made intra-abdominal surgery a less risky undertaking, the surgeon could perform an extensive dissection (if necessary) and dispense with the need for a colostomy. Nevertheless, the Paul-Mikulicz operation still has an occasional place, as in the seriously ill, enfeebled patient or when resection unexpectedly proves necessary and the bowel has not been prepared.

Surgeons were truly caught between Scylla and Charybdis in their attempts to deal with rectal cancer. Excision, even through an extended incision, was inadequate but more radical removal could scarcely be contemplated since the operation was already dangerous and an open invitation to infection, frequently overwhelming. Yet contemplated it was. Henry Widenham Maunsell, a New Zealander, in 1892 introduced a combined 'pull through' operation which could be used for growths in the upper rectum and lower sigmoid. First, he mobilized an appropriate length of bowel through an abdominal incision, then he invaginated the tumour-bearing area through the dilated anus and lower rectum. The 'prolapsed' growth was amputated externally from below and the reunited bowel returned through the anus as if reducing a prolapse[18].

John Percy Lockhart Mummery approached the problem rather more cautiously as he was acutely conscious of the danger of surgical shock and wanted to devise a simple technique that would be safe for a general surgeon. The solution he reached was to perform a preliminary laparotomy to assess the spread of the growth and its operability; at the conclusion of this he fashioned an inguinal colostomy. The next week or so while waiting to perform the perineal part of the operation were spent in daily washouts of the distal bowel through the colostomy. In this way he managed to achieve a fairly extensive excision which healed aseptically. Yet this was not a routine operation since the indications stated by Lockhart Mummery were, first, when he was uncertain whether the bowel above a constricting growth could be effectively emptied from below, and second, when the sphincter muscles were involved and would have to be removed[19].

The first deliberate attempt at combining the abdominal and perineal approaches into one operation was made by Joseph Bloodgood of Baltimore in July 1905. He believed that surgeons were wrong to content themselves with an inguinal colostomy or a sacral anus and therefore set out to fulfil the requirements of complete removal with restoration of continuity through a combined operation[20]. (On September 18, 1883, Vincenz Czerny of Heidelberg had started to do a sacral excision of the rectum. When he found this to be impossible he had opened the abdomen to remove the growth. The patient of this unintentional combined operation died the next day[21].)

However, the man who really put abdomino-perineal excision on the map was the English surgeon William Ernest Miles[22]. His decision to choose this technique was founded on his painstaking research into the lymphatic spread of rectal and sigmoid growths, but the operation very nearly failed to make good as it was associated with severe shock and a high initial mortality. Because of this some surgeons did the operation in two stages, the first being the formation of a colostomy with or without some degree of mobilization of the rectum. Fortunately it was saved by the physiological, biochemical, and associated scientific consolidation of surgical advances. The majority of surgeons preferred to do the abdominal end first, but a few started in the perineum before scrubbing up again and moving round to the abdomen. Eventually someone thought that there could be no harm in having two teams working above and below at the same time and in 1934 Martin Kirschner (the first man to succeed in removing a pulmonary embolus) of Heidelberg showed beyond doubt that it was a good thing[23].

11

More abdominal diseases

A lthough the young man whose bowels were described by Giovanni Battista Morgagni[1] may have been afflicted with ulcerative colitis (some say it was Crohn's disease), the disease did not lose its cloak of anonymity until 1859 when Samuel Wilks of Guy's Hospital gave a recognizable description[2]. Even then it seemed reluctant to assume its identity, accepting a variety of names descriptive of its main features – membranous, hyperplastic, mucous, obstinate and ulcerative. But once surgeons realized that, whatever they might call it, the colitis was not an infection, they began to treat it along the lines they would use if it were in a more accessible part of the body. This meant local treatment assisted some years later when the penny dropped, by rest from the irritation of the faecal stream.

In 1891 Mayo Robson was presented with a woman of thirty-seven whose colitis and proctitis with ulceration was only getting worse on medical treatment. He resolved to cure the condition. On June 28 he brought the sigmoid colon to the surface and four days later opened the bowel. He then embarked on a course of irrigations with boracic acid solution. On December 3 he closed the artificial anus and after an unspecified time the patient reported back fit and well. In future, he said, he would never hesitate to open the bowel in any part of its course and give local treatment[3].

Without wishing to pour cold water over his initiative, we may be fairly sure that, having played into his hands once, the natural course of the disease caught him out in the end. As it probably did Skene Keith, too. Keith's terse report was in a letter to the editor of the *Lancet* in the spring of 1895: 'In June of last year I performed an inguinal colotomy in the right side of a patient who was passing large quantities of blood with membrane, one complete cast of the bowel being twenty-two inches in length. A month ago I closed the colotomy opening.'[4]

The idea of bringing the appendix to the surface to create an appendicostomy for introducing medication and for straight-through washouts of the colon came from Robert Fulton Weir of New York who announced 'a new use for the useless appendix'. His first patient, a man of thirty-one with intractable ulcerative colitis, was improved after operation in 1901[5]. Appendicostomy rapidly became the chosen method of surgical treatment and held the field in Great Britain until the early 1940s, though in the United States it was superseded by ileostomy rather sooner. As a rule irrigations were carried out twice a day with sodium bicarbonate the favoured solution; to ensure a free through-flow a firm rubber tube was inserted into the rectum. Between times the patient wore a fine rubber tube in the stoma to prevent stenosis. An appendicostomy might be closed after some months or it might become a permanent fixture. Nevertheless, whatever success it enjoyed and its comparatively long survival as a method of treatment were owed, once again, to the naturally remittent course of the disease.

C.C. Allison of Omaha in 1909 put the case for caecostomy rather than appendicostomy[6]. His reason was that irrigation was not the sole object and in most cases diversion of the faecal stream was the essential part of treatment. But this argument failed to impress since an appendicostomy was so easy to manage.

The opening moves towards excisional surgery and ileostomy were made in the first two decades of the century. Lilienthal's operation was, in retrospect, the more significant but because it came before its time, it had less influence. Brown was groping in the direction events wanted to go and so he earned more credit.

Howard Lilienthal of Mt Sinai Hospital, New York, had a patient, a woman of twenty-three, who had had a left inguinal colostomy performed elsewhere. When her symptoms abated, the colostomy was closed but before long the diarrhoea, haemorrhage and passage of foul mucus returned and she came to Lilienthal. On December 30, 1899, he fashioned a right iliac colostomy to rest the entire colon and to provide an opening for washouts. On March 6, 1900, as the patient had greatly improved the ileum was anastomosed end-to-end to the sigmoid. At first she passed numerous liquid stools per anum but gradually she settled down to two formed motions daily, and her general condition improved still further. However, the colon continued to discharge copiously through its right iliac stoma and the woman insisted on having it dealt with. So on June 15, Lilienthal removed the entire colon and stump of ileum[7].

John Young Brown of St Louis in 1913 reported on ten ileostomies, only one of which was in fact for ulcerative colitis (the others were for late and inoperable malignancies of the rectum (three), amoebic dysentery (three), obstruction by bands (two), and one case of extensive tuberculous colitis). The patients had previously been treated by appendicostomy or caecostomy, but as soon as the large bowel was washed out it filled up again from the small bowel, thus thwarting Brown's endeavours to obtain complete physiological rest. Accordingly he closed the distal ileum and fixed an irrigating catheter in the caecum. Then he inserted a stiff rubber drainage tube into a more proximal part of the ileum. When he felt the colon had healed, he restored continuity by anastomosing ileum to either ascending colon or sigmoid[8].

Despite having only one patient with ulcerative colitis in a very small series, Brown made his point and ileostomy became the accepted surgical treatment in the United States, though in its early days it carried high immediate mortality and morbidity rates since patients were not referred until the coffin-lid was almost due for nailing down. Furthermore, the physiological problems arising out of an ileostomy were very imperfectly understood. But as time passed and one set of problems was overcome, another came to darken the prospect.

It was originally intended that the ileostomies should be temporary, since they appeared to cure the disease – in the short term. However, when the bowel was reunited the colitis seemed fated to return, and the behaviour of both local and remote complications (such as iridocyclitis [inflammation of the iris and ciliary body in the eye] and arthritis) was unaffected. Then, the final blow to any hope of restoring continuity came with the realization that the chronically diseased bowel was more than normally liable to malignant change. There was no alternative; the colon had to be removed. In the 1930s this was approached most tentatively as a four-stage procedure with several weeks between the stages. First, an ileostomy was fashioned. Second, the right colon was removed (the proximal end of the remaining colon was brought to the surface). Third, the left colon was removed (the sigmoid was brought to the surface). And fourth, an abdomino-perineal resection was performed. By the 1940s the arrival of chemotherapy and the antibiotic drugs and improvements in anaesthesia and surgical physiology enabled the second and third stages to be done together. But before continuing the main theme of the story, we shall return to Britain for a discussion held at the Royal Society of Medicine in 1940[9].

Lionel Norbury, the opener, spoke in favour of appendicostomy, though sometimes a caecostomy was called for since, as he said, 'appendicostomy is of little use when the patient is moribund.' In his opinion colectomy was unnecessary in the earlier stages and dangerous in the later; but he did admit he was speaking without experience.

The next participant, Heneage Ogilvie, was vehemently opposed to letting the patient become toxic and exsanguinated. He had performed a small number of planned three-stage operations (exclusion with ileostomy, excision, and restoration of continuity), but if there was no hope of the patient's being able to defaecate per anum again, he saw no need to excise the colon.

And so the ball was tossed backwards and forwards. William Gabriel and Lockhart-Mummery (he had acquired a hyphen) sided with Norbury, and Arthur Hurst with Ogilvie. The only person to recognize that – certainly until the arrival of some wonder drug – the ileostomy should be permanent, was Rupert Corbett. He believed that ileosigmoidostomy was dangerous and uncertain in its results. As he expressed it five years later: 'Once an ileostomy, always an ileostomy.' For the sake of the skin he delayed opening the bowel for twenty-four to forty-eight hours when possible and then inserted a Paul's tube. To protect the skin subsequently he used zinc cream on tulle gras, but 'the early fitting of an adequate box is a great help.'[10]

The determination to retain the services of the natural anus died hard, and understandably so at a time when the concept of stoma care still lay in the future. Mark Ravitch at Johns Hopkins had an idea that seemed perfect in theory, but in practice it turned sour. In two patients with ulcerative colitis (plus three more mentioned in an addendum to his paper published in 1948[11]) he performed complete colectomy with ileo-anal anastomosis; the anal end was most ingenious. The mucosal lining of the lower part of the rectum (the upper part having been removed with the colon) and of the anal canal was stripped off and the ileum drawn down through the bare tube and stitched to anal skin. Ravitch believed that the sensory endings in the retained muscular layer of the rectum would permit normal function to be restored, and indeed he reported the gradual return of sphincteric tone with eventual complete continence. Other surgeons were not so fortunate; all that most were able to achieve were desperately unhappy incontinent patients who had in the end to be given abdominal ileostomies. (Ravitch also recommended the operation for familial polyposis of the large bowel. A straightforward ileo-anal anastomosis had been performed for this condition by Rudolf Nissen of Berlin on a ten-year-old boy in 1933, although we are not told about the eventual outcome[12].)

For the ultimate steps in the excisional surgery of ulcerative colitis we cross the border into Canada where, in Montreal, Gavin Miller was gradually working his way towards panproctocolectomy. Seven years before his 1949 report[13] he had been forced to do a primary resection in a very sick girl whose colon was in imminent danger of perforating in many places (in other words he had combined the first and second stages of the three-stage procedure). She had responded dramatically. Next, in 1945, he had performed ileostomies on two patients with fulminating ulcerative colitis. They had both died; however, before this happened he had sent colonic washings to the biochemist who reported a high protein content which, Miller suggested later, might have contributed to death.

Bearing these two experiences in mind, and drawing encouragement from the recent development of the Koenig-Rutzen stoma bag[14] (the forerunner of acceptable stoma appliances) and from the fact that several years earlier he had successfully performed several one-stage hemicolectomies with ileostomy for ulcerative colitis, Miller decided to remove as much of the colon as possible at one stage. His first patient was a man of twenty-two, again with fulminating disease who again made an impressive recovery. The ileostomy was brought out through a stab wound to the right of where the umbilicus had been, and the distal sigmoid segment was exteriorized in the left lower quadrant. The intact rectal stump thus left behind kept the way open for a subsequent abdomino-perineal resection. However, in their report on sixty-nine patients (with three deaths) Campbell Gardner and Miller said they had performed this five times and then only because of some special indication such as failure to gain weight, bleeding or discharge, indicating involvement of the recto-sigmoid stump. As time passed and their experience and confidence grew, Miller's team came to adopt abdomino-perineal resection as a routine. Initially they waited three months or so between the two stages, but before long they performed the first one-stage panproctocolectomy[15].

Apart from technical considerations and ignorance of the natural history of ulcerative colitis (and of other diseases), an important factor in the reluctance of surgeons to adopt the permanent ileostomy was inadequate post-operative care.

Lester Dragstedt of Chicago was, by 1941, convinced of the good done by an ileostomy provided it was so fashioned that irritation and digestion of the abdominal wall by the outflow was prevented. To achieve this, he exteriorized about six inches of ileum (taking care to preserve its blood supply). He closed the wound loosely, tied a small Pezzar catheter into the lumen of the ileum, and then carefully wrapped a rectangular split-thickness skin graft around the exteriorized ileum – this was sutured only to the skin of the abdominal wall around the stoma. Dragstedt obtained complete takes with no excoriation of skin in the four patients he reported on[16]. But eight years later Clarence Monroe and John Olwin, also of Chicago, were unhappy about the tendency of the graft to contract. In one of their patients the exteriorized ileum shrank from three-and-a-half inches to a quarter of an inch long in eighteen months, which was highly undesirable as a long ileostomy at that time facilitated the collection of faecal material. So Monroe and Olwin decided to use a full thickness skin graft to wrap around the bowel. The graft took almost completely in the patient they reported on, and when it was fully healed they found peristalsis could be stimulated by pulling the ileum an inch or two from the abdominal wall[17]. This then halted the flow of faeces for about four hours and encouraged the hope that eventually the patient might be able to do away with the cup-type prosthesis the two surgeons had designed for him.

Yet skin grafting was not to be the answer to good surgical care of a stoma, for Bryan Brooke of Birmingham showed in 1952 that grafts of whatever thickness were not infrequently followed by ulceration, stenosis or even a fistula. His solution was deceptively simple: he evaginated the end of the ileum and sutured mucosa to skin[18]. This prevented stenosis and many of the other complications that could plague a patient with a poorly fashioned stoma.

Crohn's disease proved even more elusive than did ulcerative colitis. Although the literature, especially the German, from the turn of the 19th century was full of references to obscure non-specific granulomas, the condition did not aspire to becoming a clinical entity until 1932. In that year Burrill Bernard Crohn and his colleagues in New York described a disease they called 'regional ileitis'[19]. Unfortunately the disease did not take kindly to being unmasked and, as if to show its displeasure, slowly revealed that anatomical restriction to the ileum was a sad misconception. It can appear anywhere along the gastro-intestinal tract from mouth to anus; moreover, 'it is apparent that, in conjunction with a great increase in the overall occurrence of Crohn's disease in our experience in the last 10 or 15 years, there has been a disproportionate increase in the frequency of involvement of the large bowel, either alone or along with small bowel lesions. At the present time [1971] we see Crohn's disease roughly as commonly in the large bowel as in the small'[20].

Once established, the disease lost no time in emphasizing one aspect of its unpleasant nature; it responded little, if at all, to medical measures, and surgery came quickly on the scene. The first procedure tried by Crohn's surgical colleague, Albert Ashton Berg, at Mt Sinai Hospital was primary resection with side-to-side anastomosis of ileum and transverse colon[21]. They continued with this for a few years, though as early as 1933 a short-circuiting operation had been suggested by Crohn himself as well as by surgeons in other hospitals. John Homans and George Hass at Peter Bent Brigham, for instance, did so because they were unhappy about two patients who had undergone resection[22]. Howard Clute at the Lahey Clinic actually performed the operation on one patient. 'A loop of ileum, proximal to the area of inflammation, was anastomosed to the transverse colon and the abdomen closed.' At the time of the report, the patient was doing well and gaining weight[23]. Regrettably, details are sparse, but it seems probable that the anastomosis was a simple side-to-side without transection of the ileum. Clute did, however, say that resection could be carried out later if the symptoms persisted.

By 1936, Harry Koster and his colleagues in Brooklyn, perhaps influenced in their thinking by a false analogy with ulcerative colitis, urged that if a short-circuit were done there should be no delay over subsequent resection. Delay, they said, was 'fraught with the danger of rapid progression of the lesion, necrosis and suppuration in the mesentery and possibly peritonitis from the perforation of such an abscess or even of the intestine itself.'[24]

Three years later, R. Lee Clark and Claude Frank Dixon at the Mayo Clinic made it plain that the diseased segment should be isolated; that is, the short-circuit should be accompanied by transection of the ileum. The bowel was later resected if required, but with increasing surgical experience this was found to be needed less and less frequently owing to the excluded intestine becoming 'dried up' and atrophic[25].

Other centres, such as the Lahey Clinic, preferred a two-stage Mikulicz type of operation in which ileum and ascending colon were brought onto the surface of the abdomen and, together with affected mesenteric lymph nodes, were resected extraperitoneally. The ileostomy was so arranged in relation to the colostomy that the ileum could be drained through a small catheter. Intestinal continuity was subsequently restored. Although the results were reasonably satisfactory, the numbers were small: in a ten-year survey Samuel Marshall could report on only thirty-five operations of this type with one death (from pulmonary embolus)[26].

Another unpleasant side to the character of Crohn's disease that emerged as time went by was a marked tendency to recurrence, no matter what variety of surgery was used. When the corticosteroid drugs made their appearance, they were initially used in the surgical treatment of the disease to get the patient into better shape to withstand surgery, but later (beginning in 1960) Sidney Charles Truelove and his colleagues at Oxford applied them topically through a drip into the distal barrel of a double barrelled ileostomy in cases limited to the colon[27]. The object of the exercise was to see if continuity could subsequently be restored without producing a relapse. The results were mixed, though not without encouragement in certain chosen cases.

The attempt of John Simon of St Thomas's Hospital in 1851 to treat a boy with ectopia vesicae – a congenital condition in which the wall of the lower end of the abdomen and the front of the bladder fail to develop resulting in the interior of the bladder gaping onto the outside world – was the first essay into diverting the urinary stream. His technique was most ingenious as he passed a thread through the rectum and into a ureter about two or three inches from its end; thus the two threads (one from each ureter) emerged through the anus. Then, by tightening the threads, the ureters gradually ulcerated the rectum. This was successful and for many months a considerable amount of urine was passed into the rectum. The second part of the operation – closing the end section of the ureters – could not be done as the boy died as a result of the ureters becoming choked with chalky deposits[28].

On June 19, 1878, Thomas Smith of St Bartholomew's Hospital operated on a boy of seven with the same condition. Having first identified the ureter on the left side by passing a catheter up it, he implanted it into the colon with half an inch protruding into the lumen. Urine was excreted with the faeces for a year before suppuration intervened and 'it could not be ascertained that urine passed with the faeces.' On August 28, 1879, the performance was repeated on the right side and fifty hours later the boy's misery ended. At the post-mortem examination it was found that the left kidney had been destroyed by infection spreading up the ureter[29].

Not much happened after this until 1909 when J. Verhoogen and A. de Graeuwe fashioned a new bladder and urethra out of isolated caecum and appendix in patients whose bladders had been totally removed – an appendicostomy provided the outlet through the abdominal wall[30].The mortality rate was, regrettably, prohibitive.Then, just two years later, Robert Calvin Coffey of Portland, Oregon, overcame the worst of the problems posed by infection, leakage and obstruction by leading the ureters into the lumen of the sigmoid colon through a short tunnel in the bowel wall[31]. (Surgical science had advanced since Bernhard Bardenheuer had tried the same plan in 1886[32].) The use of a catheter to keep the ureter patent had already been suggested, but again it was Coffey who popularized its use in 1925[33].

Various technical improvements followed, thus making total cystectomy (removal of the bladder) a practical proposition. However, when in the 1930s pelvic exenteration appeared on the horizon surgeons had to think again.At first they stuck to what they knew and saved a length of sigmoid colon into which they implanted the ureters.The distal end of the sigmoid was sealed off and the proximal end brought to the surface where, unfortunately, its closeness to the colostomy made it a nuisance; the idea of having faeces and urine discharging through the same stoma (a wet colostomy) was an impossibility before the Koenig-Rutzen bag became available.

But a wet colostomy – or wet caecostomy – had problems of its own. Ascending infection was a constant danger and chloride and urea were absorbed from the urine – especially with caecostomies.Then chance took a hand when Heinz Emil Haffner was unable to use the caecum when operating on a patient with a massive rectal cancer; instead he resorted to isolated terminal ileum[34]. Eugene Bricker of St Louis, who had developed the technique by 1950, thought at first that the ileum would act as a reservoir but when he realized it was merely a conduit he adapted the Koenig-Rutzen bag into a suitable receptacle[35]. Ileal conduits then became the procedure of choice whenever bladder function had been destroyed, though a less demanding alternative should the patient be weak at the end of a major operation was to bring the ureters to the surface as cutaneous ureterostomies even though these had the disadvantage of being difficult to fit with appliances.

And, finally, we come to the Ultima Thule of abdominal surgery.The operation of hemicorporectomy was reported from three centres in the United States during the 1960s. It consisted in amputation of the entire lower part of the body at the lumbar or lumbosacral level with the creation of stomas for the urine and faeces.The first team to attempt the feat was from The Grace Hospital, Detroit, and was led by Charles S. Kennedy who had first considered the operation in 1948 but, after discussion with the patient's relatives (but not the patient herself)

had decided not to go through with it. Nevertheless, the horrible manner in which the woman died made him feel that the operation might have a use in selected cases. In 1959, a man of seventy-four came to him with cancer of the rectum for which he performed an abdomino-perineal resection on June 23. The post-operative course was stormy, but eventually he was discharged only to deteriorate. Surgical palliation of the cancer was deemed impossible, so Kennedy discussed the matter with Alexander Brunschwig, a leading proponent of pelvic exenteration, who gave him the encouragement to try a hemicorporectomy. This Kennedy did, after obtaining the patient's permission, on February 13, 1960. The operation lasted thirteen hours; the spine was separated between the third and fourth lumbar vertebrae; a colostomy and cutaneous ileostomy were fashioned for faeces and urine, respectively. The man died on the eleventh day after operation from left heart failure, possibly due to a transfusion error. But the procedure had been shown to be technically feasible[36].

The first successful hemicorporectomy was performed by Bradley Aust and Karel Absolon of the Minnesota Medical School. The patient was a twenty-nine-year-old man who had been born with a congenital deformity of the lower end of his spine (myelomeningocele) which had been repaired soon after his birth, but he had been devoid of sensation and completely paralysed below his hips ever since. Then he developed an extensive cancer in a bedsore that demanded drastic treatment. After a colostomy had been created at a preliminary operation, amputation was carried out between the fifth lumbar vertebra and the sacrum on October 17, 1961. The operation lasted six and a half hours[37]. Aust said later, in a discussion of Miller's paper[38], that he had been extremely worried about the outcome since the main burden fell on the rehabilitation team rather than the surgical. For this reason he withheld publication for a year until the man could get in and out of bed and a wheelchair unaided. Subsequently he approached five other suitable patients but with no takers.

The experience of Theodore Miller of the Memorial Cancer Center, New York, was somewhat better as four of eighteen possible patients agreed to hemicorporectomy. All had been treated fully by operation, radiotherapy and chemotherapy but were in a hopeless state although the disease was confined to the pelvis – an essential requirement. At the time of his report in 1966[38], his first patient was able to walk with the aid of a prosthesis eighteen months after operation. Another was clinically free from disease and able to drive a car and earn his living. In all four patients severe pain had been relieved by the amputation, and when questioned by people not belonging to the team, all said they were glad they had had the operation. As Seneca remarked, 'It is thanks to death that I hold life so dear.'

12

Hernias

American surgeons travelled widely and many of them spent the two years after qualification in Viennese or German clinics, where the recognized leaders of surgical thought and practice were then to be found. They were thus able to form a fairly complete picture of the state of surgery and, on their return to America, to incorporate the best of all they had learned into their own practice and bring fresh intelligence to bear on the work initially carried out in Europe. The Germanic influence was most keenly felt at Johns Hopkins University, which, in the few years since its opening in 1876, had built up a world-wide reputation for academic achievement. The men chosen to head the medical staff of the attached hospital and medical school – the latter not formally opened until 1893 – were all young, brilliant, and destined to make a lasting impression on their various fields of medicine. William Stewart Halsted was the surgeon, William Osler the physician, Howard Atwood Kelly the gynaecologist, and William Henry Welch the pathologist. Between them, they completely revolutionized medical education in the United States and their combined resources gave the student a unified picture of disease as it affected the patient. They broke away from the prevailing habit of relying on books and lectures, and instead they emphasized bedside teaching and the important part in diagnosis and research played by the laboratory.

Until this time, medical education in the United States had been unsatisfactory; there were institutions from which an aspiring doctor could obtain a diploma in as short a period as two years, and on the occasions when an outstanding teacher appeared he was unable to integrate his work into the pattern of medicine as a whole and was hindered by an almost complete lack of laboratory facilities. At Johns Hopkins all this was rectified, and in addition a high standard of education was demanded of the students before admission; how high may be judged from the remark of Osler that it was just as well he had got in as a professor for he was quite certain he would never have done so as a student!

Halsted, the surgeon of this progressive group, was a remarkable man who left the imprint of his scholarship and his love of surgery on many operative advances. Born in New York in 1852, he was educated at Yale where, true to the legend often surrounding medical students, he distinguished himself more on the athletic field than in the lecture theatre. After qualifying in 1877, he worked for a year in the New York Hospital and then went to Europe, where he studied chiefly in the clinics of Billroth and von Bergmann. There he was most impressed with the technical efficiency of the operators and contrasted it with the practice to which he was accustomed. Some years later he recalled the experiences of his trip:

'I was impressed with the fact that our surgeons were greatly handicapped in most of their operations by lack of proper instruments, particularly of artery clamps.... Rarely had I seen in our country, prior to my first visit to Europe, more than one artery clamp at a time left hanging in a wound. Clamps were too few for this – four to three or even two being considered ample for an operation. Few hospitals, in New York at least, possessed as many as six artery clamps in 1880. I recall vividly an operation in Vienna, performed by Mikulicz in Billroth's clinic in 1879. Americans, newly arrived in Austria, were greatly amused at seeing perhaps a dozen clamps left hanging in a wound of the neck while the operator proceeded with his dissection, and were inclined to ridicule the method as untidy or uncouth. Slowly it dawned upon us that we in America were novices in the art as well as the science of surgery.'

When he returned to New York, Halsted rapidly became popular as a surgeon, serving on the staffs of a number of hospitals and all the time striving towards the ideal in surgical perfection. During this period he twice demonstrated his self-confidence in ways which, had they not been successful, would have been damned as foolhardy in the extreme. In 1881 his sister gave birth to a baby and was literally at death's door from haemorrhage. Halsted happened to be present and without hesitation withdrew blood from his own vein and injected it into hers. Then, before twelve months had elapsed, his mother was seriously ill with gall-bladder trouble. The consultants who examined her refused to countenance an operation, but so convinced was Halsted of its necessity that he performed the operation himself and successfully removed a number of stones. This was the first time he had ever operated on a gall-bladder.

A few years later he became interested in the problem of local anaesthesia, and this nearly resulted in the premature termination of his career. The Incas of ancient Peru knew that if they chewed coca leaves and applied the spittle to the skull of a patient they could reduce the pain of trephining. In 1855 the chemical substance responsible had been extracted from the leaves by a German chemist; four years later another German, Albert Niemann, isolated the substance in a pure form and called it cocaine[1]. In the years that followed occasional papers appeared dealing with cocaine, but it was not until 1878 that von Anrep demonstrated its anaesthetic properties on animals and suggested that it might be used in human beings[2]. Real interest was first shown when Carl Koller, at an Ophthalmological Congress at Heidelberg in 1884, read an account of his success in anaesthetizing the conjunctiva and cornea[3]. The news of this reached Halsted in New York and at once he saw the great future for cocaine if it could be proved safe for injecting into the tissues around a nerve, thus making the whole area supplied by the nerve insensitive to pain. In those days such an anaesthetic would have a considerable advantage over inhalation anaesthesia, which was still risky in certain patients.

Halsted, Richard Hall and their colleagues working at the Roosevelt Hospital experimented on themselves and by injecting a diluted solution of cocaine were able to achieve the desired result, though the anaesthesia was of rather short duration[4]. Out of this work was to develop the extremely valuable procedure of regional block anaesthesia, together with the discovery of synthetic substances having the same anaesthetic action as cocaine but with a longer duration and without its dangers. It is now a well-known fact that cocaine readily causes addiction and has the most demoralizing effect upon anyone so affected; it was, therefore, a supreme tragedy that the men who were striving to relieve human suffering should be ignorant of this terrible danger. Their achievement for humanity was accomplished at the expense of personal disaster, for most were utterly finished and ended their days in abject misery. Halsted stood out from among them and by a phenomenal effort of will he overcame the addiction, though his health was temporarily ruined and he had to retire from practice for over a year.

After his recovery in 1887 Halsted was invited by his old friend, William Welch, to come to Baltimore, where the latter had already started on his life's work in the beautifully equipped laboratory at Johns Hopkins. There Halsted spent two years studying the problem of intestinal stitching and by experiments on dogs showed how the anastomosis could be made more secure[5]; he also did research on the thyroid gland from the surgical viewpoint. In 1889 he returned to active practice as associate professor of surgery at Johns Hopkins and a year later was appointed professor and chief surgeon to the hospital. Halsted was a perfectionist, always seeking better and safer ways to operate. He never hurried and was one of the first surgeons to advocate and practise the essentials of good operative technique, namely, that all bleeding points must be carefully and completely secured, asepsis must be complete, and that the tissues of the body must be handled with extreme gentleness and when cut must be sewn together again with accurate approximation.

He was thought by his fellow surgeons to be a little too pernickity over the control of haemorrhage, since he sometimes required up to four-and-a-half hours to remove a breast (an operation that can be attended by the most bothersome bleeding), whereas the time usually taken was only an hour-and-a-half. To enable the bleeding from small blood vessels to be controlled with the minimum of damage, Halsted invented an improved form of artery forceps with much finer points than hitherto; they could thus pick up the bleeding vessels without including more than the smallest bit of other tissue. At a convenient time the blood vessel was tied with fine silk, the ends of which were cut off short and the artery forceps removed. Whenever faced with a difficult surgical problem he would give great thought to the matter, carrying out experiments in the laboratory, or new operations on animals and, provided the condition was not such that immediate surgery was indicated, the patient had to wait. The results were well worth the waiting. Halsted's scientific approach to surgery was founded on his deep knowledge of the basic sciences of anatomy, physiology and pathology, which enabled him to foresee likely complications of new procedures and to work out means for their circumvention.

Surgical residencies, as part of the surgeon's training, were introduced by Halsted and have since become an established routine. Halsted saw the way events were shaping and made postgraduate residential training an integral part of the complete surgical education. The number of famous surgeons who were trained by him bears witness to his wisdom. He also left the imprint of his genius on the surgical technique for individual conditions, most especially hernia, cancer of the breast and diseases of the thyroid gland.

In its broadest sense a hernia is the bulging of a structure or organ through a gap in its containing tissue; the most frequent place for this to happen is in the abdomen, and we will first consider the indirect inguinal hernia, the commonest form of 'rupture', and one that occurs in the groin. Throughout history hernias have been a curse to mankind; they cause pain and discomfort in the groin and any form of straining will make the condition worse. The only adequate treatment is by surgery and this is intimately bound up with a detailed knowledge of the anatomy of the region, but until the risk of infection could be divorced from abdominal surgery, surgeons were unable to devise a satisfactory curative operation. Ever since pre-Christian days the surgeon's knife had been employed in an endeavour to treat hernias, yet, apart from causing considerable pain, nothing was achieved and if the patient survived the operation it could be guaranteed that the hernia would recur because there was no comprehension of the intricate nature of the anatomical problems involved. In these circumstances it is not surprising that patients delayed consulting a surgeon – or an itinerant herniotomist – until some complication had intervened and they were confronted with the choice between certain death and the faint hope of relief, a fact which of itself contributed to the poor results.

An idea of the meaning of a hernia can be gained by imagining the inside of the abdominal cavity to be lined with a thin membrane, the peritoneum (like a polythene bag), with the muscles of the abdomen on the outside. In the male the testicles are situated in the scrotum outside the abdomen, but in the embryo they were inside and the cause of all the bother is just the fact that they had to have some way to pass through the abdominal wall. They chose to do this in the groin in an ingenious manner that deserved to be foolproof. At the middle of the groin they traversed the inner layer of muscle through a hole known as the internal inguinal ring and then passed towards the inner end of the groin in a tunnel, the inguinal canal, formed of the muscle layers to emerge through the remaining muscle layers and continue into the scrotum covered only by skin and fat. When the testicle made this journey it brought with it the spermatic cord, which contains the vas deferens, the tube that carries the sperm. The need for preserving the spermatic cord prevents the surgeon from sewing up the two rings and so making absolutely certain that the hernia will not recur. In the female there is an imitation of the descent of the testicle, resulting in the formation of the two rings and the inguinal canal, but as there is no spermatic cord surgical cure is thus much easier to achieve.

A hernia develops when the peritoneum bulges into the internal inguinal ring, forming a little sac. The bulge at first is only felt when the patient coughs or strains, but the sac may gradually get bigger and extend down the inguinal canal and into the scrotum. It may contain fat or a small loop of bowel, though almost every structure inside the abdomen has been reported at one time or another to have been found in a hernial sac. Before the hernia becomes too serious it is possible to manipulate the contents back into the abdomen, but when this is no longer possible the hernia is said to be irreducible. The complications of hernia are due to the bowel becoming obstructed or having its blood supply cut off, events more likely to occur with large and irreducible hernias; they were frequently fatal in the past and even today are matters of serious concern.

Before 1880 every conceivable idea had been tried, except the correct one of complete removal of the sac, together with repair of the defect in the abdominal wall. Most attention had been paid to strangulated or obstructed cases, as the uncomplicated ones could be controlled by a truss without the considerable risk of operation, although this did not deter some surgeons from attempting a cure whenever they got the chance. The use of trusses, which have been known since ancient times, is confined to those hernias that can be reduced; they have no place in treatment when complications have developed. The basic operation performed throughout the ages was that of herniotomy, in which the sac was incised and the intestines manipulated back into the abdomen. The modifications of, and departures from, this technique were innumerable, for sometimes the sac was cut away and at others it was only tied off round its neck; the stump of the sac was frequently cauterized with a red-hot iron. If the hernia was strangulated, it was usual to attempt reduction without operation by standing the patient on his head and performing all manner of manoeuvres, far from gentle, to get the gut to go back; when the patient became practically moribund as a result of this, surgery was undertaken and, in order to ease the reduction, the internal ring was often incised or dilated.

While all this was going on, the wretched patient was bled, purged and given enemas of tobacco smoke; after operation, if he survived, he could expect hot or cold poultices to be applied, a considerable amount of suppuration with frequent failure of the wound to heal properly and almost certain recurrence of the hernia. The presence of the spermatic cord did not unduly disturb many operators - they simply castrated the patient, thus doing away with any necessity for its preservation. Provided only one testicle was removed, the patient was probably no worse off than his fellow sufferer who retained both. When the testicle was saved it was often lifted, temporarily, from its bed in the scrotum to protect it, and this, combined with the other surgical escapades, would place its blood supply in serious jeopardy so that subsequent atrophy was not unusual. A popular extension of charlatan herniotomists, who needless to say were itinerant, was to remove both testicles even though the hernia was only on one side. This practice led to condemnation of castration in any degree, but did not die out until the end of the 18th century.

By this time surgery for uncomplicated hernias had become so dangerous that it was rarely performed and even in complicated cases the sac was held in great fear and was only occasionally opened or excised. The main contribution of the early 19th century to knowledge of hernias was the definition of the anatomy of the region, with its complicated arrangement of the muscles and their fibrous extensions. When Listerism made abdominal surgery a reasonably safe proposition, attention was once more focused on the surgical cure of hernia.

H.O. Marcy, an American, was quick off the mark and grasped most of the principles of successful modern hernia surgery. As early as 1870 he was working on the problem, advising the use of buried catgut sutures to strengthen the abdominal wall[6], an extremely courageous and advanced suggestion, since in those days burying foreign material in wounds was to be avoided because of the danger of infection. In 1881, at an International Medical Congress held in London, he reported on a new operation he had developed in the intervening years, which consisted of very careful dissection of the hernial sac away from the surrounding structures, tracing it right back to its origin in the abdominal cavity and ligating and excising the sac as high as possible. The spermatic cord he next retracted out of harm's way and with sutures made of kangaroo tendon he reconstituted the inguinal canal, closing both inguinal rings round the spermatic cord[7]. This operation was truly remarkable on all counts and marked the turning point in hernial surgery, though unfortunately it did not receive the attention it merited and surgeons continued to stumble along until eventually Marcy's principles were rediscovered by various other surgeons whose names became attached to the operations they devised. (Marcy, incidentally, was responsible for perpetuating the unfounded rumour that Napoleon had left orders to be called at 4a.m. on the morning of the battle of Waterloo, June 18, 1815, but in the night he had had a severe epileptic fit and Larrey therefore allowed him to sleep till six o'clock[8].)

In the decade following Marcy's original work a number of surgeons made tentative attempts to cure hernia, some in the right direction, some in the wrong. An English surgeon, William Mitchell Banks, drew attention to the importance of removing the hernial sac in its entirety so that no remnant of a bulge remained on the peritoneum, a point now recognized as essential if recurrence is to be avoided. Apart from this, Banks's contribution was limited, since he was one of many who were afraid to interfere with the inguinal canal. In 1886 William Macewen, of Glasgow, decided that if the deep inguinal ring could be plugged it would prevent the hernia from recurring and he utilized the sac for this purpose[9]. Although variations of this plugging procedure were introduced as late as the 1920s it fell out of fashion since recurrences were not prevented.

Two of the three operations that were to set the style for many subsequent hernia techniques were first reported to the medical profession in 1889. They were somewhat similar but had been devised quite independently by Halsted and by Edoardo Bassini, professor of surgery at the University of Padua. Bassini's interest in this particular part of the body was probably inspired by a bayonet wound of the groin received while on active service in his youth which had left him with a faecal fistula. Be that as it may, in 1883 he was attempting to cure hernias by an elaborate plugging method. It was not long before he found that recurrences occurred unless the patient wore a truss, and so he changed over to the method he had heard described by Marcy at the Congress in London, but with a difference in emphasis. Marcy believed that the absorbable kangaroo tendon was the secret of his success but Bassini saw that it really lay in careful dissection and the complete removal of the sac, with adequate restoration of the walls of the inguinal canal; he therefore used ordinary silk for all the repair work. After operation, Bassini put his patients in a plaster-of-Paris cast and kept them in bed for six weeks. Rather regrettably, he also assessed his results at the end of this period and quite naturally was able to report very favourably on the operation[10]. Further experience on the part of other surgeons showed that recurrences did in fact occur. The disposition of the repairing stitches was inclined to weaken an important layer of fascia, the internal ring was not given enough support and a weak area was left close to the pubic bone. The restoration of the inguinal canal also went against the now understood mechanical and anatomical principles with the result that the muscles of the area failed to function properly and underwent local atrophy. Nevertheless, the Bassini operation was a marked advance in the surgical treatment of hernia.

Bassini first reported his operation in Italian in a small book that did not attract popular attention; however, in 1890 he republished it in a widely read German journal[11]. The account of Halsted's operation appeared in 1889 in America[12], but because the reputation of American surgeons at that time was not as great as that of their European counterparts, operations based on the Bassini repair enjoyed a greater and longer-lasting popularity. The feature of Halsted's operation was his utilization of the cremaster muscle and its fascia (this muscle surrounds the spermatic cord and runs down to the testicle) to strengthen the posterior wall of the inguinal canal. He also used silk stitches in reconstituting the ligaments and fascia of the area, but there was tension on the anterior wall of the canal with subsequent weakening of the muscle. His operation differed from Bassini's in another respect, since he tried to get extra strength in the walls of the inguinal canal by sewing them together deep to the spermatic cord. The cord thus no longer ran in the inguinal canal, but lay instead just beneath the skin.

In 1903 Halsted introduced a modification in which he incised the sheath of the rectus abdominis muscle (the longitudinal paired muscle in the centre of the abdominal wall) and made a flap to reinforce the weak spot at the inner end of the inguinal area, known as Hesselbach's triangle[13]. Unknown to him, this had been done a few months earlier by the French surgeon, Paul Berger, who had used the flap to strengthen the whole of the posterior wall and not just one part of it. This technique is now realized to be unsound. As with all his operations, Halsted took great care to tie off every bleeding point and was most meticulous with each stage of the repair. The incision was closed with buried stitches of fine silk and a pad of sterile gauze was placed over the wound, which was then covered with a bandage in the form of a spica; this he soaked in alcohol and finally poured a thin solution of collodion over the whole dressing, so that when it hardened the patient was in a light-weight cast. Redressing took place on the eighth day and, if all went well, Halsted allowed the patient to get out of bed on the thirteenth day, though the usual practice, apart from that of Bassini and his followers, was to enforce a three-week period of bed rest. In this departure from accepted routine, Halsted once again showed himself to be thinking along modern lines.

The third of the three techniques that paved the way for modern developments was that of Georg Lotheissen, who appreciated the importance of including Cooper's ligament in the repair by suturing it to the transversalis fascia[14]. He believed this method, which he described in 1898, to be of most use in femoral hernias but failed to appreciate its significance in the repair of the inguinal variety (a femoral hernia also occurs in the groin but in a slightly different position). It was not until 1927 that William Wayne Babcock was able to show the great benefit of this method, which strengthened the weakest area where most recurrences developed[15]. Babcock's operation, or Cooper's ligament operation, is technically more difficult than Bassini's, but it restores and preserves normal function in the region and is subject to fewer recurrences. The points of the operation are careful and complete dissection throughout with complete removal of the sac and stitching white fibrous tissue or ligament to fibrous tissue or ligament, at no time including red muscle in the stitches. The objections are technical and include variations in individual anatomical structures which may add to the difficulty and duration of the operation.

Successful operations for hernia thus depend on an accurate understanding of the complicated anatomical and functional mechanisms of the area, and as there have been well over two hundred different modifications and types of operation described since 1890, it will be appreciated that the problem of surgical cure is far from easy. Many of these modifications were minor, quite a number failed to take into account the principles involved, and some of the different techniques, such as plugging the canal, fell by the wayside, but there is one most important development with a wide field of application. This is the plastic repair, known as hernioplasty. The operations of the Bassini, Halsted, and Cooper's ligament type are called herniorrhaphies, though with the range of modern techniques available the dividing line between a plastic repair and an ordinary repair has become rather obscured.

The first attempt to strengthen the hernial defect with some sort of a graft was made in 1901 by Lewis Linn McArthur of Chicago, who used strips of fascia obtained from one of the abdominal muscles. He was able to cut the strips through the same incision that he used for operating on the hernia and, after the usual reduction of the hernia and removal of the sac, he sewed the strips in the form of stitches to reconstitute the walls of the inguinal canal[16]. McArthur's technique failed to find acceptance and the next attempt was made in 1910 by Martin Kirschner, who obtained a strip of fascia lata from the thigh about two or three inches wide and long enough to cover the inguinal canal[17]. (The fascia lata is a fibrous band that runs down the outer side of the thigh beneath the skin and superficial fat but external to the muscles.) This patch was stitched into place after the hernia had been repaired in the normal manner. Again the surgical world failed to respond and it was not until 1921 that the value of fascial grafts was generally recognized. Besides its use for hernias the principle of the technique found extensive use in other aspects of plastic surgery.

Two Toronto surgeons, William Edward Gallie and Arthur Le Mesurier, had been using patches of fascia lata to repair gaps in other muscles of the abdominal wall, usually beneath the scars of old operations. They found that these patches did not always heal strongly into place and that recurrences sometimes happened. They accordingly wondered whether a better result could not be obtained by doing away with catgut and other stitches and using strips of the fascia as stitching and strengthening material in one[18]. As a result of extensive experiments on animals, they found the idea to be workable and applied it to inguinal hernias[19]. The object of the operation was to darn the whole inguinal area with these strips of living tissue and so make them an integral part of their new home. The strips, a quarter of an inch wide, were obtained by making a long incision in the outer side of the thigh.

In 1933, James Masson invented an instrument called a fasciatome which can be introduced through a small incision at the top of the thigh and pushed along under the skin, stripping off a width of fascia as it goes[20]. It was designed to cut the end of the strip where desired and when pulled back out of the wound to bring the strip of fascia with it. The use of a fasciatome shortened the time of the operation but the gap left in the fascia lata cannot be sewn together; this is a matter of no serious importance, as it does not affect function, although in athletes and the like it is probably better to obtain the fascia by a long incision and sew up the gap afterwards. A point of the utmost importance, emphasized by Gallie, was that the fascia had to be used immediately it was removed from the thigh, otherwise it died and no advantage was gained from its use. Because it is living, it has great tensile strength and a considerable degree of elasticity. If it dies, it loses these properties and contracts, thus putting tension on the surrounding structures before it is eventually absorbed by the body.

The disadvantages of fascial grafts stem from the fact that large needles are required for the stitching and these may produce holes in the tissues which can give rise to weakness, and also that the accompanying operation on the thigh may lead to discomfort or even disability. In suitable cases the method first advocated by McArthur of using fascial strips from the external oblique was of use as it avoided the need for cutting the thigh. A further type of plastic repair was to use a patch of fascia with strips still attached to it, so that the hernia could be covered and strengthened with the patch; the strips were then sewn into tissues more removed from the site of weakness, thus putting less strain on the whole area. In 1927 Amos Koontz reported on his use of alcohol-preserved strips of fascia lata from the ox as suture material[21], but although the initial reports seemed encouraging, fascial grafts from anywhere but the patient's own body were unsuccessful as they degenerated and became absorbed.

Skin has also been used as a graft since 1889, though it did not prove so popular as other body tissues. The graft is taken from the edges of the hernia incision or from the upper part of the thigh and has the fat removed completely; it is then cut to the appropriate shape and sewn into place with silk or cotton stitches. Like fascial grafts it is a living structure with good tensile strength. It gradually becomes converted into firm scar tissue, but care is needed that no spaces are left when closing the wound because of the danger of infection. The method is again most suitable for large hernias. The final methods of repair make use of foreign materials to strengthen the inguinal canal. They act by forming a scaffolding on which fibrous or scar tissue forms. The substances used include floss silk and nylon, steel wire, polyvinyl and tantalum mesh. The last of these holds pride of place.

The surgical treatment of femoral hernias has had a similarly extensive history and the basic problems of repair are very much the same as for inguinal hernias since they also are concerned with the strengthening and healing of the muscles, ligaments and fibrous tissues of the groin. Like the inguinal variety, a femoral hernia has a sac of peritoneum, but the course it takes is different. In an inguinal hernia the bulge comes out above the inguinal ligament (this ligament runs in the line of the groin and is the dividing line between abdomen and thigh), but in a femoral hernia the bulge comes out below the ligament through a relatively weak area where the main artery and vein to the lower limb enter the thigh. The hole through which the vessels pass is known as the femoral ring, one of whose borders is a sharp-edged ligament, and this contributes to the main danger of femoral hernia, namely, that anything contained in the sac, usually a loop of bowel, is very liable to become strangulated. The close proximity of the important vessels adds considerably to the hazard of operation, a fact well known to the ancients.

Until the time of Guy de Chauliac at the end of the 14th century the two varieties of groin hernia were believed to be the same, but after he demonstrated their difference, attempts were made to relieve strangulation by cutting the appropriate constricting ring. This was soon found to be extremely dangerous and instruments were devised for stretching the ring instead. No one attempted to carry the operation any further, and if a fatal peritonitis did not ensue the patient was still left with a rupture.

To operate on an uncomplicated femoral hernia was unthinkable until 1876 when Thomas Annandale, professor of surgery at Edinburgh, operated on a patient with both an inguinal and a femoral hernia on the same side. The incision he used was the one for an inguinal operation and through this he found he could also deal with the femoral hernia by reducing it and plugging the femoral opening with the stitched-up sac[22]. He did not realize the advantage of the inguinal approach which was first fully appreciated by Guiseppi Ruggi in 1893, who utilized Cooper's ligament by sewing it to the inguinal ligament[23]. There have been as many different modifications for dealing with femoral hernias as there have been for inguinal hernias; a considerable number were found to have no advantage over existing methods, and not a few were far inferior. Fascial sutures have been used to close the femoral canal, but they are more difficult to insert than in repair of the inguinal canal.

13

Cancer of the breast

Among Halsted's many surgical interests was cancer of the breast. In 1882 he started work on the problem, and in November 1894[1] he gave to a grateful surgical world a detailed account of his radical operation for the treatment of breast cancer, which showed how clearly he had grasped the issues involved. A few days later another American, Willy Meyer of New York, described a similar operation[2], worked out independently; but although the names of the two surgeons are sometimes linked, the procedure is popularly known as Halsted's radical mastectomy. The routine removal of the smaller breast muscle (the pectoralis minor), however, did not originate with Halsted but was part of Meyer's operation.

The cancer starts within the tissue of the breast, originating in either the glandular tissue or the ducts; sooner or later, depending largely on the type of growth, it spreads in the lymphatic system to the neighbouring lymph nodes which are situated in the axilla (armpit), above and below the clavicle (collar-bone), in the neck, beneath the breastbone where this is joined by the ribs and also more deeply within the chest. Dissemination by the blood stream to other parts of the body is usually a later event. This may seem a most formidable enemy for the surgeon to conquer, but Halsted assumed, with the knowledge at his disposal, that spread to the axilla was the first and most important happening. He believed that if he could remove the breast and the lymph nodes in the axilla, with the intervening lymphatic vessels all in one piece at an early enough stage of the disease, he would stand a good chance of curing the cancer. Had Halsted's assumption been correct there is no doubt his operation would have been a success in a great number of cases; unfortunately, we now know that when the patient comes to operation the lymphatic spread is often considerably more extensive.

Many surgeons at that time knew and talked about what should be done and a very few made tentative efforts to put it into practice, but no one had yet had the courage and initiative to devise in all details a suitable operation that fulfilled the necessary requirements and could be taught to other surgeons. There was far more to the technique than just slicing off the breast: bleeding could be excessive, therefore careful, patient haemostasis was required; exquisite dissection was demanded to remove the lymph nodes without damaging the important nerves and blood vessels; gentleness and a sure knowledge of what he was doing were essential, for the patient was often in poor condition and the surgeon had no modern aids such as blood transfusion to call upon in the hour of need. Halsted possessed in full measure all the necessary qualities.

If Halsted's operation for the condition was new, breast cancer most certainly was not. From earliest times surgeons either left it alone, removed the breast with a clean sweep of the knife, or cauterized the tumour. Marcus Aurelius Severino, at the beginning of the 17th century, has been credited with the first removal of an enlarged axillary lymph node during the course of the operation, and Jean Louis Petit, at the end of that century, with continuing the incision into the axilla to dissect out the lymph nodes. He may also have removed the fascia and some of the tissue of the larger muscle (pectoralis major) beneath the breast. And, as we have seen, Larrey removed Fanny Burney's breast in 1811. By the 1860s it was becoming obvious that the operation had to be extensive, and a most important paper was written by Charles Hewitt Moore of the Middlesex Hospital, London, in 1867[3]. He emphasized that adequate surgery should include removal of the breast and all surrounding skin, the pectoralis major muscle and the lymphatic tissue and that they should all be excised in one piece. With the inadequacy of current operations, this paper enthused Christopher Heath of University College Hospital, London, to remove the axillary nodes whenever he found them enlarged[4]. The suggestion was also taken up by German surgeons, notably by Volkmann, who thought it might be well to explore the axilla in every case, but Ernst Küster was the first to advocate the systematic cleaning out of the axilla. Volkmann, and perhaps Billroth, occasionally removed the small pectoral muscle with all or part of pectoralis major, but the operation was incomplete[5].

Although his significant paper appeared in 1894[1], Halsted had previously published a brief account of his operation in 1890[6], but as the emphasis in this paper was on an aspect of surgical management, the radical nature of the technique was unappreciated. And it certainly was radical. He wrote, 'we regularly clear out the infraclavicular and usually the supraclavicular region and remove a part, at least, of the pectoralis muscle'. This was in addition to clearing out the axilla. Furthermore, like Moore, he laid great emphasis on removing the entire dissection in one piece so that the knife would not cut across the path of the cancer and thus increase the risk of cancerous cells being left behind. The large bare area left at the end of the operation 'often heals by the so-called organization of the blood clot.' Halsted concluded by giving some interesting figures for the local recurrence rates of different surgeons: Billroth, 82 percent of 170 cases (1867-76); Volkmann, 60 percent of 131 cases (1874-8); Bergmann, 51-60 percent of 114 cases (1882-7); while his own figure was 6 percent of 50 cases (1889-94). The general opinion was that if no local or glandular recurrence had appeared in three years, then it had been a radical cure.

The main modifications subsequently made to his operation concerned the shape of the incision. Many have been proposed but the one most commonly used was an incision that started further down the chest and more towards the middle, surrounding the breast elliptically rather than circularly, and continuing further into the axilla. Operations to extend Halsted's radical mastectomy in an attempt to remove cancerous lymph nodes other than those in the axilla took about fifty years to come to fruition even though Halsted himself, or his colleagues, had dipped their toes in the water. Originally, to reach the supraclavicular lymph nodes, he had had to divide the collar-bone, but by 1898[7] he had found the division to be unnecessary. He continued, 'Dr. H.W. Cushing, my house surgeon, has in three instances cleaned out the anterior mediastinum [the front part of the inside of the chest] on one side for recurrent cancer. It is likely, I think, that we shall, in the near future, remove the mediastinal contents at some of our primary operations.' He added that Cushing had introduced the pulse, or ether, chart. The operation took from two to four hours and was concluded by covering the wound immediately with a skin graft taken from the thigh. We shall meet Harvey Cushing again as he was destined for greatness in the field of brain surgery.

With an operation as extensive as Halsted's, it was essential for an accurate diagnosis to be made before surgery was undertaken, since it would be a crime to submit a woman to mutilation who only had an innocent tumour and not a cancer. In the late stages there was no doubt as to the diagnosis, but in the early ones, in which operation might be expected to have the most beneficial results, accurate clinical diagnosis was often impossible and the nature of the growth could only be known with certainty by studying it under the microscope. The removal of tissue from the body for microscopic examination is known as biopsy and nowadays is a common preliminary to surgery when a diagnosis is uncertain. It was introduced, in 1878, by a Berlin gynaecologist, Carl Ruge, and his Halle colleague Johann Veit, and its use initially was limited to growths within the uterus[8]. Howard Kelly, of the gynaecology department of Johns Hopkins, realized that the biopsy technique could have great value to other branches of surgery, and so it became common practice at the hospital to excise obscure lumps and have a look at them under the microscope.

Elsewhere in the world it took much longer for surgeons to appreciate the benefits of the method. One of the snags encountered was that it usually took a few days for a pathologist to prepare and stain a microscopic section of the lump and to give a report. Halsted had warned against excising pieces of malignant growth in the breast for microscopic examination unless operation followed immediately; if it did not, there was the danger that the damage to the growth would cause it to spread. He was able to give this paradoxical warning because a new rapid technique, known as the frozen section method, had been developed at Johns Hopkins in 1895 by T. S. Cullen[9]. As soon as the surgeon removed the suspicious tumour, or part of it, it was rushed to an adjoining room where the pathologist froze it with carbon dioxide and was able to cut a sufficiently thin section, stain it, mount it on a microscope slide, and send a report back to the surgeon within three or four minutes. The advantages of this technique for many conditions were slow to be appreciated by most surgeons and it did not come into general use for another ten years.

For more than one hundred and fifty years it has been known that breast cancer spreads to the internal mammary chain, a group of lymph nodes lying inside the chest to the side of the breastbone, but it was believed that this happened late in the disease. Surgery was considered impracticable, although attempted by Cushing, because of the dangers attendant upon opening the chest. In 1927, W. Sampson Handley reported that 'during the last 6 years I have inserted radium tubes as a prophylactic in nearly every primary breast operation.' He exised the internal mammary lymph nodes in five patients but he felt it made the operation too long and too severe. 'I believe that by the time the axillary glands [lymph nodes] are enlarged, the disease has frequently, and perhaps usually, obtained access through the inner ends of the intercostal spaces to the internal mammary glands, and that in quite early and still operable cases these glands contain microscopic deposits of cancer cells.'[10] The idea was not pursued – until 1946.

Then, Sampson Handley's son, Richard S. Handley, and A. C. Thackray, both of the Middlesex Hospital, decided to see just how often the internal mammary chain really was affected[11]. Their results showed that about a third of all operable breast cancers had already spread to the chain, and this surprising finding made surgeons wonder whether something should not be done about it during all operations on the breast. At first radiotherapy was tried, as it was still thought that surgery would be too difficult, yet the results were not entirely satisfactory. Therefore, in spite of the hazards, attempts were made to remove the lymphatics by surgery. In the event, this did prove to be feasible, though it was a major undertaking. But, in 1950, Owen H. Wangensteen, of the University of Minnesota, described a yet more extensive operation, in which he split the breastbone and removed the internal mammary chain on both sides, together with lymphatics deeper in the chest and those situated above the collar-bone[12]. His operation was preferably done in two stages and carried a high operative mortality rate of about 13 percent. However, the tissues were not removed in one piece. It was left for

Jerome A. Urban, of New York, to devise an extended operation that removed everything, breast and lymphatics, in one block and he achieved this by opening the chest and deliberately entering the pleural cavity[13]. His operation did not include removal of the lymph nodes above the collar-bone, but his operative mortality was more reasonable than that of Wangensteen, being about 1 percent. The procedure was most applicable to early cases.

Another bomb was thrown into the therapeutic arena by Robert McWhirter of Edinburgh, who treated cancer of the breast by simple mastectomy (removal of the breast only) and radiotherapy of his own technique to the lymphatics, thus returning to a practice of the mid-1930s. He started this method in 1941 and in his hands the results for any stage of the disease were as good as, if not better than, those obtained by Halsted's radical mastectomy[14]. He came in for some devastating criticism, seemingly because the reasons underlying his method were misunderstood or not accepted. It does, however, make one wonder to what extent the results of any treatment are influenced by the inherent behaviour of a particular tumour in a particular patient.

Cancer of the breast in the female and cancer of the prostate (an accessory sex gland lying just below the bladder) in the male are sometimes hormone-dependent. By this is meant that they retain some of the characteristics of the tissues from which they are derived, and their growth is therefore influenced by hormones circulating in the body. In advanced forms of these two cancers, when secondary deposits have developed elsewhere, it is possible to give some relief and slightly longer life by altering the hormonal environment. This may be done by suitable drugs or by surgical removal of the glands that produce the hormones. In 1889, based on his observation that the breast atrophied when ovarian function had been lost, Schinzinger proposed spaying in the treatment of breast cancer[15]. Whether or not he knew of Schinzinger's idea, George Beatson, of Glasgow, in 1896 removed both ovaries for advanced disease[16]. However, the brilliant conception was ignored for nearly fifty years until, in 1940, Charles Huggins of Chicago[17] revived the idea and pioneered the operations of removal of ovaries or testes, depending on the sex of the patient, for advanced breast or prostate cancer. Because the adrenal glands also produce the responsible hormones, he explored the possibility of removing these as well. The patients upon whom he operated between 1943 and 1945 all died (the longest survival being 116 days)[18], as the glands produce other hormones essential to life, but in 1951, when cortisone became available to maintain life, he reintroduced the procedure[19]. Whether the adrenals were removed as an alternative to, at the same time as, or subsequent to removal of the sex glands, it was never curative; a welcome palliation of symptoms, when all other treatment had failed, was the most that could be expected.

Following the relative success of these operations, the next possibility to suggest itself was the removal of the pituitary gland within the skull. This was done under the direction of Howard Christian Naffziger in America in 1951 for a different sort of cancer (malignant melanoma)[20], and later that year a great neurosurgeon, Herbert Olivecrona of Stockholm, who did much to further the procedure, performed his first removal of the pituitary gland for malignant disease elsewhere in the body[21, 22]. In a high proportion of cases the signs of the disease regressed, even though many patients were seriously ill and in a far advanced stage, but one of the striking features was the disappearance of pain. The pituitary might be removed as a primary operation in late stages, or alternatively, after the ovaries and adrenals had been excised and the inevitable relapse had occurred. In either instance, there was an expectation in about half the patients of a further remission that might last for a year or more, and death could come more easily. A factor limiting the usefulness of the operation was the need of a specialized neurosurgical team.

14

Epilepsy, trigeminal neuralgia and pain

T
he earliest major surgical operation ever performed had remained virtually unchanged since prehistoric man carved a circle of bone from the skull with a flint knife. The instruments used for this procedure of trepanning, or trephining, became more elaborate as time progressed, but the reasons for its performance scarcely altered. Resort was had to trephining in cases of fractured skulls to relieve pressure on the brain, and in epileptics to let the devil out; but infection and haemorrhage made the outcome dismal and quite effectively protected the brain itself from intrusion. Brain abscesses were common and it was usual to drill a number of holes over the skull until the effort was rewarded by a flow of pus. Not unnaturally this sort of hit-or-miss surgery contributed to the appalling results. Only when Lister put surgical practice on a sound footing did it become apparent that, to achieve anything constructive inside the skull, the surgeon must know exactly where to find the disease.

At the beginning of the 19th century the craze for phrenology, or the study of lumps and bumps on the head, had given impetus to finding out what part of the brain did what, but before long this method of approach was found to be utterly futile. Paul Broca, in 1861[1], was the first to show that certain areas of the brain were concerned with particular movements and although he is sometimes considered to be the 'father' of neurosurgery, it was the work of two Germans and an Englishman that really made the uncharted reaches of the brain accessible to the surgeon's art. Since it was too dangerous to experiment on human beings, the brains of animals were mapped out by electrical stimulation, Gustav Fritsch and Eduard Hitzig using dogs[2], and David Ferrier, of Yorkshire, a variety of farmyard inhabitants[3]. In 1874[4,5] Ferrier made a map of the function of the monkey's brain and for want of any better guide the monkey maps were applied to the human brain, a state of affairs that continued for a further thirty years, with modifications from studies on the orang-utan and gorilla.

The only occasion when the human brain was stimulated for purely experimental purposes in these early days was in 1874 when Roberts Bartholow, a Cincinnati surgeon, had charge of a patient with a hole in his skull produced by a cancer of the scalp. Through this hole Bartholow pushed needle electrodes into various parts of the brain and, by watching the movements that resulted, he obtained some extremely valuable information[6]. The price paid by the heroic patient was death from meningitis, an end that in any case would not have been long delayed.

Surgery of the brain got away to a slow start; previous experience was horrifying and the guide to localization sketchy and second-hand from animals. In 1879 William Macewen, professor of surgery at Glasgow, diagnosed a tumour in the dura mater over the frontal area of a patient's brain and removed it with an outcome entirely satisfactory[7]. Two years later he performed his second brain operation, this time for an abscess which he located successfully, but the patient failed to recover. Distressed, though quite undeterred, Macewen went on to perform two more successful operations[8], both for clots of blood pressing on the brain, before any other surgeon had the courage to invade this treacherous field. For five years Macewen stood alone. However, with so complicated a subject more was needed than a demonstration of successful surgery; it was necessary for techniques to be worked out in detail; the possible extent of operations and the indications for intervention had also to be determined. These tasks Macewen left for others, since he was, at heart, a general surgeon doing his best for whatever case was on the operating table and as there was no one else better qualified to operate on his neurological cases, he took them in his stride. The magnitude of his results can be found in his book *Pyogenic infective diseases of the brain and spinal cord*[9], published in 1893, where he recorded nineteen patients with brain abscesses operated upon, eighteen of whom were cured. This came at a time when surgeons were wallowing in mortalities of 100 percent for this disease and although the picture improved over the next few years to give a mortality rate of about 50 percent – a figure that remained the average until the advent of penicillin and other antibiotics – no one was able to produce results even approaching those of Macewen. He undoubtedly owed his success to his genius in discarding the unnecessary aspects of Listerism and operating under conditions that bore a marked resemblance to asepsis.

The general pattern followed over the next few years was set by the first surgeons to emulate Macewen. In 1884 a brain tumour was successfully removed by Francesco Durante of Rome[10]. Later that same year, a young man of twenty-five, from Dumfries, was admitted to the Hospital for Epilepsy and Paralysis in Regent's Park, London, complaining of twitchings, weakness of his left arm and leg, vomiting and headache. Alexander Bennett diagnosed the cause as a tumour in the motor area of the right side of the brain and persuaded Rickman John Godlee, a nephew of Lister, to operate. The operation went off quite satisfactorily, but not even the close relationship to Lister could prevent the wound from suppurating, and the patient died twenty-eight days later, relieved of his original symptoms[11]. Even though these operations showed that neurosurgery could be performed with some hope of success, no one emerged to take the reins and guide this new subject along scientific lines until, in 1886, the deficiency was supplied by Victor Horsley.

Before undertaking any operation on the brain, Horsley decided on his exact course of action by laboratory experiments[12]. Then, armed with his astute diagnostic ability, he moved into the wards, where he carefully selected suitable patients for surgery. Over a period of months he performed ten brain operations for a variety of tumours and for epilepsy; only one, a patient with a tumour, died from operative shock. All the others recovered with considerable improvement in their health[13]. Horsley's report attracted attention and, in America, Robert Weir operated twice, losing one patient from shock and the other from recurrence of the growth a few months later[14, 15]. At the end of 1887 William Williams Keen, of Philadelphia, operated successfully on a patient who survived in good health for seven years[16]. Then the floodgates opened. In the next ten years literally hundreds of surgeons carried their knives and fingers into the brain, either because everyone else seemed to be doing it or from a misguided assessment of their own ability.

Volkmann and other surgeons who had done outstanding original work elsewhere in the body, tried their hands on the brain only to find the technical and physiological problems beyond their powers. The majority of would-be neurosurgeons had their ambitions most effectively dispelled by their first (and only) harrowing experience. Until 1905, about half the patients were lost on the operating table through shock or haemorrhage. In a third of tumour cases the surgeon was unable to find the growth, and even if he did there was only an even chance that he would be able to remove it. This he would do with his bare fingers, thus predisposing to haemorrhage, shock and infection. There was little else left to go wrong. In the hands of a small number of competent surgeons the results for tumours were better, though not exactly encouraging; the mortality rate varied from 30 to 80 percent, depending on the type and location of the growth.

Nevertheless, from the beginning, surgeons were not unmindful of a need to develop the basic techniques. Drilling holes and enlarging them with chisels was most unsatisfactory, so Wilhelm Wagner[17] decided to cut a bone flap with a mallet and chisel, a dangerous undertaking but a step in the right direction. Then, after various modifications along these lines, the final solution came from Leonardo Gigli who reverted to the use of drilled burr holes which he joined up by passing a flexible wire saw through one hole and out the other, thus enabling a flap of bone to be removed with safety[18].

By his unceasing experimental work in the laboratory, Victor Horsley did more than anyone to extend the scope of the new science in its early days and give it a sure foundation on which to build. A most important contribution was his introduction of 'Horsley's wax' which was applied to the bone edges of the cut skull to control the extremely troublesome bleeding. He had first used ordinary modelling wax in animal experiments and, as this proved satisfactory, he set about devising a wax that could be rendered aseptic and thus suitable for human use. The result was a preparation consisting of seven parts of beeswax and one of almond oil.

The surgical treatment of epilepsy enjoyed a great popularity with the early 'neurosurgeons'. By 1893 a few hundred cases had been reported with a surprisingly low mortality rate, in some hands as low as 7 percent. The inspiration for operating on patients with focal epilepsy (the type then amenable to attack) came from the work on localization of function in the brain, except that the surgeons applied the information the other way round. If a fit started in a patient's right leg, the epileptic focus was in the motor area on the left side of the brain, and so the surgeon planned his approach accordingly. In his first operation for epilepsy on May 25,1886, Horsley confirmed this reasoning by electrical stimulation of the appropriate brain area, observing that the muscles that twitched were those in which the fit had started[13]. He was thus able to be certain of removing the correct part of the brain.

This patient's epilepsy had been due to an old head injury with scar formation in the motor area, which made it fairly easy to find the affected region and cut it out, but in one of Keen's patients the fits had started in the left hand and when Keen opened the skull he could see no apparent cause in the brain. He found the 'hand center' by electrical stimulation and with great courage removed it[16]. His efforts were rewarded by a marked lessening in the number of fits with the only disability a slight paralysis of the patient's left hand: a small price to pay.

Although the results of the surgical treatment of epilepsy were quite good, very few surgeons attempted the operation more than once. This makes the record of Charles McBurney, famed for his work on appendicitis, all the more praiseworthy: by 1893 he had operated on nine patients with epilepsy without a single death[19]. A remarkable feature of the work of these pioneers was the way in which they would remove vast chunks of brain with apparent unconcern, exploits that would be viewed with considerable apprehension by later surgeons.

The surgical attack on epilepsy was brought to a fine art by the work of Wilder Graves Penfield in Montreal. Born in Washington in 1891, Penfield qualified from Johns Hopkins in 1918. From 1921 to 1928 he worked in New York. He then became professor of neurology and neurosurgery at McGill

University and founded the Montreal Neurological Institute, which was opened in 1934, the same year that he became a Canadian citizen. By the most meticulous and painstaking research, Penfield, dubbed in his time 'the greatest living Canadian', furthered the science of the localization of function within the brain, and by his brilliant surgery restored many epileptics to a life free, or almost free, from fits. In 1952 the crown was set upon his distinguished career when he received the Order of Merit.

On the other side of the world in 1945, in Johannesburg, Rowland A. Krynauw began operating on children who were paralysed down one side and had severe epilepsy or mental disturbances[20]. Except for selected areas on the under part, he removed the whole of one side of the brain, with astoundingly good results that gave freedom from fits and improvement in the mental condition, together with some degree of alleviation of the paralysis. Other surgeons, for example Walter Dandy in 1928[21], had performed operations of a similar extent, but these had been for tumours, which more obviously demanded heroic measures.

In 1940 William van Wagenen of Rochester, New York, reported on a rather incredible approach to the problem[22]. His reasoning was based on his observation that tumours or cerebrovascular accidents in the area of the corpus callosum reduced the number of fits or stopped them completely. (The corpus callosum is the most important of the bands of fibres joining the two cerebral hemispheres.) His first operation to sever the band took place on February 6, 1939, and at the time of his report he had operated on ten patients mostly with much improvement. What probably happened was that by severing the pathways in the corpus callosum, the spread of the epileptic wave to the opposite hemisphere was limited. In successful cases, the patients did not seem to lose consciousness or to have generalized convulsions. However, when the seizures originated from multiple sites the operation was usually without effect.

The first organized attack on nerves to relieve pain was for trigeminal neuralgia or 'tic douloureux', an agonizing condition in which one side of the face is wracked by paroxysms of severe pain. The cause is in the trigeminal nerve itself and that is where treatment must be directed. In the 17th century an attempt had been made at cutting the nerve, but by a mistake in anatomy the nerve to the facial muscles was cut and the wretched patient was left with his pain and a paralysed face into the bargain. Thereafter drugs and other medical measures were employed though there was the rare exception, such as the occasion in 1821 when John Lizars of Edinburgh cut one of the lower branches of the nerve from within the mouth; the pain of the operation was almost unendurable but the patient went back to his work in the fields greatly pleased with the result[23]. In 1858 John Murray Carnochan devised a method for dealing with a branch of the nerve in its course outside the skull[24], and in 1862 Joseph

Pancoast devised a radical operation in which he divided the trunks of the two main branches of the nerve as they emerged from the base of the skull[25]. These two operators were followed by other surgeons who temporarily removed parts of the cheekbone to get better access. But none of these operations was attended by permanent success, and it became obvious that the attack would have to be directed to the Gasserian ganglion (a relay station on the nerve, also known as Meckel's ganglion, or the trigeminal or semilunar ganglion) within the skull.

In 1890 William Rose of London attempted such a procedure, but the operation proved excessively difficult since he had entered by the small hole through which one of the branches of the nerve emerges and was only able to remove part of the ganglion[26]. A year later Horsley approached the problem with consummate genius. He suggested cutting the nerve before it reached the ganglion, anatomically an easier operation. Experiments on animals and cadavers showed the best way of approach to be through the temporal bone. However, it was most unfortunate that the first time he tried the operation he chose a very ill patient, who died of operative shock[27]. Although the technique itself was a success, Horsley did not use it again, but it was subsequently resurrected by another surgeon some years later.

A few months after Horsley's unlucky operation, a New York surgeon, Frank Hartley, renowned for his boldness in tackling difficult and dangerous operations, achieved a permanent cure. He entered the skull through the temporal bone and removed the ganglion in its entirety[28]. It so happened that another surgeon, Fedor Krause, of Berlin, was also working on the problem and, entirely unaware of Hartley's operation, carried out a similar procedure six months later[29].

Although at the turn of the 19th century neurosurgery had established itself in the surgical world, the outlook was rather dim as many surgeons had tested their skill and failed; only a handful had emerged with the right mental and physical equipment for the work. The task of consolidating neurosurgery as a specialty was to rest in the competent hands of one man, Harvey Cushing. His contribution to the subject was immense and it is little exaggeration to say that neurosurgery and neurology were advanced every time he picked up his scalpel to operate or his pen to write. His articles were a model of perfection, clear, complete in every detail, and beautifully illustrated with his own superb drawings. In 1905, when associate professor of surgery at Johns Hopkins, he stated the requirements necessary for a surgeon to become proficient in the specialty. These included a thorough grounding in medicine and pathology followed by the close study of neurology in the wards and experiments in the laboratory. He saw most clearly that if there was to be advancement in neurosurgery, there must be 'concentration of thoughts and energies along given lines'.

Cushing's first essay in the field, and one that brought him early fame, was his treatment of trigeminal neuralgia by removal of the Gasserian ganglion[30]. His modification of the Hartley-Krause operation gave him a mortality rate in a large series of cases of 5 percent, or about half the average for the time. By adopting the earlier method of temporary removal of part of the cheekbone and combining this with the temporal approach, he was able to avoid the very common complication of tearing the middle meningeal artery; this grooves the inside of the temporal bone, and easily became damaged when tension was put on the dura mater. Alas for Cushing, all his work was soon brought to naught; in fact, had he been a little less stubborn he would have realized he was barking up the wrong tree, for the operative solution to the problem had been provided shortly after he began his series of operations by another American, Charles Harrison Frazier of Philadelphia[31]. In 1901 William Spiller, a neurologist, had suggested to Frazier that it might be possible to relieve the neuralgia by cutting the trigeminal nerve behind the ganglion, just as Horsley had done on that ill-fated occasion eleven years previously, though it is uncertain whether Spiller knew of this operation. At all events Frazier carried out this easier and safer procedure with entirely satisfactory results.

For six more years Cushing plodded on, insisting that removal of the ganglion was the only way to effect a permanent cure[32]. He reasoned that if only cut, the nerve was quite likely to join up again; however, fate took a hand in the proceedings when on one occasion Cushing was forced to cut the nerve, being unable to remove the ganglion because of a neighbouring tumour[33]. The patient recovered and had no further bother with neuralgia. Thereafter Cushing was a staunch supporter of operating on the nerve and not on the ganglion, reconciling his conscience to this volte-face by advocating total removal of part of the nerve, thus making reunion impossible, and by giving himself the credit for the approach used by Frazier.

The further advances in the treatment of this condition were due to Frazier, who, although a brilliant neurosurgeon, was definitely second fiddle to Cushing; he also had a peculiar habit of not reporting on his technical advances till many years after their inception. For instance, one of the complications of the operation was corneal ulceration and in 1915, Frazier devised a very delicate and selective operation, leaving intact the nerve fibres supplying the cornea; the paper describing this was published in 1925[34]. And in 1919 (reported in 1934) he began also to spare the motor part of the trigeminal nerve[35] which is concerned with the muscles of chewing and swallowing, though he had actually been preceded in this refinement by Cushing who, in 1916, in one patient had saved the motor nerve[36], and by Max Peet of Ann Arbor in 1917[37].

Cutting the nerve fibres carrying the sensation of pain was the chosen operation until 1951, in which year Palle Taarnhøj of Copenhagen removed a small tumour that was pressing on the nerve and causing neuralgia[38]. Unlike previous surgeons, he did not cut the nerve as part of the operation. Nevertheless, the patient was relieved of his pain, and thus the operation of decompression of the trigeminal nerve came into being. This meant that in cases not caused by tumour, Taarnhøj simply relieved any pressure that normal structures might be causing. Modifications were introduced by other surgeons and all had the great advantage that ordinary sensation of the face was left undisturbed; when the nerve was cut the affected side became anaesthetic. Of considerable interest is the view, held by a number of neurosurgeons, that the Taarnhøj operation does not, in fact, achieve its success by decompression but by elimination of the reflex that gives rise to the pain.

A similar doubt assailed Robert Pudenz who saw no apparent reason for the success of the decompressive operations, arguing that the only factor common to the differing types was operative trauma. So he seemingly stood the whole situation on its head by adopting the technique of posterior root compression, operating on his first patient in December, 1953[39]. If the pain involved the second and third divisions, he applied gentle compression with a small bit of a dental roll; if it was limited to either division alone, he used the back of a blunt dissector. Twenty-nine patients were completely relieved of pre-operative pain (though it recurred in a small number), and there was no postoperative facial anaesthesia.

Severe and intractable pain in other parts of the body can also be relieved by the neurosurgeon, and this was first done by Robert Abbe who, in 1888, cut the appropriate nerves as they emerged from the spinal cord. The patient, a man of forty-four, had intractable brachial neuralgia. After nerve stretching and then amputation of the arm, he underwent intra-dural division of the posterior roots of the sixth and seventh cervical nerves under ether anaesthesia on December 31, 1888. The wound was packed but not closed and then on January 2, 1889, the eighth root was divided without anaesthesia – there was pain only when the root was handled; happily after all this the patient was improved[40]. The next step was to be a large one and took the point of the scalpel right into the spinal cord, there to divide the nerve tracts. William Gibson Spiller, in 1905[41], thought this might be possible, yet it was not until 1911 that he managed to persuade Edward Martin, professor of surgery in the University of Pennsylvania, to undertake the delicate and potentially hazardous operation. Martin was successful[42], and within a few months three other surgeons performed similar procedures, quite unaware of Martin's work. In 1920 Frazier published his first results[43] and the operation then became popular; but because it was not always successful in cases of pain in the upper part of the body, surgeons later carried the knife higher up the spinal cord, into the brain stem, and finally into the frontal lobes of the brain itself.

15

Tumours of the brain, hydrocephalus and psychosurgery

Victor Horsley aroused interest in the spinal cord as well as the brain when he removed a tumour from the cord in 1887[1]. This was the first occasion such an operation had been done successfully, though we find Macewen indulging in some friendly rivalry tinged with jealousy since, in 1883, he had removed part of the vertebrae (an operation known as laminectomy) to relieve pressure on the spinal cord. Macewen's operation was on a lad with a curvature of the spine that was causing distressing symptoms. By removing the overlying part of the spine and a fibrous mass of tissue underneath, he obtained a good cure[2,3]. He followed this operation with five more, in which results were good in three patients with fractures, but in two with tuberculosis the disease was aggravated and proved lethal a short while after operation[4]. When Horsley published his case of a true neoplasm, Macewen tried to minimize his glory by pointing out that he had really been the first to remove a 'tumour'. It all depends on what is meant by 'tumour'. The mass removed by Macewen did not fall into the pathological classification of new growths, whether benign or malignant, whereas Horsley's did. The honours may therefore be considered evenly divided.

The plight of patients with tumours of the spinal cord was terrible; the kidneys became infected, bedsores were the rule and pneumonia often developed. Simple relief of the pressure on the cord would suffice to make their end more comfortable if it could not cure, but in the years following Horsley's operation attempts at surgical relief were few and far between, probably because 50 percent of patients subjected to operation died as a result and only about a quarter derived any benefit from the procedure. Why the results were so bad after the initial successes is difficult to see.

The study of brain tumours was to be Harvey Cushing's main concern for the rest of his life, once he had sorted out his difficulties over the operation for trigeminal neuralgia. At first both Charles Frazier and he were advancing along similar lines and the rivalry gave rise to some amusing and sarcastic interchanges in the medical literature, until gradually Cushing demonstrated his superiority. A factor of considerable importance to his success was his early training at Johns Hopkins where he had been house surgeon to Halsted and had learned the elements of good surgical technique from this most meticulous and painstaking surgeon, attributes essential for the delicate surgery of the brain. In 1900 he had visited Europe and studied for a time at the Berne clinic of Theodor Kocher, another master of the surgical art. On his return he introduced the idea of taking the patient's blood pressure during operation, a measure that gives a valuable indication of the degree of shock[5]. Thus Cushing was well equipped to pursue his inclinations with skill, learning and that indefinable something that makes for genius.

Following its explosive start, surgery for brain tumours subsided to an extent almost threatening extinction. Operations were few and far between and attended by uniformly bad results, which was not really surprising since localization was still in its infancy and only those tumours in the motor area of the brain could be located with anything approaching accuracy. As the skull cannot expand, anything growing inside causes an increase in pressure which produces a vicious headache, vomiting and disturbances of vision progressing to blindness; therefore, even if the tumour could not be found these effects could be relieved by allowing the brain to expand. This was first done by removing a flap of bone, opening the dura mater, and closing only the skin over the top. As this was usually the last resort after a surgeon had attempted and failed to find the tumour, the place where it was done might be anywhere on the skull. The result was a soft bulge that sometimes assumed quite alarming proportions. Realizing the limitations of brain surgery, Cushing decided that, rather than attempt removal of the tumour, it would be far better to devise an operation for decompressing the brain. His solution was simple and consisted of removing the flap of bone from under the muscles of the temple or those of the back of the skull; the muscles would prevent subsequent unsightly bulging, yet would allow the brain to expand sufficiently to relieve the symptoms[6]. The operation, known as palliative decompression, became the accepted procedure for a few years. However, it *was* only palliative; the tumours were still inside the skull continuing their destruction or compression of brain tissue. Some inspiration was urgently needed to give a lead on their removal in the majority, and not only the minority, of cases.

Having got a reasonably satisfactory palliative operation to fall back on, Cushing devoted more time to the problem of actual removal and in 1910 he was able to report on sixty-four patients in a quarter of whom he had achieved good results from removal of the tumour[7]. Unlike his predecessors who used their fingers, he dissected out the tumours very gently with a piece of gauze and saved the patient a considerable amount of shock and haemorrhage. However, he had found it necessary to do the palliative operation in two-thirds of the patients, half of whom were restored to a fair state of health. The total mortality was 10 percent. Events were thus beginning to shape in the right direction and, with the knowledge that tumour surgery was not quite as disastrous as had been feared, Cushing continued to operate and to search for a more adequate technique.

The answer did not elude him for long. In 1911 he published an account of a method that was to revolutionize neurosurgery and, although not making it foolproof, resulted in a lowered mortality rate and opened the way to more extensive operations. The curse of brain surgery was bleeding, extensive and almost uncontrollable; but due to the different texture of the tissues it was not possible to stem it in the same manner as elsewhere in the body. Cushing's solution was to devise little clips of silver wire which he picked up in forceps and gently and accurately used to compress the bleeding point, leaving the wire permanently in place[8]. At the same time he introduced small stamps of muscle for the control of haemorrhage in the brain and dura mater, situations where even the clips could not be used. Thus with his haemostatic armamentarium completed by simple, yet extremely effective, devices there was no holding him, and in 1915 he published the results of his operations on one hundred and thirty tumour patients with the astounding mortality rate of 8 percent[9]. Surgeons like Horsley (who died a year later of heat stroke in Mesopotamia) and Krause were still almost fumbling with rates of 40–50 percent. Cushing's paper heralded the turn of the tide.

The structure inside the skull that attracted Cushing's particular fancy was the pituitary gland, an organ that has earned for itself the title of 'conductor of the endocrine orchestra', as it is intimately concerned with the regulation of hormones within the body, and affects the function of all the glands that make life liveable and continuable. Cushing had thus selected a subject worthy of his genius. He began his research by work on the actual function of the pituitary, and as a result of experiments on animals deduced that it was essential to life[10]. Then he turned his attention to the surgical attack on tumours of the gland and, as early as 1909, performed the first operation for acromegaly, a condition in which there is overactivity of part of the pituitary, resulting in enlargement of the bones of the face and extremities. He entered the skull by a roughly semicircular incision on the forehead, and progressing through the bony structures at the top of the nose was able to remove half the gland with a small, sharp, long-handled spoon[11]. The young patient eventually returned to his occupation of farming.

In 1912, the year he became professor of surgery at Harvard, Cushing published his classic work on the disorders of the pituitary, in which he recorded an operative mortality rate of 14 percent for tumours in the gland[12]. Over the years this was gradually reduced and the rate for 1927 was only 4 percent[13], a truly magnificent achievement. The method of approach was different from his first case, as he adopted a route that did not involve opening the skull; instead he went in through the nose by the endonasal transsphenoidal approach. This remained the popular route until the late 1920s. The alternative mode of entry was much more likely to result in severe haemorrhage or brain damage at the hands of the average surgeon, since it consisted of raising a large bone flap from the forehead and lifting up the front of the brain to gain access to the pituitary lying beneath and somewhat behind. This had first been performed by Frazier in 1913[14] with considerable success, and he predicted that it would be the operation of the future; but almost immediately afterwards, he himself was using the endonasal operation as a routine. His prediction did eventually come true in the 1930s when, as a result of Cushing's later work, it was found to be safe and to give better exposure.

We cannot leave Cushing's contributions to neurosurgery without mention of tumours of the acoustic nerve. These occur on the nerve of hearing in the posterior part of the brain and any attempt at surgical removal had previously been attended by so shocking a mortality that surgeons considered them, and others in the area, to be unsuitable for operation. Cushing disagreed, and after a few years' preliminary skirmishing, with good results, he produced in 1917 another classic book, this time on tumours of the acoustic nerve[15]. The operative mortality rate recorded here was more astounding than anything he had achieved before: 11 percent compared with an average of 75 percent reported by other (and competent) neurosurgeons.

In the early days of brain surgery the two chief anaesthetic agents available both had their drawbacks. Ether increased the tendency to bleeding, and chloroform had a depressant effect upon the patient and lowered his blood pressure. Ethyl chloride was good for starting off the anaesthetic and was used as such by Cushing, but there was a definite need for a satisfactory form of anaesthesia. Research was renewed on methods of giving substances rectally, and in the first decade of the century ether vapour in air or oxygen was used; however, it was subject to the disadvantage that the absorption rate could not be controlled and therefore the degree of anaesthesia was variable. In 1913 oil-ether rectal instillations became popular owing to the work of James Gwathmey[16], but the same objections applied. Local anaesthesia was another available possibility, although the idea of performing a long and tedious operation on the brain under a local anaesthetic rather horrified surgeons, who did not take kindly to it until Cushing, in 1910, showed that it had very great advantages over the general anaesthetics then in use; its only disadvantage in the early days was its occasional inadequacy.

Cushing continued to use the local form as a routine practice, but later a satisfactory mode of general anaesthesia was slowly developed, based on barbiturate drugs given intravenously[17] and the use of a tube passed down inside the windpipe[18], thus enabling breathing to be controlled by the anaesthetist and doing away with the need for the mask and other apparatus to be gathered round the patient's head.

A great handicap to neurosurgeons had been their inability to localize about a third of the brain tumours, which meant that unless they were extraordinarily lucky a palliative decompression was the only solution. Strangely enough, it was Halsted who was indirectly responsible for suggesting the method whereby nearly every tumour could be located. He was always remarking on the way shadows of gas in the intestines would 'perforate bone' in x-ray pictures of the abdomen, and so persistent were his comments that an idea took root in the mind of Walter Dandy, a neurosurgeon at Johns Hopkins and one-time house surgeon to Cushing. Dandy had been trying to inject fluid contrast media into the ventricles, or spaces, of the brain, but as this had proved toxic to animals he was still searching for something suitable. He reasoned that if intestinal gas showed through bone, it should be possible to outline the ventricles by the injection of air. This he did in 1918[19] with eminently satisfactory results, and so was born the method of pneumoventriculography, in which any alteration in shape due to the presence of a tumour, or other space-occupying lesion, shows up clearly on an x-ray. A further diagnostic method was introduced in 1927 by Egas Moniz, who outlined the pattern of the blood vessels by injection of a radio-opaque fluid[20].

Another important technical advance of Cushing's generation was the harnessing of electricity for surgical operations. Electrosurgery with the use of a diathermy knife began in the 1920s, and in 1928 Cushing introduced it into neurosurgery[21]. The surgeon holds an insulated handle with a needle protruding from the end, and the circuit is so arranged that it is completed when this needle touches any part of the patient's body. The 'knife' cuts by burning and is the modern counterpart of the old-fashioned cautery, with the exception that it can be used most delicately and selectively. Besides its use for cutting tissues within the body, it can also coagulate bleeding points, and the benefit of this instrument to brain surgery and surgery of other organs, such as the liver and kidney, where haemorrhage is likely to be troublesome, was immense. Although Cushing had reduced the mortality rate from brain surgery to amazingly low levels, he was able to reduce it still further with electrosurgery.

Hydrocephalus, or 'water on the brain', is a disease occurring in many forms, in some of which there is an obstruction to the normal free circulation of cerebrospinal fluid inside and around the brain and the spinal cord. Depending on the form and the site of the obstruction, there are a number of operations that can be undertaken to relieve the condition, either bypassing the obstruction or actually draining the fluid to some other part of the body. These operations provide an example of procedures devised a long time ago, but which did not become workable propositions until plastic tubes were invented to replace the irritant materials used previously.

The first and seemingly obvious way to drain the fluid, in the light of the dangers of attacking the brain directly, was to perform lumbar puncture – admittedly only a temporary measure. This was carried out in 1891 by Heinricus Quincke[22]; he was followed seven years later by the American Alexander Hugh Ferguson who drained the cerebrospinal fluid by passing a length of silver wire from the spinal canal through the spinal column and into the peritoneal cavity[23]. Then, in 1905, Walther Kausch led a rubber tube from the brain into the peritoneal cavity[24], and in the same year Cushing repeated Ferguson's operation, but used a silver cannula[25]. Nevertheless, the suggestion had already been made (in 1895) by Gärtner that it was a physiologically sound strategy to establish a connection between the ventricles and either the venous or the lymphatic systems of the head and neck[26].

The idea was not put into practice until 1908 when it was attempted on both sides of the Atlantic. The more successful was Erwin Payr, of Leipzig, who took a graft of either saphenous or temporal vein to connect a lateral ventricle to the longitudinal sinus (a venous sinus within the skull); all three of his patients died within four months but at autopsy no reflux of blood or thrombosis of the longitudinal sinus was detected[27]. In 1911, he reported on another eight patients in whom he had connected a lateral ventricle to the internal jugular vein using, as graft, the formalin-fixed, paraffin-treated anterior or posterior tibial artery of dogs or calves[28]. The results were excellent in three patients. A less successful procedure devised at Johns Hopkins deserved better as its provenance was impeccable. The surgeon was R.D. McClure and the idea had been suggested by Alexis Carrel, an experimental surgeon par excellence, and, encouraged by Cushing, they agreed that the vascular graft should contain valves and in their experimental work on six dogs they chose a segment of external jugular vein. The one operation, on July 23, 1908, was on a ten-month-old baby; the graft was a portion of a cephalic vein from the father's arm. The baby stood the operation well, but died some hours later from a sudden rise in temperature[29].

Some of the operations that were tried had temporarily successful results, but there were so many unknown factors that one by one they went out of fashion. Then in 1948 the drainage of brain or spinal canal into the peritoneal cavity (where the fluid is easily absorbed) was reintroduced by William Cone[30], and a year later Donald Matson used a plastic tube to drain the spinal canal into a ureter[31], thus resurrecting another old operation previously done with rubber by Bernhard Heile in 1925[32]. In 1951 Matson adapted the operation for draining the brain[33]. The ureter is the tube carrying urine from the kidney to the bladder, so

135

both of these procedures had the disadvantage that a kidney was sacrificed and, also, the excess cerebrospinal fluid was drained into the bladder, where it was voided in the urine; this loss of fluid meant that the body chemistry was liable to be upset, a consideration that did not apply when drainage was into a part of the body where reabsorption could take place.

In all the operations the plastic tubes are passed just below the skin to get from the brain or spinal canal to wherever they are going and, to overcome the need for further operations in a growing child, the tube is sometimes telescoped. However, this is a minor difficulty compared with other problems, of which the most serious is the danger of the tube's becoming blocked. In an endeavour to prevent this, Griffith R. Harsh III, of St Louis, Missouri, in 1952 devised an operation suitable for use in females only. To avoid the plastic tube having to lie free in the peritoneal cavity, he stitched it to the frond-like fimbria of a Fallopian tube[34].

Other ingenious operations include those of William Nosik, who in 1950 drained the brain into the mastoid cavity[35]; of Joseph Ransohoff, who in 1952 utilized the pleural cavity[36], and of Robert Pudenz, who in 1955 led a plastic tube into the right auricle of the heart[37]. Perhaps the best-known procedure is one in which use is made of the Spitz-Holter valve. This was invented in 1956 by John Holter, a Philadelphia engineer, and given to Eugene Spitz, a neurosurgeon, for use in Holter's son who had already undergone several operations with only temporary benefit. The valve is designed to drain the fluid from the brain into the heart at a set pressure and in a one-way flow.

Although as far back as 1891 a Swiss surgeon, G. Burckhardt, had operated on six mental patients to their considerable benefit[38], interest in surgery of the brain for the relief of afflictions of the mind, so-called psychosurgery, did not come into prominence until 1935. In that year an International Congress on neurology was held in London at which some experimental work on the behaviour of chimpanzees after removal of their frontal lobes was reported. This so impressed Egas Moniz, professor of neurology in Lisbon, that he decided a similar operation would help human patients. Accordingly he invented an instrument to cut the connections between the frontal lobes and the rest of the brain without doing any other damage. Then, in 1936, he persuaded his colleague, Almeida Lima, to put theory into practice and was able to record almost complete cures in certain mental conditions of which the chief symptoms were anxiety and worry[39]. In the United States, Walter Freeman and James Watts performed the operation later the same year[40] and went on to improve both the technique and the assessment of the results. Subsequent enthusiasm was not, however, world-wide, for surgeons in Great Britain, France, and Germany were somewhat sceptical, though in other countries, such as Brazil and Italy, the reception was more cordial.

In 1937, Mario Fiamberti approached the brain from below through the roof of the orbit, instead of going in through the skull above[41]. A number of other approaches were also devised in the endeavour to achieve consistent results, and the most significant was that of James Lyerly who, in 1938, introduced an 'open' method[42]. In this, the brain is exposed from above and the surgeon works with direct vision, unlike the earlier operations in which the cutting was done blind, and in which uncontrolled bleeding often led to a period of coma after operation. Lyerly's work was not recognized until 1948, when James Leonard Poppen of Boston reported his success with a large number of patients, using an essentially similar approach[43]. The open technique not only made the blind methods largely obsolete but also helped to reduce the operative mortality. Although about a third of the patients were improved, an undesirable feature in most was the loss of drive, initiative and depth of personality; there were, however, a few patients who, being released from self-consciousness and fear, showed a greater accomplishment than before operation.

16

Specialization

I n the closing years of the 19th century, surgeons were making a journey into an unknown of an entirely different nature from that of the brain. Before this time they had confined their activities to dealing with manifestations of disease that could be seen; injuries were repaired and growths were cut out, and the knife was used only for obvious physical disorders. It was, therefore, a tremendous step forward when the surgeon invaded the realms of disease hitherto considered the perquisite of the physician and demonstrated that surgical skill could heal the body when certain parts were not functioning properly. Cushing played a role in the evolution of what is known as physiological surgery by his operations on the pituitary gland; these lowered the gland's ability to function and so were useful in the management of diseases such as acromegaly. However, the first step had been taken by the surgeons who operated on one of the instruments in the endocrine orchestra, the thyroid gland.

The man who raised thyroid surgery out of a bloody morass was Theodor Kocher, professor of surgery at Berne. He achieved his success by concentrating his energies on this one subject in an age when specialization was frowned upon, and it was probably during Cushing's visit to his clinic that Cushing became inspired to study his own particular subject in all its many aspects. Kocher's grounding in general surgery was excellent and, owing to his beautifully delicate technique and rigid adherence to asepsis, he was also able to make considerable contributions to abdominal surgery; he studied the functions of the brain and spinal cord, and in 1880 devised an operation for the radical removal of the tongue in cases of cancer[1]. It is small wonder, with such a remarkable record, that Kocher has earned a place as one of the founders of modern surgery. His clinic was a model of perfection, smoothness and precision;

the next patient would always appear in the theatre at the precise moment he was required and all would be in readiness. At the operation it was a rare thing for Kocher to find he had made an incorrect diagnosis. His surgery was a joy to watch; neat, almost bloodless and, if anything went wrong, he was always complete master of the situation.

A goitre is a swelling of the thyroid gland due to a lack of iodine in the diet or to a blockage of its synthesis, and is most prevalent in the mountainous districts of the world. Thus, residing in Berne, Kocher had plenty of opportunity to study the disease. Only a few years before he appeared on the scene the general opinion about operating on goitres was definitely unfavourable since the gland is one of the most vascular in the body, and if haemorrhage failed to kill the patient on the table, subsequent sepsis and secondary haemorrhage almost certainly would. Kocher, who was the first to operate on the gland[2], completely altered this picture and, in 1883, recorded over one hundred operations, with a mortality rate of 13 percent[3]. The extent of his specialization is shown by a further report fifteen years later of more than six hundred thyroid operations with only one death[4].

It was this work that led directly to the beginning of physiological surgery, and with it to the attack on thyrotoxicosis or Graves's disease, a state in which the thyroid is overactive and leads to generalized overactivity of the body. In florid cases, the sufferer is nervous, thin, sweats and flushes easily; the heart rate is increased and palpitates, but often the most striking feature is the prominent staring eyes. Kocher had shown that in cases of goitre, which causes no symptoms apart from those directly attributable to its size, surgery could be undertaken with safety. The step from this to removal of part of the gland in thyrotoxicosis may now seem obvious and simple, but for Ludwig Rehn, of Frankfurt am Main, it was literally a step into the unknown. He was, in 1880, the first to remove part of each lobe of the gland for exophthalmic goitre[5], though Kocher later developed the operation and did much research into the disease.

The complications of any surgical attack on the thyroid are illustrated by a comparison of the techniques of Kocher and Billroth. Kocher (who operated under local anaesthesia) always performed an immaculate dissection, removing the entire gland with very little damage outside its capsule. Sometimes his patients developed myxoedema, in which the subject becomes lethargic with a puffy, dry skin owing to lack of thyroid secretion; it was therefore necessary to give these patients thyroid extract (first used by George Murray in 1891[6]) to restore them to a 'normal' state. Billroth, on the other hand, was more rapid in his work, having less regard for the tissues, and sometimes he accidentally removed the neighbouring parathyroid glands, with the result that the patient developed tetany – cause and effect was confirmed (though it had already been demonstrated experimentally) by von Eiselsberg, who was working in Billroth's clinic[7]. The tetany was found to be controllable with calcium in 1909. As his rougher dissection left pieces of thyroid tissue behind, Billroth's patients did not develop myxoedema. A further complication is for the nerves to the larynx to be unavoidably cut, resulting in voice changes.

The importance of surgery for simple goitre was soon appreciated, but operations for thyrotoxicosis did not become popular until the end of the first decade of the 20th century, when Charles Mayo[8] and Halsted[9], who both improved Kocher's operation, and Kocher himself reported on large numbers of cases with good results. A young Australian surgeon, Thomas Dunhill, achieved brilliant results. In his 1907 paper Dunhill noted that the mortality rate was high when chloroform was the anaesthetic so in seven patients he had operated under local, all with uneventful recoveries[10]. In 1908, he reported on thirty-two operations for thyrotoxicosis in twenty-five patients – there was one death (the thirteenth case!) due to the removal of both lobes – some of the patients had been seriously ill and two had advanced myocarditis[11]. And, in 1909, he reported on one hundred and thirteen patients, of whom eighty-eight had had thyrotoxicosis, with the one death he had previously reported[12]. Dunhill advocated early operation with a second operation later, if necessary, and showed that even the most severe case was able to benefit from surgery, a fact that inspired confidence in other surgeons. In 1909 Kocher received international recognition for his work and was awarded the Nobel prize.

Harvey Cushing had brought home most forcibly to the surgical profession the value of concentrating thought and energy along given lines. Initially he had had difficulty making his colleagues appreciate the wisdom of dividing surgery into specialties, for it was widely agreed that a surgeon worthy of the name should be able to undertake any operation. Experience with brain surgery proved the error of this, and although the separateness of the more specialized specialties such as ophthalmology had been accepted for a number of years, it still took some time for the lesson to become generally learned. By the beginning of the 20th century surgery was at the crossroads; the progress achieved in fifty years had been remarkable and it was apparent that if further advances were to be made surgeons with a particular interest in one subject would have to devote themselves to its development. Nevertheless, the idea of specialization met with stiff opposition, since the majority of surgeons were unable to see how the patient would benefit, and they believed that the only benefit accruing to the surgeon would be purely financial – provided, of course, that he picked the right specialty and made a name for himself before other competitors flooded the market. This antagonism and shortsightedness was the product of several factors. First, during the 1890s there were quite enough people at the top of the profession who repeatedly affirmed that surgery had achieved as much as was humanly possible and that no new fields remained for conquest.

Second, the training of the surgeons of this generation had been in general surgery and new problems were accordingly attacked by resort to general principles. It was not immediately realized that many problems of the new specialist surgery demanded fresh sets of principles. Third, the time had not long passed when 'specialists' had been unqualified itinerant lithotomists, herniotomists and the like, and the association of ideas in all probability affected the reasoning of those who were opposed to specialism. These unqualified practitioners were at the worst charlatans and quacks, and at the best well-meaning and often skilful men who for some such reason as lack of education had been unable to qualify in the examinations of the day. The specialties, however, did not have their origins in this type of practice, but gradually evolved from developments within the framework of orthodox medicine and surgery.

The eye had excited the curiosity of surgeons for centuries, and many had been the fanciful theories propounded to explain the phenomenon of vision. Although the anatomy and physiology had been worked out in a fair degree of detail by the middle of the 19th century, it was still impossible to study the behaviour of the eye during life, and without this the majority of diseases remained a mystery. An instrument was needed that would permit a clinical examination of the interior of the eye, but the optical properties of the internal structures proved a stumbling block. The problems were finally overcome by Hermann von Helmholtz, professor of physiology and pathology at Königsberg, who in 1850 invented the ophthalmoscope[13]. His original design was soon improved by the incorporation of a rotatable disc holding different lenses for eyes of differing refractions – in the early model the examiner had to insert the lenses separately. The illumination was provided by daylight, gas, or oil flame until 1886, when the electric ophthalmoscope was introduced. The instrument revolutionized the approach to eye conditions and very soon its benefits were applied to ophthalmic surgery by Albrecht von Graefe, one of whose many contributions to the new specialty was iridectomy for acute glaucoma[14]. In this operation, part of the iris is removed, with the object of relieving the great increase of pressure that builds up inside the eye and causes intense pain and often leads to blindness. The reasons why this operation is sometimes successful are rather nebulous, and today it is only used in certain types of the disease, having been superseded by techniques that increase the drainage of fluid in the eye. In England the possibilities of the ophthalmoscope were but slowly realized, and although Spencer Wells had drawn attention to its value[15], it was the neurologists who eventually popularized the instrument because of the importance of eye changes in the diagnosis of many brain diseases. The next important discovery, after which ophthalmology has never looked back, was the power of cocaine to produce local anaesthesia in the eye[16].

Helmholtz was a truly exceptional person: as a child he read Greek and Arabic works in their original languages and when his future career was under discussion, he expressed an ardent desire to be a physicist. His father pointed out the impecunious nature of the pursuit and put him in for medicine. This was indeed fortunate for medicine, since his discoveries could have only been made by a medical man who was at the same time a brilliant physicist. Besides his invention of the ophthalmoscope he confirmed and expanded the colour theory of vision[17] propounded by Thomas Young[18] and later, when professor of physiology at Bonn, he described the basic principles of the physiology and physics of sound[19]. In 1871 his childhood wish came true when he was appointed professor of physics at Berlin.

The window of the eye is the cornea which enjoys a privileged position when damaged and grafting is required, as being a window is its only 'function'. Since normally the cornea has no blood supply, antibodies cannot reach the graft to kill it. One of the problems after operation, though, is to prevent tiny blood vessels from growing into the graft, as this results in a clouding of vision. However, corneal grafting really only became a practicable proposition with the formation of eye banks, where corneas are stored by special freezing methods. Needless to say, the idea was not new.

Early in the 19th century some experimental work was done using animal eyes, but infection and clouding invariably developed. To deal with this, Arthur von Hippel of Giessen, in Germany, in 1879 tried using glass with a gold rim, which could be taken out and cleaned, but it was not a success[20]. However, a real advance was made by Henry Power of St Bartholomew's Hospital, London, whose experiments, started in 1872, showed conclusively that human cornea had to be employed and that animal grafts were doomed to failure[21]. Then in 1905 and 1906, Eduard Zirm of Olmütz performed the first successful operations by two differing methods[22, 23].

Since that time, techniques have been refined to a quite incredible degree. For instance, José Barraquer of Bogota, Colombia, who had been working on corneal surgery for nearly twenty years, in 1965 reported on the way he was reshaping the cornea. Previous methods designed to alter the surface of the patient's cornea had all been abandoned, but what Barraquer did was to remove the outer layer of the cornea, quick-freeze it, and grind it to a predetermined shape in much the same way as a spectacle maker grinds his lenses to meet the patient's prescription. The newly shaped layer of cornea was then stitched back into the eye. Barraquer had done this operation more than a hundred times on patients with severe astigmatism or other refractive errors, and on those who were visually handicapped after extraction of their lenses for cataract, before he decided to use donor cornea and thus reduce the risk of damaging the patient's own cornea. In 1968 he described his new technique for removing the outer layer of the patient's cornea, being very careful about exact diameter and thickness. Then after complex mathematical calculations he froze and ground the layer of donor cornea to the precise shape and size needed. This was inserted in the recipient's eye and covered with the outer layer removed at the start of the operation. After a month the bandages were removed; the patient was able to see better than before the operation, though it took some months before the maximum improvement was reached[24, 25].

Return was also made to introducing artificial windows into the cornea as a last resort when corneal grafting procedures had failed. Progress was possible when plastics became available as these were sufficiently inert to be accepted by the cornea, but even so the success was all too often only temporary and the plastic was rejected. To overcome this, Beneditto Strampelli of Rome in 1963 devised the operation of osteo-odonto-keratoprosthesis[26]. One of the patient's teeth was removed together with part of its socket; a section of this was cut in such a way as to form a thin ring with socket bone on the outside and tooth tissue on the inside. This ring was implanted into the cornea, which had been prepared at an operation about three months previously to make it extremely vascular and receptive. The underlying idea was that the cornea would accept the socket bone quite readily, as it is part of the patient's own body; a strong fibrous union would be formed. Then, the plastic window was glued with ordinary dental cement into the centre of the ring; this was also efficient as it is well known that teeth accept foreign materials as fillings without giving trouble. The surgical technique is, however, extremely difficult and the slightest mistake can lead to failure.

By his work on the ear and hearing, Helmholtz had played an important role in another specialty that was developing in the last quarter of the 19th century. Otorhinolaryngology, or the study of the ear, nose, and throat, was, during its evolution, often divided into the three regions by virtue of the discoveries taking place. As with the eye, a formidable obstacle to progress was the inability to see inside these three organs; direct sunlight was an unsatisfactory form of illumination and naturally was unable to penetrate beyond angles. In the middle of the 18th century mirrors became popular, and candles were sometimes used to supply the light, but unless bulky and unmanageable apparatus was employed it was still impossible to see round corners. Friedrich Hofmann, a general practitioner in Burgsteinfurt, Germany, in 1841 discovered that by using a concave mirror with a hole in the middle it was possible to concentrate the sun's rays into the ear, and by straightening out the ear canal with a suitably shaped cylindrical tube he could see the drum through the central hole of the mirror[27]. This simple instrument enabled a young Viennese otologist, Adam Politzer, to relate the post-mortem changes in the ear to the clinical appearances during life and so establish criteria for the diagnosis and classification of ear diseases. His atlas, published in 1865, was remarkably complete[28].

For some years it had been an occasional practice to incise the eardrum in certain cases of chronic ear disease and deafness; this was done by blindly passing a knife down the ear canal. Now that it was possible to see the drum, a Halle surgeon, Hermann Hugo Schwartze, realized that the operation was more suited to cases in which pus collected behind the drum (suppurative otitis media) and, moreover, that he could choose the most appropriate time and perform the incision under direct vision. One danger of otitis media is the spread of infection to involve the mastoid bone, situated behind the ear; and so in 1873 Schwartze revived the previously unsuccessful operation of simple mastoidectomy[29] which was later improved by Emanual Zaufal in 1884[30]. Having exposed the bone, Schwartze used a mallet and chisel on the hard exterior and then, with a sharp spoon, he removed all the honeycomb of bone that forms the mastoid process; he needed great care to avoid going too deeply and so injuring the underlying dura mater. In this operation, which is carried out in acute cases, the middle ear with its little bones is left undisturbed, but in the operation of radical mastoidectomy, which was developed in 1888 by von Bergmann[31] and in 1889 by Ernst Küster[32], and is indicated in chronic suppurative ear conditions, the middle ear and the mastoid are converted into a single cavity.

In otosclerosis, the commonest cause of conductive deafness in the young adult, the small bones of the middle ear become hardened and fixed. Before 1938, operative procedures had usually been successful only in the hands of their originators, but even so a great deal of pioneering work had already been done by Gunnar Holmgren of Stockholm[33], who started his experimental work in 1917, and by Maurice Sourdille, of Strasbourg, who in 1924 began his series of operations which were done in three stages in an attempt to avoid the dangers of infection and labyrinthitis[34]. In 1938 Julius Lempert of New York devised a one-stage method which other surgeons were able to copy with reasonably good results[35]. Using a magnifying glass and an ordinary dentist's drill, he made a hole inside the ear itself and was able to restore a limited amount of hearing. This operation, known as fenestration, is a highly delicate and specialized undertaking, as shown by the fact that in 1943 a survey in America reported on some fifteen hundred fenestration operations, of which twelve hundred had been done by two surgeons[36]. It called for a lot of postoperative care and could leave the patient with an unwelcome degree of vertigo.

Fenestration did, nevertheless, mark the beginning of a new phase in ear surgery, as surgeons realized that much was possible if the internal structures could be magnified and brightly illuminated. Special operating microscopes were invented, and plastic operations on the eardrum and other parts of the internal ear became a practical proposition. The basic principles underlying these plastic operations were stated by Fritz Zöllner of Freiburg im Breisgau, Germany, in 1951[37] and by Horst Wüllstein of Siegen, Germany, in 1952[38]. Consequently, in 1952, Samuel Rosen of New York proposed a new operation for otosclerosis by means of which the affected bone, the footplate of the stapes, was mobilized[39, 40]. However, the conception was not really new, since Jean Kessel, in 1876[41], followed by a handful of other surgeons in the closing years of the 19th century, had also tried mobilization, but had been unable to obtain an adequate exposure. Rosen lifted out the whole of the lower part of the drum and folded it back on the top part, thus allowing unimpeded vision. He also invented special instruments for the operation, the great advantage of which is that the normal anatomy of the ear is restored and the patient is left with normal, or nearly normal, hearing.

The examination of the larynx, or voice box, had met with conspicuous lack of success ever since the early attempts were made at the beginning of the 19th century. This was again owing to the lack of satisfactory illumination, but in addition the nature of the instruments caused the patient's throat to contract. Before this time most cases of voice trouble were considered to be due to tuberculosis or syphilis, and as the same unsatisfactory treatment served for both it mattered little that the vocal cords could not be seen. However, as medicine and surgery advanced and had more to offer, it became imperative for the larynx to be visualized so that an accurate diagnosis could be made. By a fantastic combination of circumstances, the right man was available to achieve this object.

The famous Spanish tenor and singing teacher, Manuel Garcia intended his son, also Manuel, to follow in his vocal footsteps and as a boy young Manuel showed every promise. But, probably because of over-training while his voice was breaking, he developed into a rather inadequate baritone. He joined his father as a teacher and approached the job from a new and scientific angle. Determined to know everything possible about the voice, he made many anatomical dissections of the larynx of human beings and animals, even going to the extent of removing the larynx and trachea and blowing air through the vocal cords to see how they behaved. This did not satisfy him as his great desire was to see the vocal cords in action in life. In 1850 he moved from Paris, where Jenny Lind had been one of his many famous pupils, and settled in London as professor at the Royal Academy of Music (Sir Henry Wood, who had studied at the academy, called him the finest teacher of his day). Four years later, while on holiday in Paris, he saw in his mind's eye the arrangement of two mirrors that would enable him to see the vocal cords. He at once sped to an instrument maker and bought a long-handled dentist's mirror and an ordinary hand mirror.

When he got home he heated the dental mirror in water and dried it (to prevent its steaming up in his mouth) and placed it against his uvula, flashing sunlight onto it with the hand mirror: 'I saw at once, to my great joy, the glottis open before me and so fully exposed that I could perceive a portion of the trachea. When my excitement had somewhat subsided, I began to examine what was passing before my eyes. The manner in which the glottis opened and shut, and moved in the act of phonation, filled me with wonder.' The fact that he achieved his aim at the first attempt should fill us with wonder also, for as any medical student can testify, it is no easy matter to see the vocal cords of even a co-operative person (usually a fellow student) at the first try. The miracle came about because his throat could tolerate instrumentation and also because his singing training had taught him to relax his throat and keep the back of his tongue down. A few months later he presented a paper to the Royal Society in London, in which he described his method of mirror laryngoscopy and detailed the actions of the different parts of the larynx during singing[42]. This, however, attracted little attention, as the method of examination was not considered to have much practical application and the physiological studies were overlooked, probably because Garcia was not a member of the medical profession.

In Vienna the idea was received more warmly by Ludwig Türck, and in the summer of 1857 he used the method to examine his patients[43]; but a cloudy autumn deprived him of his source of light and he gave up using laryngoscopy. In the meanwhile, Türck had had a visitor from Budapest, one Johann Czermak, who had shown great interest in the mirrors and returned to his home town with the bright idea of adopting the concave mirror with the little hole in its centre used by ear surgeons to shine a light on to the mirrors[44]. Czermak used a lamp as his source of light, and at first held the mirror on a holder between his teeth; later he had it fixed to a head band and in this form it has become popular among cartoonists as the sign of a doctor. To Czermak must undoubtedly go the credit for making laryngoscopy a practical and acceptable form of examination, even though there was a most acrimonious argument between himself and Türck over the matter of priority. This, incidentally, did as much as Czermak's tours of demonstration to bring the method to the notice of the profession. Eventually a commission was appointed to settle the squabble, which it did to the financial satisfaction of both parties.

The next development came in 1895, when Alfred Kirstein of Berlin devised a glorified tongue depressor which enabled the larynx to be seen by direct light[45]. The object was to allow operative instrumentation to take place within the larynx, since reflected light was suitable only for examination purposes. It was not entirely successful, and the forerunner of modern direct laryngoscopy instruments was produced by Gustav Killian of Freiburg in 1897[46]. This consisted of an illuminated split tube, rather like a rounded duck's bill, which was passed directly over the back of the tongue, and through which the larynx was seen by direct vision. By introducing another tube through his laryngoscope, he soon found that he could get beyond the larynx into the trachea, and even into the larger branches within the lungs. Thus he founded the science of bronchoscopy, which was developed to a high degree of perfection by a Philadelphia laryngologist, Chevalier Jackson, who had, by 1907, established himself as the master of removing foreign bodies from the air passages[47].

Laryngoscopy made practicable the diagnosis of laryngeal cancer. However, in the early days mistakes were common, and one that was of historic importance occurred when Crown Prince Frederick of Germany (who was married to Victoria, Queen Victoria's eldest daughter) developed hoarseness in 1887. His own physician called in Karl Gerhardt, the professor of medicine at Berlin, who diagnosed a small tumour of the posterior end of the left vocal cord, but was unable to say whether it was benign or malignant. A few weeks later the hoarseness became worse and Gerhardt made several attempts to destroy the tumour with an electric cautery. As there was no improvement and the cautery wound failed to heal, the respected surgeon Ernst von Bergmann was invited to give his views. He suggested removing the tumour by open operation through the Adam's apple. Frederick was not in favour, so yet another opinion was sought and Morell Mackenzie was sent from England by Queen Victoria at the request of her daughter, the Crown Princess Victoria. Mackenzie examined the royal patient and was unable to pronounce upon the growth, but asked for a piece to be removed and examined under the microscope by Virchow, the renowned pathologist. The first specimen showed no evidence of malignancy, but as it was small another piece was removed which again showed no malignancy. Unfortunately it soon became evident that Frederick was seriously ill and everyone then became convinced that his condition must be malignant.

However, research in the mid-20th century raised doubts about the final diagnosis. The lesion was at a part of the vocal cords where cancer is relatively uncommon and the two most likely explanations now seem to be either that the repeated cauterizations induced malignant change, if such eventually took place, or that they set up a destructive inflammation of the laryngeal cartilages. At all events, Frederick soon required a tracheostomy to enable him to breathe. After the tube had been in place for some time, von Bergmann appeared again and insisted it needed changing. This he proceeded to attempt but was unable to get the new tube into the trachea, possibly because the original incision had been made a little to the right instead of in the mid-line. Fritz Bramann, the surgeon who had carried out the initial tracheostomy and who had some four hundred of these operations to his credit, had to come to his chief's rescue. The traumatized wound inevitably became infected and Frederick died after he had been emperor for ninety days. Morell Mackenzie was utterly ruined and returned to England in disgrace. The blame for the emperor's death was his, and this despite the fact that had he recommended removing the growth by means of an open operation the chances of survival would have been only 5 or 10 percent. Mackenzie died four years later during an attack of asthma, the victim of incompetence and international jealousy. The leading laryngologist of his time, the man who put his specialty on the map in England and showed the way for Europe, had an uncomfortably raw deal.

17

Gynaecology

The same problem of difficulty in examination that faced ophthalmology and otorhinolaryngology – that of seeing what was going on – also presented itself to gynaecology, but for entirely different reasons. A hundred and fifty or so years ago gynaecology, or the study of diseases of the female reproductive organs, was in the doldrums, owing to an astonishing degree of false modesty on the part of women, even though they might be in severe pain, and to surgeons showing no inclination to carry out an examination. It was even thought that a gynaecological examination would induce a lax moral sense in the patient. The speculum had been used since Roman times for making internal examinations, yet, except in France, it had to be rediscovered by surgeons of the Victorian era. Operations for removal of the uterus and attempts to cure leakage of urine from the bladder into the vagina, through a vesico-vaginal fistula, caused by damage during childbirth, had been performed in the past, but at this period of history the only operation carried out with any degree of frequency, and with varying results, was for cysts of the ovary, which were either tapped through the abdominal wall to remove the fluid or removed by open operation (see Chapter 4). Such was the respect in which the peritoneum was held that at the beginning of the antiseptic era, some surgeons, amongst whom was Spencer Wells[1], adopted a procedure whereby the cyst was removed but the cut end of its stalk was fixed outside the abdomen while the abdominal wound was being closed, instead of being returned inside the peritoneal cavity. When aseptic techniques were established this method was abandoned.

In the United States, in Alabama, lived a surgeon by the name of James Marion Sims who shared the popular distaste for examining the female organs and sent any female patients with genital disease to be dealt with elsewhere. In the 1840s his hand was forced when a woman fell off her horse and was brought to him complaining of severe internal pain. For the examination, he made her kneel with her head down below her shoulders; the only abnormality he could find was a retroversion of her uterus, meaning that instead of being angulated in a forward direction it was bent over backwards. He corrected the displacement and the good lady was relieved of her symptoms. However, in the light of modern knowledge, the retroverted uterus had almost certainly been present before the accident and had nothing to do with the pain, which was caused by muscle spasm and had been relaxed by Sims's internal manipulations.

The incident had a profound effect on Sims. In the special position in which he had examined the woman, the whole vagina was filled with air, making inspection of this organ and of the neck of the womb a surprisingly easy matter. He realized that this would simplify the treatment of local conditions, especially of that very distressing complaint, vesico-vaginal fistula, which so far had been considered incurable. For the next four years he worked hard at perfecting an operative technique, during which time he improved the exposure by using a spoon handle to hold open the vagina, later developing this domestic implement into the duckbill-shaped speculum that bears his name[2].

It was in no small measure due to the fortitude of his patients that in 1849 he finally succeeded in effecting a cure: the lucky woman had already been operated on thirty times. Other surgeons had achieved cures in isolated cases, but Sims's cure was not fortuitous and could be performed by any experienced surgeon, hence its importance. His technique was to freshen the edges of the fistulous opening and then to stitch them together with silver wire[3]; where he and others had previously failed was in the use of silk sutures, which cut out and therefore did not hold the wound edges together for long enough. His final point was the introduction of a catheter into the bladder, so that the diversion of urine would not interfere with healing. Subsequently, in 1857 Maurice Collis of Dublin, who died at an early age from a blood infection contracted while operating, introduced the only important addition to Sims's original technique. He separated the bladder wall from the vagina and sewed up the hole in each structure individually[4,5]. This modification was improved in 1896 by Alwin Karl Mackenrodt[6]. Sims also introduced a more dignified position for the patient, in which she lay on her left side with her right shoulder falling forward, her left leg slightly flexed and her right leg drawn well up. This also gives adequate exposure and is now known as Sims's position[2].

In 1855 Sims founded, in New York State, the first hospital in the world for diseases of women. When the American Civil War broke out, he left America and for six years lived in London and Paris, where his services were much in demand and where he did an immense amount to advance gynaecology.

In Great Britain the leading exponent of this new specialty was Robert Lawson Tait, whose wholehearted methods and overbearing personality aroused a great deal of opposition, which was also brought to bear on those who followed his surgical teaching. This is scarcely surprising as the subject was still considered rather indecent and the way in which these surgeons entered the abdomen to operate on and remove the organs that made a woman a woman was a bold move. Their colleagues and the public required educating to the correctness of gynaecological surgery. They did, however, make mistakes, and one of these was their misplaced emphasis on retroversion of the uterus. This condition was believed to be the cause of a vast number of female ailments and, before the days of asepsis, was treated with all manner of pessaries, which mostly kept the womb perched on a long wooden stem and accounted for the high rate of couch-borne semi-invalids among the fair sex. Clifford Allbutt's invective in his Gulstonian Lecture of 1884 to the Royal College of Physicians was truly stinging:

'She is entangled in the net of the gynaecologist, who finds her uterus, like her nose, a little on one side, or again like that organ is running a little, or it is as flabby as her biceps, so that the unhappy viscus is impaled on a stem, or perched on a prop, or is painted with carbolic acid every week in the year except during the long vacation when the gynaecologist is grouse shooting, or salmon catching, or leading the fashion in the Upper Engadine.'... The patient's mind is 'thus fastened to a more or less nasty mystery, it becomes newly apprehensive and physically introspective and the morbid chains are riveted more strongly than ever. Arraign the uterus and you fix in the woman the arrow of hypochondria, it may be for ever.'[7]

James Young Simpson was most impressed with retroversion and in his lectures in the early 1870s blamed the condition for the large number of woman who were unable to walk. He then went on to show how this regrettable state of affairs could be rectified[8]. This was part of his campaign to overcome the prevailing tendency to diagnose female complaints as hysteria or neurosis, and to give gynaecological diagnosis a sound basis. He succeeded, but the pendulum swung violently in the opposite direction and when abdominal surgery became safe, such was the importance attached to correcting retroversion that the surgical honour of gynaecologists was at stake. Innumerable operations were devised for slinging, tying, stitching, or otherwise returning the uterus to its rightful position. It is recorded of a certain Liverpool gynaecologist, William Alexander, that in 1911 he was asked to demonstrate his suspension operation[9] to a group of visiting surgeons and accordingly sent his assistants to the four quarters of the city to find a suitable subject. They returned, unable to produce even one woman who had not already had Alexander's operation performed upon her! However, the tide was beginning to turn, and shortly after this date retroversion of the uterus found its correct level of importance. It is now mainly corrected as part of an operation for other conditions.

Tumours of the uterus did not enjoy such popularity in treatment. In pre-aseptic days the innocent fibroid was treated either by removing the ovaries, thus producing an artificial change-of-life, or by removing the uterus through the vagina, but neither was performed at all frequently. One or two surgeons, such as Simpson and Spencer Wells, attempted an abdominal approach, but if the fibroid formed an integral part of the wall of the uterus, rather than being attached to it by a stalk, they were usually forced to remove the whole organ and as a result most of the patients died. Satisfactory abdominal removal of fibroids, therefore, had to wait for more accurate diagnosis of the nature of the fibroid and for safe aseptic surgery. Lawson Tait had in 1874 successfully performed the abdominal operation and his further endeavours in this direction increased the antagonism towards gynaecology, which was commonly referred to as wholesale castration of the female species.

A follower of Tait's principles was John Bland Sutton, appointed assistant surgeon at the Middlesex Hospital in 1886. His colleagues soon became thoroughly displeased with him because of his partiality for pelvic operations and when in 1890 he performed his first sub-total hysterectomy for fibroids, in which he removed the body of the uterus, leaving the cervix behind, Matthews Duncan called him a criminal mutilator of women[10]. Admittedly the operation carried a high mortality rate, but it did much to relieve chronic invalidism and only by perseverance could the results be improved. When, in 1896, Bland Sutton was appointed to the Chelsea Hospital for Women, he was able to devote himself to pelvic operations, and ten years later had reduced the mortality rate to 2 percent, thus giving gynaecological surgery a sure foundation.

Malignant tumours of the uterus were a very serious problem, for they constitute a high percentage of cancers among women. The poor state of affairs existing over female examination did nothing to help early diagnosis, even if surgery had been able to offer much hope of cure. It is therefore to the credit of Thomas Addis Emmet of New York that as early as 1868 he drew attention to the lacerations of the cervix occurring during childbirth, pointing out that unless repaired by surgery they were liable to progress to cancer[11, 12]. Simpson appreciated the dangers of cancer of the cervix and recommended its amputation if the growth could be detected before it had spread[13]; otherwise existing treatment was of no avail.

The next advance was made by Wilhelm Freund of Breslau, who in 1878 devised an operation whereby the whole uterus was removed[14], but once again if the cancer had spread beyond these confines the operation could not hope to cure. Like other cancers, one of the ways in which this type spreads is through the lymphatic vessels to lymph nodes. In 1895, Emil Ries, a pupil of Freund, dissected out these nodes as part of an experimental operation on cadavers[15]. Within a short space of time, many other surgeons were carrying out this extension of the technique. Ernst Wertheim of Vienna, particularly, was interested in the operation, performing it a great many times until he became extremely proficient, and made it so popular that it became known as Wertheim's operation although his original technique underwent considerable modification. He disposed of the notion that cancer of the uterus was an unusual disease and one that could be cured by removal of the affected part only; he applied the principle, already learned in other regions of the body, that to obtain the best results it was necessary to remove as much as possible of the surrounding tissues as well as the tumour[16,17]. There were, and still are, two most important obstacles in the way of the surgeon, namely the ureters which drain urine from the kidneys to the bladder, for if these were accidentally cut the outcome of the operation was seriously prejudiced. At first Wertheim passed small catheters into the ureters before the operation and tried to keep them out of danger by adopting the popular vaginal approach. But as he soon discovered, he was unable to obtain a satisfactory removal of tissue in this manner and therefore abandoned the vaginal method for the abdominal operation, discontinuing the catheterization of the ureters as he was now able to locate them more clearly[18].

Wertheim was most concerned with the problem of sepsis which was the bugbear of all uterine operations at this period, and he tried various way of cauterizing and removing the cancerous tissue to reduce the incidence, finally adopting a method of packing the vagina with disinfectant gauze and only cutting into this organ as the very last stage of the operation. Unfortunately, even by 1911[19], all this fine work was attended by a mortality rate of from 10–20 percent, and with the wide adoption of radiotherapy the operation was almost discarded except in a few centres. But, as so often happens, the wheel turned full circle until surgery, radiotherapy and chemotherapy all have a place determined by the individual case. With the perfection of the technique it was possible to extend the scope of the operation as indicated by the spread of the cancer, but this made increased demands on the skill of the gynaecologist who had to be able to encroach on the preserves of the urological and abdominal surgeons, besides having to have a working knowledge of the principles of radiotherapy and chemotherapy.

The origin of caesarean section which belongs to gynaecology's sister specialty, obstetrics, is lost in antiquity and initially was performed immediately after the death of a mother in an endeavour to secure a live baby. The name derives from an ancient law, the lex regia, of Etruscan times, when Numa Pompilius, the second of the seven legendary kings of Rome, decreed that no woman dying in childbirth was to be buried without first having the child re-moved through the abdomen. It was Pliny who circulated the story that Julius Caesar was born in this way and thus took his name from a derivation of the word caedo, 'I cut'. In fact Julius Caesar's mother was alive many years later. Caesarean section may have been performed in 1500 on a living woman who survived, but except for other isolated instances in desperate circumstances it did not achieve importance until the time of aseptic surgery. In the middle of the 19th century the type of caesarean section performed, in which the uterus was opened directly in its upper segment, cutting through the peritoneum, was attended by high mortality due to almost inevitable infection. To combat this, the womb itself was sacrificed and removed. However, in 1825 Ferdinand Ritgen of the University of Giessen reported that an extraperitoneal approach had been tried four years previously[20].

In 1876 Edoardo Porro, of Milan, followed the extraction of the baby by removing the ovaries, cutting out the body of the uterus and sewing the upper end of the stump of the cervix into the abdominal wound, where it eventually healed[21]. Porro's early operations of this nature were desirable because the uterus was diseased, but as the results were an improvement on those in which the uterus was healthy and therefore left behind, the procedure was adopted also for healthy wombs. As the general technique improved, it was found possible to cover the stump with peritoneum and return it to the pelvic cavity. But with the progress of aseptic surgery, this unnecessary mutilation ceased and classical upper segment caesarean section came into its own largely owing to the work of Max Sänger of Prague, who improved the technique[22]. Even so, at this date (1882) there was a mortality rate of 50 percent owing to late cases and inadequate technique. In spite of this the operation became so popular that in 1890 it was performed far too frequently and without sufficient justification. As the novelty wore off, it settled down to be used only when indicated to save the mother's or baby's life and held the field until the 1920s.

With the lower segment caesarean section, which was then beginning to challenge the classical approach, the incision is made low down in the uterus in the pelvic cavity; it has the advantage over the upper segment section in that the uterine wound can be covered with peritoneum, thus reducing the likelihood of adhesions later in life. The prototype of this operation was first performed successfully by Theodore Gaillard Thomas, of New York, in 1870[23]. However, it received an unenthusiastic reception as it was considered unsafe owing to the possibility of injuring surrounding organs; also, the delivery of the baby might damage it or the mother. Nevertheless, its possibilities were recognized, and after a long uphill struggle, during which many modifications were tried, it finally ousted the upper segment section from popularity. British surgeons were even slower than their Continental colleagues to adopt the operation; in 1921 Eardley Holland[24] and Munro Kerr[25] published results showing its superiority, yet ten more years were to elapse before the lower segment operation was used at all frequently in Britain. As in the early days of upper segment operations, it too tended to be abused, being performed for the convenience of mother or surgeon without due attention being given to its necessity.

18

Orthopaedics and x-rays

The concept of orthopaedics has expanded more than that of any other specialty since 1741 when Nicholas Andry coined the name from two Greek words meaning 'straight' and 'child'. His concern was with crippled children whose deformities he attributed to unbalanced action of the muscles[1]. For the next hundred years the art of preventing and correcting these deformities was largely manipulative and did not involve surgery. Such operations as were performed consisted of subcutaneous tenotomies (the making of incisions in the skin through which superficial tendons were cut) to allow the deformity, for instance wry neck or clubfoot, to straighten itself. The treatment of fractures was in the hands of general surgeons and, owing to infection, amputation was the order of the day should a joint become diseased or injured. From its modest beginnings orthopaedics has developed into the branch of surgery dealing with diseases and injuries to bones, joints, muscles, tendons, and ligaments.

The orthopaedic advances of the first half of the 19th century were in pathology, although a few surgeons were anticipating future events by performing conservative operations on joints. In Scotland, James Syme, Lister's father-in-law, was one of the early surgeons who tried to save limbs by excising injured or diseased joints rather than resorting to amputation[2]. In Hanover, his contemporary, Georg Friedrich Stromeyer, who performed similar operations[3], had an unforeseen influence on British orthopaedics when he operated on a young doctor, William John Little, for a clubfoot. Little was eternally grateful for his cure, and on his return to England resolved to help the crippled to the best of his ability. In 1837, he founded an infirmary which did so well that eight years later it became known as the Royal Orthopaedic Hospital. Little himself was a physician at heart, although he did a tremendous amount of work in studying the various deformities and the methods of treatment by manipulation, splinting and subcutaneous tenotomy[4].

Even before the arrival of antisepsis, surgeons were beginning to attack the bones themselves in an effort to cure deformities, and in 1852 Bernhard Langenbeck treated a hip deformity by making a small skin incision and cutting through the neck of the femur – a subcutaneous osteotomy[5]. The first surgeon to attempt this type of operation in England was Little's son, Stromeyer Little (the reason for his Christian name is obvious), who in 1868 enabled a little girl with deformed knees to walk by partly cutting through the lower end of the femur with a chisel, until the bone could be broken and straightened. The other knee was only affected by ligamentous shortening and was straightened by manipulation[6].

These operations demanded a great deal of courage on the part of the surgeon (and of the patient) in view of the terrible risk of infection. The chisels were of the carpentry variety, if not actually the property of carpenters, and only bevelled on one side; they produced erratic cuts in the bone and could not be used with any degree of precision. Nevertheless, in 1873, with the benefit of antisepsis, Billroth was using these inadequate instruments to correct knock-knees, usually the result of rickets, by cutting through the top part of the tibia and removing a v-shaped section[7]. Then in another five years the answer was provided by William Macewen who was well aware of the shortcomings of the carpentry chisel, and also of its possible dangers. The surgeon was unable to observe its behaviour inside the bone, or to see how deeply it had penetrated, and if accurate results were to be obtained both these uncertainties had to be eliminated. Macewen therefore devised a chisel with a cutting edge bevelled on both sides and with distances marked on the blade; this instrument he called an osteotome. In his instructions to his instrument makers he was careful to specify the sort of metal to be used, in order to avoid the unwelcome complication of the chisel's breaking or chipping[8].

The osteotome marked a very real advance in orthopaedic surgery, but it was not the only contribution of this remarkable 'general' surgeon to orthopaedics, for in 1879 Macewen performed the first bone-grafting operation. By experiments on dogs he showed that the periosteum, or limiting membrane around bones, was not necessary for the regeneration and survival of bone. When a young boy came to him with a useless arm he was able to put the experiments to practical use. Two years previously a bone infection had destroyed five inches of this boy's humerus. After making a suitable incision, Macewen packed the gap with pieces of bone that he had saved when doing osteotomies on the tibias of other patients. The gods must have been smiling more than usual on Macewen that day, since it was really pure chance that the bone chips were placed where they became subjected to the stresses and strains of muscular action, and so grew into a solid bone, giving the boy a useful arm that differed little from normal.

Although this magnificent operation showed what could be done, bone grafting did not come into popular use until many years later, when the metal plating of fractures gave the necessary impulse to the use of bone grafts for other purposes.

Four years later, in 1883, Thomas Annandale, professor of surgery at Edinburgh, opened a knee joint for what proved to be a torn cartilage. Previously the cause of this type of joint derangement had been unknown, and because surgeons would not operate owing to the danger of infection, the field had been left wide open for manipulators, often untrained, to try their luck. They had little success. Annandale found the torn cartilage, stitched it back into its proper place, and thus enabled the patient to return to his job as a collier with a satisfactorily functioning knee[9]. The operation brought this common condition into the fold of orthodox surgery where it could be cured, so putting the collective nose of the manipulating fraternity somewhat out of joint.

One of the conditions for which an orthodox manipulative technique is very often curative is congenital dislocation of the hip: in this the upper margin of the hip socket is poorly formed and the head of the femur rises out of the joint when the child gets old enough to walk. It is a disease of considerable antiquity, being described by Hippocrates, and is possibly the reason why the angel was able, with apparent ease, to dislocate Jacob's thigh when the two were wrestling (Genesis, 32, v. 24). However, in more recent times there was great difficulty in distinguishing a dislocated hip from a fractured femur, and it was only with the advance of anatomical knowledge and clinical examination in the early 19th century that congenital dislocation became recognized again, although it was thought to be incurable.

The first satisfactory form of treatment was introduced by Adolf Lorenz, who devised a special method of manipulation, which ideally should be started before the child begins to walk. Lorenz came of peasant stock and, after a very hard childhood and an abortive attempt on the part of an uncle to lead him into a Benedictine monastery, he went to Vienna where, with the aid of a scholarship, he studied medicine, determined to make a name for himself as a surgeon. After qualification he taught anatomy for a while before taking up surgery. Then came a bitter blow: he was sensitive to carbolic acid; his hands became inflamed and the skin of his face was so tender that he had to grow a beard. Unable to continue with surgery, he decided to take up orthopaedics, and in a few years had achieved considerable fame as a manipulative surgeon.

In 1897 he began to manipulate young children with congenitally dislocated hips on an apparatus that gradually pulled their legs into a sideways split, in which position they remained for months[10]. This treatment produced children with hips that would stand up to almost normal strains. With severe cases, or those not discovered till the patient was some years old, manipulation did not succeed and operation was required. Surgery had, in fact, preceded manipulation since Albert Hoffa of Berlin had operated for the condition in 1890[11], and so, when antisepsis gave way to asepsis, Lorenz was able to return to operative surgery and contribute to the development of the variety of procedures that were being introduced.

Subsequent to manipulation or surgery in congenital dislocation and for a large number of other conditions, including fractures, immobilization of the part is necessary, and is provided by a plaster-of-Paris cast. This is made out of roller bandages impregnated with calcined gypsum which, after dipping in water, sets hard. A particular advantage is seen in fractures of the limbs, since the broken bones can be held in perfect position while the bandages are being applied, and after the cast has set this alignment is maintained. The name, plaster of Paris, derives from the quarries in Montmartre, where gypsum has been worked for many hundreds of years although its use in surgery is of much more recent date. Waxes and resins had been used to stiffen bandages in ancient Greece, and the Arabians towards the end of the first millennium AD used lime prepared from certain sea shells. The surgeons of the Middle Ages, with their complete disregard for the obnoxious, compounded casts of egg white, flour, and animal fat; after a few days the stench from these ingredients, combined with putrefying flesh, must have been truly appalling. Casts then went out of fashion and attention was directed to ordinary splints until the end of the 18th century when a report came from Persia of an Arab soldier who had had his leg encased in plaster of Paris, which had simply been poured round it. This form of plaster casting without bandages had apparently been used by the Arabs for centuries[12], and a few years later was adopted by one or two European surgeons, but failed to make any impression on the profession as a whole.

A Dutch army surgeon, Antonius Mathijsen, while garrisoned at Harlem in 1851, had had the bright idea of doing what the ancients had done and impregnating bandages with the stiffening substance[13]. At first he tried it on material cut to the shape of the limb, but as this was not satisfactory he used roller bandages instead. He recommended padding the limb before applying the bandages, and as one of the advantages of the method in his own particular sphere of activity, he said that if water was not available on the field of battle, urine would serve as an admirable alternative[14]. At last an eminently suitable means of immobilization had been discovered, bringing fame and honours to its inventor although, as was almost bound to happen, objections were raised as to cost and durability, but with the rapid adoption of the bandages these were soon shown to be unfounded.

The importance of keeping at rest injured structures, or those that had been subjected to surgery, was also exercising the mind of John Hilton, and in the opening years of the 1860s he delivered a series of lectures on 'Rest and pain'[15] at Guy's Hospital. This had a marked effect in drawing attention to the postoperative care of the patient and deeply impressed Hugh Owen Thomas of Liverpool. The results Thomas obtained convinced him of the truth of Hilton's theories and he made it his guiding principle in the treatment of fractures and diseased joints, to prescribe enforced, uninterrupted and prolonged rest.

Thomas's father had left the island of Anglesey, where the family had been bonesetters for generations, to settle in Liverpool where his skill soon became recognized. When young Hugh showed a leaning towards medicine his father decided to regularize the situation by giving him an orthodox medical education. After qualifying, Thomas became assistant to his father, but as he was unable to adapt himself to the ways of a bonesetter, however clever, he set up practice on his own account in another part of town. In a short while he had established a great reputation for himself, working for very long hours, without holidays, and having no dearth of injury cases among the dock workers and labourers, many of whom were in straitened circumstances and were treated for nothing. In 1875 Thomas published *Diseases of the hip, knee, and ankle joints*[16] which showed his original approach to the subject. By his insistence on rest he achieved a great advance in the treatment of tuberculous joints which were usually treated by amputation or excision of the joint when the disease had become chronic, but with rest the gross crippling changes did not develop.

He possessed a high degree of mechanical skill combined with infinite patience and these qualities enabled him to devise simple and efficient tools. He employed a blacksmith and a leather worker to make splints to his own basic design, which were subjected to prolonged trials on his patients. They were efficient and simple, possessing all the essential features for keeping the joint rested and in good position. Originally intended for use in joint diseases, the splints proved so useful and adaptable that they became indispensable in fracture treatment and in orthopaedic surgery, both as splints, per se, and for applying traction to the limb by means of weights and pulleys.

Thomas always wore a yachting cap with the peak tilted over his left eye, as the eyelid had been deformed by an accident in his youth. He smoked incessantly. Although his practice grew to include the more well-to-do classes in Liverpool, the fame that was his due failed to come in full measure during his lifetime. Robert Jones, a nephew, who was trained in his uncle's practice, later brought Thomas's methods to the notice of the world.

In the second half of the 19th century, amputation for joint disease was giving way to excision, an operation that left the patient with a stiff and unstable joint. In many cases, especially in the lower limb, it was better to arthrodese (fix) the joint permanently in a useful position – a procedure originally devised to stabilize joints that had lost their support as a result of some form of muscular paralysis. Eduard Albert, professor of surgery at Vienna, carried out the first arthrodesis in 1875[17], and by 1894 Robert Jones had performed fifteen arthrodeses on knees and ankles for severe instability resulting from poliomyelitis. In 1908 he published an account of an operation, performed in two stages, for paralytic clubfoot[18].

Another method by which the after-effects of poliomyelitis can be overcome is to transplant the tendons of unaffected muscles in such a way that they take over the function of those paralysed. In 1881 Karl Nicoladoni attached the peroneal muscles at the side of the leg to the Achilles tendon of the gastrocnemius (calf) muscle which was paralysed[19]. The operation was an initial success and the patient, a sixteen-year-old boy, was able to bend his foot downwards again, but unfortunately Nicoladoni was called away to take up a new post, and owing to lack of necessary care and rest, success was turned to failure. Nine years later B. F. Parrish of New York performed a similar operation, believing himself to be the first. This time the limb was put in a plaster-of-Paris cast and the operation was a permanent success[20]. Tendon transplantation then became popular, although it was not performed in England until 1897, when Frederic Eve of the London Hospital was the surgeon[21]. The lost time was soon made good and in 1903 Jones and Alfred Herbert Tubby produced a book in which the whole question of surgery for paralysis was discussed, and the indications for arthrodesis, tendon transplantation or the two methods in combination were set out[22].

In 1895 a discovery was made that had far-reaching effects on medicine and surgery, opening up an entirely fresh field of diagnosis and study of disease and leading to a new form of treatment. The way had been well prepared for the discovery of x-rays, starting in the 17th century with the researches of Otto von Guericke, burgomaster of Magdeburg, into electricity and the production of a vacuum[23], and culminating with the work of 19th-century scientists, among them William Crookes, on the cathode ray. Then, late in the evening of November 8, 1895, the professor of physics in the University of Würzburg, Wilhelm Conrad Röntgen, was working alone in his laboratory on cathode rays when by chance he noticed that the Crookes partial vacuum tube, through which he was passing a current at about 10 000 volts emitted a radiation that threw a greenish fluorescent light onto a barium platinocyanide screen some feet away. He immediately carried out tests that proved conclusively that the cathode rays could have nothing to do with this phenomenon. Next, he placed various objects, such as cardboard, wood and paper, in the path of these new rays to see whether they would be penetrated. None was a barrier; but when he put his own hand in their path he saw that the rays cast a shadow not of the whole hand but of the bones. His next move, therefore, was to throw the shadow onto a photographic plate, and the privilege of having the first x-ray photograph ever taken went to his wife, the bones of whose hand soon became famous all over the world. This discovery may well seem to have been fortuitous, but some months later Röntgen said that he had actually been looking for invisible rays.

This was no idle boast, for a few other scientists were already on the verge of the discovery and Röntgen was alert for any variation from expected happenings in his experiments. However, although he knew there was probably something to find, he must have been absolutely astounded by what these new rays could do.

In the weeks that followed, Röntgen worked like a man possessed to discover all about the rays, eventually publishing his results at the end of the year in a paper on a new kind of ray[24]. He referred to them as 'x', the unknown, and x-rays they have remained ever since. The news about the rays very soon got into the popular press, and before ten days of the new year (1896) were passed, the whole world knew of Röntgen's magnificent achievement. The interest was immense, doctors were plagued with requests for x-rays to be taken, and some fantastic speculations as to their properties were rife. So seriously were a lot of these taken that people feared intrusion into their innermost secrets, or at any rate intrusion into secrets hidden by their clothes, should pocket machines become available, and firms were not slow to cash in on the beliefs, advertising x-ray-proof waistcoats and, for the ladies, x-ray-proof underwear. In America there was a move to prohibit the use of x-rays in theatre opera glasses.

The scientific world also showed its gullibility by reporting that the shadow of a bone cast with x-rays onto the brain of a dog made the animal hungry[25]. But, taken by and large, medical men realized the true possibilities and limitations of the rays and set about adapting them to medicine and surgery. The first obvious application was to the study of bones and their diseases and to the location of foreign bodies, such as bullets, which would show up in x-ray pictures[25]. Robert Jones was one of the first to use x-rays and demonstrated a bullet in a boy's wrist before operating for its removal[26]. The speed with which x-rays found a place in surgery was quite amazing; within a matter of months there was an extensive literature on the subject; stones in the urinary bladder and gall-bladder had been demonstrated, and experiments were started on introducing radio-opaque substances into the body to show up the outline of hollow internal organs. The trouble here was that the substances also had to be harmless, but iodine was soon found to be suitable and now forms the basis of many compounds used to show up internal organs or abnormal hollow tracks, such as sinuses and fistulas, within the body. The stomach soon attracted attention and it was suggested that air would be best for giving an outline, as poisoning was a real danger if chemical substances were introduced into the alimentary canal. However, a barium compound was eventually produced that was absolutely safe, though possibly the 'barium meal', a paste-like concoction, was not, until modified in relatively recent times, to everybody's taste.

From the use of x-rays as a diagnostic aid it was but a short step to employing them for treatment. Bacterial diseases, such as tuberculosis, were an obvious target, but unfortunately experiments failed to show any beneficial effect, and so doctors turned the rays on cancer, in which group of diseases radiotherapy now has its widest application. It is a strange fact that although x-rays and other radiations are used to treat cancer, they can also cause the disease by injudicious exposure. This was most tragically not realized by the early doctors who, completely unprotected, worked to perfect the machines and extend the scope of the new specialty. Some of the first patients also suffered from the effects of overexposure, which led to their hair falling out or to an intractable dermatitis; but the scientists and doctors whose lives were lived among x-rays suffered most, many dying from leukaemia or contracting skin cancer, usually on their hands. Nowadays, radiology and radiotherapy are exact sciences, and great care is taken to protect both doctor and patient from their harmful effects.

The sensation caused in the orthopaedic world by the discovery of x-rays was almost equalled by the temerity of a Guy's Hospital surgeon. William Arbuthnot Lane was actually converting simple fractures into compound ones by operating to set the broken bones. The horror of the elder surgeons, whose minds functioned along pre-Listerian lines, was such that Lane became subjected to an inordinate amount of criticism, at times bordering on the abusive. In the 1890s in England, compound fractures were still considered dangerous because of the risk of infection; simple fractures may have been uninspiring, but at least they were safe. Yet even simple fractures did not always heal well, and the patient might be left with a shortened deformed limb or the bones might unite by fibrous tissue, not by bone, leading to instability. This often meant that the patient was unable to return to his normal work; a serious matter for him but of no great concern to the surgeon, who felt he could do no better. Some surgeons did feel they could do better. Hugh Owen Thomas and Robert Jones were greatly concerned for the injured patient, and besides improving the treatment they also achieved far better functional results. Yet in spite of their care there remained a proportion of fractures that did not heal adequately. Arbuthnot Lane decided to operate and make sure that the fracture was properly set and in good alignment by using a form of internal fixation. Unable to interest his senior colleague in the matter he waited until this gentleman was on holiday, and then pounced on all the fractures that came to the hospital, taking them to the theatre and operating. Fortunately he was entirely successful and the patients made trouble-free recoveries.

At first Lane used silver wire to hold the broken ends together, but, as this proved rather unsatisfactory, in 1893 he employed steel screws[27]. In one of his early cases, a fracture of the tibia and fibula, manipulation under anaesthesia and subsequent splinting had failed to produce healing; but when Lane operated he found that interposed between the broken ends were pieces of torn muscle and chips of bone. Not unnaturally, bony union was impossible under these circumstances and only by open operation could the fracture be treated properly. After removing the muscle and bone chips, Lane had to use powerful lion forceps to get the bones in alignment. He then drilled small holes across the fracture line and inserted the screws to maintain the reduction, in much the same way as a broken chair leg might be repaired. Some time around 1905, Lane introduced his bone plates, which were strips of steel of suitable length with two or more holes at each end to take the screws that fixed the plate to the bone[28].

In point of fact Lane was not the first surgeon to use any of these internal splints. Lister, in 1877, had successfully repaired with silver wire the fractured patella (kneecap) of forty-year-old Francis Smith who had fallen off his horse. The operation took place at King's College Hospital (which was then in Lincoln's Inn Fields) on October 26[29]. Smith was seen again five years later when movement and walking were very fair and still showing improvement. Despite this success the method had not been generally adopted. Billroth had used wire and his teacher, Langenbeck, had employed metal plates, yet the reasons leading up to their use had precluded their further development. These methods were the product of the observation that old ununited fractures sometimes healed if they became infected and pus formed round them. As such, the readoption of wiring and plating needed an entirely new approach, along a new line of thought. Lane supplied the necessary requirements and his success was due to his superb operative technique.

It was vital that there should be no chance of infection, and so Lane devised the 'no-touch' technique. At no time during the operation must anything touched by the hand come in contact with the wound area. Before operation the site was prepared and shaved; then, in theatre, it was painted with iodine. The gowns of Lane and his assistants and all the towels that were to be used were boiled and then soaked in 1in 20 carbolic acid. The gowns were worn wet over a long mackintosh apron extending from neck to ankle. After the skin incision had been made, the towels were clipped to the edges of the wound and folded backwards so that the patient's skin was covered, leaving only the wound itself open to view. Lane had designed special instruments with long handles, so that his fingers never came nearer than four inches to the wound. Needles were threaded and stitches tied, using forceps only. This technique was elaborated before the days of rubber gloves and face masks, yet when these aids to asepsis were introduced Lane did not relax one bit from his scrupulous attention to its detail. He did, however, dispense with the uncomfortable wet gowns when the method of sterilization by steam under pressure came to be the accepted practice.

The 'no-touch' technique was not the sole source of Lane's success. He was a master craftsman who knew exactly what he was doing and had an intuitive grasp of the mechanics of the human frame, putting in the screws and plates precisely where they were needed. In fractured necks of femurs he sometimes, with uncanny accuracy, inserted a screw up through the neck, to the amazement of visitors who could scarcely grasp the anatomical relations of the bone during the operation. With this procedure he was many years in advance of Smith-

Petersen, who invented the well-known tri-fin nail that bears his name and which is carefully introduced under x-ray control. Lane always used long incisions as he did not hold with trying to perform operations through an inadequate exposure. He was exceedingly gentle with the tissues and insisted on complete control of haemorrhage, introducing toothed artery forceps to England. Unlike many of his contemporaries, who still believed that speed was expected of a good surgeon, he operated with unhurried precision, yet should the condition of the patient demand it, his fingers could work like lightning.

Lane thrived on criticism or else he would certainly have retired from the field a disillusioned man. Surgeons, impressed by his results, would buy his type of instruments and return home sure that they could then repeat Lane's performance. In most cases they could not. Unable to secure asepsis, infection ruined their results, but instead of blaming themselves for inadequate attention to the minutest detail practised by Lane, they blamed Lane himself for introducing such an operation. The arguments and criticisms continued for nearly twenty years until a body of surgeons appointed by the British Medical Association investigated the problem. By this time the lessons had been learned and Lane emerged triumphant. In 1913 his services to surgery were recognized and he was created a baronet.

Lane is now chiefly remembered for his work on fractures, although he had many interests in other branches of surgery with memorable operations to his credit. He was a courageous surgeon and never allowed himself to be bound by the opinions of his time if he believed them to be wrong and felt that he could do better. On occasion he had employed bone grafts without much success, but it was indirectly due to his work that they came into use.

Other surgeons, dissatisfied with Lane's metallic plates, wanted some substance which, while serving the same purpose, would not be so troublesome in their hands. Foremost amongst them was Fred Houdlett Albee of New York who, in 1911, made use of grafts, cut with a specially designed power-driven saw, from the patient's tibia. His first report concerned their use in tuberculous disease of the spine, in which the grafts permitted immobilization of the affected vertebrae, thus preventing further deformity and giving the rest necessary for healing[30]. In Albee's operation the graft was inserted between the surgically split spines of the vertebrae. After operation, the patient had to lie on a plaster bed for a number of weeks and then wear a spinal brace for about a year, to ensure complete fusion of the graft into the spine. Many types of spinal fusion have since been developed and the indications have increased to include other spinal conditions for which immobilization of the vertebrae is required. Albee later brought bone grafts into use for the treatment of various deformities and ununited fractures[31].

Metals are now used in surgery mainly for the treatment of fractures, the reconstruction of diseased joints and as prostheses for joint replacement. The opening moves were made in 1931 when Marius Nygaard Smith-Petersen, a Boston surgeon, introduced his nail, which has three fins running along its length, for internal fixation of the extremely troublesome fractures of the neck of the femur[32]. However, yet again it will surely come as no surprise to learn that the hip had been nailed in 1878 by Langenbeck[33] and by Lister soon after, and that in 1907 Fritz Steinman of Berne had used a pin that could be inserted to allow traction to be applied to a fractured leg[34]. Sven Johansson, a Swede, modified the Smith-Petersen nail in 1932 by having a hole made through its length, which enabled it to be inserted along a marker wire[35], thus making an extensive open operation unnecessary. Seven years later, Smith-Petersen devised a cup made of vitallium metal for fitting over the head of the femur in cases of osteoarthritis of the hip joint[36].

The stimulus of World War II led to the emergence of a large number of plastic substances and it was inevitable that many should be tried in surgery. In 1950 the Judet brothers, Jean and Robert Louis, of France, removed the head of the femur from a hip joint and replaced it with an artificial one made of acrylic plastic[37]. Thus were the floodgates opened for the joints in both upper and lower limbs to be replaced by a wide variety of metals and plastics.

But to return to the beginning of the 20th century by which time the specialty of orthopaedics had blossomed into an extensive art in which deformities were treated by open operation on bone, and by operations on tendons and ligaments. Thus far the only injuries to have come within the scope of the orthopaedic surgeon had been fractures, but the horror that was to descend upon the world in the second decade of that century produced a vast array of casualties demanding treatment and rehabilitation for their mutilated bodies. A much wider field was thus opened up for the healing potential of orthopaedic surgery.

19

Fields of battle

The battlefields of history supplied the young surgeon with the raw material for his training. A period of military service was an essential element in the background of any aspiring surgeon before the 18th century and many famous doctors were, by profession, military surgeons. Then, with the foundation of hospitals and the advancement of knowledge, experience could be gained in civil practice, and slowly this led to a forsaking of the more hazardous school. Yet war continued to provide a stimulus. In the past one hundred and fifty years the discoveries and developments of surgery have been adapted to military use; many of the problems peculiar to war wounds have been overcome and, in turn, the lessons learned applied to peacetime practice.

Sepsis, the curse of generations of surgeons, both civil and military, was not a serious problem to the ancients largely because the wounded bled to death or died from exposure before medical aid arrived. Homer estimated the mortality rate of those wounded in the Trojan War to be 75 percent. As the number of surgeons attending the armies in later centuries increased, more wounded survived only to succumb to infection. The natural inclination of war wounds to be infected was enhanced by the general treatment provided. This amounted to amputation, the extensive use of the cautery and the application of a variety of noxious medicaments, all carried out with complete disregard of elementary hygiene.

Matters did not improve with the passage of time. The destructive power of weapons of war steadily increased while the surgical care that could be offered remained virtually static. Occasionally, attempts were made to introduce an element of humanity onto the battlefield as, for instance at Dettingen in 1743 where the French and English agreed that the hospitals of both sides should be regarded as sanctuaries for the sick and wounded and mutually respected. This good intention scarcely survived the campaign. During the Napoleonic Wars the chief surgeons of both the French and the English armies made heroic efforts to care more humanely for the wounded, but they were up against the military machine: casualties were a confounded nuisance interfering, as they did, with the battle plans of the generals.

The next major conflict, and the first since the arrival of anaesthetics, was the Crimean War. At the start the medical arrangements were a thorough disgrace – though the blame did not lie with the Army Medical Department, a civilian organization with its staff devoid of military authority. (Not until 1898 did the Department become the Royal Army Medical Corps with officers and men having substantive military rank.) The trouble lay with the various military departments responsible for seeing that the Medical Department's requisitions were met – which they either were not or only after a delay and then, as like as not, incompletely. The consequences were appalling, worthy of the worst of the Dark Ages. Verminous, dying of cholera, dysentery and fever, men lay in battle-stained uniforms on damp, muddy floors. They were attended by pensioners recalled to the colours and asked to volunteer and not by fit men recruited from the depots as requested by the Director General of the Medical Department. Furthermore, their number fell well below the requirement.

Drugs were almost nonexistent. Leeches, when the orders were supplied, came in stoppered, airtight bottles and were thus dead and useless. Chloroform was considered unnecessary, as the howls of the patient showed he was still alive, and pain anyway was a good thing, as it helped towards recovery! Diet for these seriously ill men consisted of salt-pork or beef, hard biscuits and shocking coffee. The wounded who were fit enough to stand the journey were evacuated to the base hospital at Scutari, where the filth and horrors were repeated and operations – that is, amputations – were performed in the midst of the sick and the dying who were the inmates of what passed for wards. Then, after the war had been in progress for some months and death had claimed more from disease than from enemy action, an angel of mercy appeared in Scutari.

The indomitable courage, the boundless energy and sincere love for humanity that made up the personality of Florence Nightingale led her to the Crimea with thirty-eight specially chosen female helpers in October, 1854[1]. The military authorities did not welcome her arrival. Nevertheless, she overcame the obstructions put in her way, cleaned up the hospital and brought organization to the chaos of the administration. With her own money and that collected in a public appeal, launched by the London *Times*, she established kitchens and a laundry. With stores that she had had the foresight to bring with her, she clothed the patients and restored their self-respect. She instituted a routine of round-the-clock nursing care for the patients. A Hospitals Commission had already been sent out from England, and in February 1855 a Sanitary Commission was also sent to investigate the sanitation of the hospital buildings. They found that such sewers as existed were choked and flooding back into the wards, and were contaminating the water supply[2]. At this period, in England, Edwin Chadwick was revolutionizing public health and, working on his principles, the Commission 'saved the British Army'. In the first six months of 1855 the mortality rate in the hospital was reduced from 42 to 2 percent, an achievement bordering on the miraculous, but one that caused a breakdown in Miss Nightingale's health.

The outstanding medical character on the other side of the Crimean front line, where similar atrocious conditions prevailed, was Nikolai Ivanovich Pirogoff, the leading Russian surgeon of his day. In 1847 he had been the first man to use ether anaesthesia on the battlefield, and in the Crimea he employed plaster of Paris on a large scale. Although female nurses, who may have been camp followers but were at least organized, had been employed in wartime one hundred and fifty years previously, their presence was not really felt until the Crimean War, and it was a strange fact that both sides made effective use of their services. Pirogoff, through the interest and influence of the Grand Duchess Helena Pavlovna, had managed to get Russian nurses sent to the Crimea where they proved their worth. To a surgeon with his advanced ideas, the appalling conditions must have been most disheartening. Nevertheless, he was able to make some headway against the terror of sepsis by endeavouring to operate as early as possible and then entrusting the patients to the care of the nurses[3].

With an eye to the future, a certain Italian by the name of Cavour had brought Sardinia into the war on the side of England and France, earning the gratitude of these two powers. As Italy was then under the domination of Austria, Cavour's next step was to induce Sardinia to declare war on Austria, and he further en-sured the support of France by giving her Savoy and Nice. The battle that gave Italy her independence took place at Solferino in 1859, where the combined forces of Italy and France massacred the Austrians. Present at the battle was Henri Dunant, a wealthy Swiss banker. He was so appalled by the sight of over 40 000 men lying wounded and left to die with no medical attention that he wrote of his experiences and appealed for some form of organization to prevent such a happening in the future. The book[4] had a wide circulation and reached the hearts of many powerful persons.

The outcome was the Geneva Convention of 1864, where delegates from sixteen countries drew up rules governing the welfare of the wounded and the protection to be afforded to hospitals and medical personnel. Thus did the Red Cross come into being. Dunant spent his entire fortune on the enterprise and was reduced to pauperism. Later he became mentally unbalanced, but finally he achieved worldwide recognition in 1901 with the award of the Nobel Peace Prize; the money he gave to charity.

Another famous conflict of this period was the American Civil War, again notable for its horrors and lack of medical services. This was the country where almost twenty years previously anaesthesia had been given to the world, yet the old prejudices still governed the actions of surgeons and they preferred to amputate without an anaesthetic while the casualty was still in a state of 'battle tension' (an old belief was that in this state the heart was better able to stand the strain of surgery), and they were unwilling to run the risk of an anaesthetic reducing the surgical shock which was believed to contribute to success. Drugs were in short supply, especially in the South. Surgeons were in short supply on both sides. Scarcely out of medical school, doctors were mobilized in an attempt to stem the tide of death, but antisepsis lay in the future and many casualties were done a disservice by surgeons who operated with filthy, infected instruments, not infrequently borrowed from some kitchen table. Nevertheless, the diseases of war – dysentery, tetanus (lockjaw), typhus and typhoid – claimed many more of the dead than did the weapons of war, although a gentleman with a medical degree, Richard Jordan Gatling, made a brave attempt to even matters by inventing the machine gun. This emphasized how the killing power of weapons was increasing with no commensurate gain in surgical care.

A manual of military surgery for surgeons in the Confederate Army, by J. J. Chisholm, included the recommendation that curare be used for the treatment of tetanus[5]. Spencer Wells had previously used the drug on three occasions in 1859[6], but although sometimes employed in the following years, it was too dangerous and only in more recent times has it been restored to an important place in the treatment of the agonizing muscle spasms of this disease.

In Europe the Prussians and the French got so annoyed with each other, largely owing to some crafty misrepresentations on the part of Bismarck, that in 1870 they went to war. In the campaign that led up to the siege of Paris, antiseptic principles were used for the first time under battle conditions by William MacCormac, the British chief surgeon of the Anglo-American Ambulance Corps. His American counterpart was James Marion Sims. Prominent among the French surgeons was Louis Ollier, who used plaster of Paris to treat wounds as well as fractures. By this means he ensured that the wounded limb would have complete rest, so enabling Nature to proceed unhindered with her job of healing. If there was much swelling of the tissues around the wound, he used constant irrigation instead of plaster owing to the increased danger of infection taking hold in the swollen areas.

The surgeon-general of the Prussian forces was Friedrich von Esmarch, who is remembered by the rubber bandage bearing his name that is used for binding round a limb from the distal end upwards to force the blood out and enable operations on the limb to take place in a relatively bloodless field[7]. His greater contribution to the surgery of war was his insistence that every soldier should carry a first-aid kit and, equally important, should know how to use it. When Paris finally fell after five hungry months of siege, the triumphant booming of guns heralded the arrival of the new German Empire on the European scene. The significance of this did not escape the British authorities; war was now a really serious matter and the death knell of an archaic system was sounded when it was announced that commissions in the British Army could no longer be bought.

The years at the end of the 19th century were occupied with skirmishes and campaigns in distant parts of the world. For some time the Italians had been trying to 'protect' Abyssinia but in 1896 Menelek II, an able and independent ruler, took exception to the intrusion and a large Italian force which was sent against him was soundly defeated at Adowa. On their return home, a number of Italians found themselves at a disadvantage in life, owing to the Abyssinians' unfortunate habit of cutting off the hands of their prisoners. Giuliano Vanghetti saw the possibility of utilizing the muscles in the stumps as a source of power for artificial limbs and devised a scheme whereby the muscle ends could be attached to a system of levers[8, 9]. But he was a physician and surgeons took no notice of his work until 1905, when Antonio Ceci put the idea into practice[10, 11].

The operation was improved upon by Vittorio Putti of Bologna in 1911[12, 13], and again in World War I by Ferdinand Sauerbruch who also introduced a glove type of artificial limb[14, 15]. The technique of kinematization is to make a hole through the end of the muscle and arrange the skin to line the hole. Through this a rod is passed. An operation of such ingenuity deserved a better fate, but it was abandoned owing to the very real problem of how to attach living tissue to the levers, the heaviness of the artificial hand and, in the early days, to bad surgical technique.

[Children born with congenitally deficient arms pose a rather different problem that was highlighted when, in the early 1960s, there was an explosive increase in their numbers. This was traced to their mothers' having taken thalidomide as a preventive measure against morning sickness in the early stages of pregnancy. These children needed a new type of artificial arm and fortunately Ernst Marquardt was already working in Heidelberg on one powered by compressed carbon dioxide gas carried in a small cylinder[16]. Even toddlers under three years old could be taught how to work the prostheses to feed themselves and to play. Alas, though most amputees are prepared to learn how to use these and other prostheses of similar ingenious design (for instance, those making use of electrical impulses generated by the forearm muscles – when these are present), it is a sad fact that quite a number prefer a hook, claw or other simple device when faced with the tasks of everyday life.]

At the southern end of the African continent, the age-old pattern was repeated in the Boer War (1899–1902): disease killed 14 000 soldiers of the British Army; 8000 died of typhoid fever alone, a slightly greater number than were killed in action. Unfortunately, by one of life's tragic twists, a vaccine became available just too late to have an impact. The professor of pathology at the Netley Military Hospital, Almroth Wright, had perfected a vaccine made of dead typhoid bacteria. Once proof of its safety and effectiveness had been shown by a trial in 1899 in the Indian Army, he had recommended that it be adopted by the British Army[17]. Nevertheless, its use in the Boer War was haphazard and voluntary, so denying it any hope of providing adequate protection against the disease. No records were kept and the frightful incidence of typhoid fever led the authorities to assume that the vaccine was of no value. During the two years following the war fierce argument surrounded the vaccine, until finally sense prevailed and a Royal Commission pronounced in its favour. Since then, efficient sanitation, careful control of water supplies and compulsory vaccination have virtually removed typhoid fever from among the hazards facing a disciplined army.

The major surgical lesson learned from the Boer War was the importance of early and adequate operation for the majority of wounds, although a significant exception to this general principle was in connection with wounds of the abdomen. Since the early days of antiseptic surgery, controversy had raged over the problem of whether to open an abdomen in an emergency or to leave it alone and let Nature take her own course without hindrance. Experience in the Franco-Prussian war, in which there was a mortality rate of nearly 100 percent from gunshot wounds of the abdomen, had led James Marion Sims to believe that surgery was indicated, but those surgeons who operated were unable to achieve good results. In civilian life, where the emergency arose because of some disease inside the abdomen, the general improvement in surgical technique and the arrival of asepsis led to exploratory operations when required, and these gave much better results than leaving the patients alone. The emergency of war wounds had to be dealt with under conditions far from ideal, and often many hours after wounding by which time the abdomen was well and truly contaminated by bowel contents. Nevertheless, in the 1890s surgeons took up their position in one or other of the camps and became abstentionists or interventionists. Surgeons favouring intervention were fewer and came mainly from America and Germany. French and English surgeons on the whole abstained, and this was the official policy in the military campaigns of the early part of the 20th century.

In the Boer War an attempt was made by William Stevenson, professor of military surgery at Netley, to change this policy to one of intervention for patients in whom the intestines were believed to be injured. This he advocated because the results of operating on patients with perforated stomach ulcers in civil life were good. The results in war injuries proved to be appalling. Sir William MacCormac, who was now the consulting surgeon to the Field Force in South Africa, felt constrained to comment:'In this war, a man wounded in the abdomen dies if he is operated upon and remains alive if he is left in peace.'

The interventionists won a decisive victory in the Russo-Japanese War of 1904–5 owing to the discovery that time was the vital factor. Abstention was the Russian order of the day, but this failed to take into account the presence of Princess Vera Ignatievna Gedroitz, who had trained and qualified in Germany, the home of the interventionists. She displayed remarkable courage and initiative by equipping a railway carriage as an operating theatre close to the front line, where she received casualties within three or four hours of wounding. She achieved a staggering degree of success with abdominal wounds and was thus able to convince the Russians that if these casualties could be operated on within a short time of wounding and under suitable conditions, they did far better than if left alone[18]. The interventionist policy received general acceptance after the outbreak of World War I, but it was emphasized that good organization was vital in ensuring the rapid evacuation of casualties to a suitable surgical unit.

A major consideration in the surgery of World War I was the constant fight against infection. In the first few months of the war the nature of the wounds was not understood and surgeons were working in the dark. Treatment consisted in excision of the wound with drainage through rubber tubes (which frequently became blocked), washing out with an antiseptic and eventual closure by secondary suture when the wound was deemed to be free of infection. At first small in-and-out wounds were thought to be sterile and were closed there and then by primary suture. The lesson that every wound was infected was quickly learnt when foul discharges began leaking from wounds closed in this manner. Increasing experience showed that the two main problems were how best to deal with infection and how best to manage the wounds surgically.

Before the war carbolic acid was still relied on for washing out wounds in casualty departments and perchloride of mercury was used in the dressings. Disaster attended this practice in France – both were poisonous in the strengths needed and the action of perchloride of mercury was nullified by serum. Various other antiseptics, such as hydrogen peroxide and potassium permanganate, were tried with better results being claimed. There was no official policy and individual surgeons used whatever they had available. However, a systematic search was undertaken by Alexis Carrel, a Frenchman, and Henry Drysdale Dakin, an Englishman (both of whom settled in America). After testing two hundred or more different substances they found that the most effective were those containing chlorine and the best was sodium hypochlorite[19]. This unfortunately was too alkaline and damaging to the tissues, so Dakin neutralized it with boric acid and Carrel christened the result 'Dakin's solution'[20]. The solution killed the bacteria and helped to dissolve dead tissue, but had the disadvantage that its effect was short-lived. The Carrel-Dakin treatment of wounds, which the two men evolved, overcame this difficulty by a system of irrigation. The technique was complicated and had to be carried out to the last detail in order to be effective. When it failed, it was often because surgeons relied too much on the antiseptic properties of the solution at the expense of adequate surgery. The contaminated wound was first thoroughly debrided, then little rubber tubes with holes in them were placed in all parts of the wound and kept in place with loosely packed ordinary gauze; the surrounding skin was protected with vaseline gauze. The tubes were all connected to a container of the solution and the wound flushed every two hours[21]; the open ends of the drainage tubes had to be left above the level of the wound and never in a dependent position (a common fault). The dressings themselves were changed daily under aseptic conditions, and a swab was taken for microscopic examination. When the bacteria had as good as disappeared and the wound looked healthy, it was closed by secondary suture. The process demanded patience with a time-consuming attention to detail. Nevertheless, it served a vital function in the treatment of contaminated wounds in World War I and Dakin's solution, which he later modified, was the most efficient antiseptic for the next twenty years.

So serious was the problem of sepsis to a generation of surgeons brought up on asepsis, that one or two seemingly desperate remedies were suggested. An example was maggot therapy. During the Napoleonic Wars, Dominique Jean Larrey, Surgeon to Napoleon's Imperial Guard, had been impressed by the cleanliness of wounds infested with maggots which consumed dead tissue and helped to promote healing. In 1917 an American, William Stevenson Baer, was also intrigued by the work of maggots when he saw two soldiers who had been lying out in no-man's-land with compound fractures of their femurs. The usual mortality rate for this condition was 75 percent and by all the laws these two men should have been dead; however, they were in fine fettle, thanks to their swarm of maggots. Baer then introduced maggot therapy, but the idea was doomed from the start since there was difficulty in getting sterile maggots and the nature of the treatment was unaesthetic in the extreme. Nothing daunted, Baer was still battling away in 1931, using maggots in the treatment of chronic bone infections[22].

Two vastly unpleasant infections, tetanus and gas gangrene, were also liable to complicate the wounds, the more so as battles were fought over cultivated and manured land, which is notorious for harbouring the bacteria responsible for these diseases. The incidence of tetanus in 1914 was 150–300 per 10 000 wounded, and the mortality rate varied between 58 and 78 percent, but with the introduction of tetanus antitoxin injections towards the end of the year it fell to 0·6–7·0 per 10 000, with a higher incidence at times of heavy fighting. The mortality rate was 42–48 per cent. This level was maintained throughout the rest of the war[23].

Gas gangrene was a more serious occurrence. Since dead muscle in the wound is particularly liable to lead to this infection, it was necessary to remove all dead and dying tissue. But on occasion the infection spread up the muscles and local surgery was insufficient for its eradication. In 1916 it was discovered that the gas produced by the disease would show up on x-rays[24], and when this was seen surgical intervention, with possible amputation, was a matter of the utmost urgency. However, the method was not foolproof as inaccuracies in the interpretation of the x-rays sometimes led to limbs being amputated when the gas was not, in fact, due to gas gangrene. After some months of war, Michel

Weinberg[25] introduced an anti-gas-gangrene serum which greatly improved the chances of those infected, although it could in no way take the place of early and adequate surgery.

After the first disastrous months the surgical management of wounds settled down for a while into debridement (in its modern meaning of scrupulous wound toilet – see p. 5) followed by secondary suture. It was vital to ensure the complete removal of all shell fragments or bullets, every little bit of in-driven clothing and any dead or dying tissue in the wound, with incision of the deep layers of fascia to prevent tension and to allow drainage to take place. This last was debridement in its original meaning of unbridling. Its importance had first been realized by Leonardo Botallo in the 16th century[26], but had been ignored until Pierre Joseph Desault re-introduced it at the end of the 18th century[27]. Desault's pupil, Larrey, applied the lessons of his teacher with great effect during the Napoleonic Wars[28, 29], but debridement then again lapsed into obscurity. In 1898 Paul Friedrich described a technique that bears a superficial resemblance to wound toilet and was based on a widely held belief that persisted until the early stages of World War II. This was that, during the first six hours after wounding bacteria were germinating locally, so by excising the edges and sides of the wound into its depths within this time limit, it should be possible to remove the bacteria and prevent infection[30].

On each occasion that the wounds were dressed after debridement a loopful of exudate was smeared on a slide, precisely labelled and sent to the laboratory where it was stained and examined under the microscope. The wound was said to be 'clinically sterile' and ready for secondary suture when the smear showed 0·2–0·4 organism per microscopic field. When debridement could be carried out at the casualty clearing station within twelve hours of wounding, and when the technique of debridement became more thorough, surgeons found that the time to clinical sterility was reduced to four to five days in soft-tissue wounds[31]. Closure at this time became known as delayed primary suture. (Lessons of war and major disaster have, it seems, to be learned over and over again; for instance, at first in World War II and more recently in the cyclonic destruction of Darwin, Australia, on Christmas Day 1974, the policy of delayed primary suture was not applied – with the inevitable consequences.)

The majority of wounds in World War I were caused by shell fire, and the jagged fragments carried particles of mud-caked clothing and equipment deep into the tissues. Add to this the unavoidable delay in the evacuation of casualties, thus allowing sepsis to become established. Every soldier was issued with a first field dressing and an ampoule of iodine; when wounded he emptied the

173

ampoule into the wound and applied the dressing *loosely* to prevent it acting as a tourniquet when the inevitable swelling began a few hours later. Larger shell dressings were carried only by stretcher bearers. The first stop for the casualty, whether by stretcher or walking, was the regimental aid post; he might arrive there within minutes or, if wounded in no-man's-land, it might be days before he could be reached by the stretcher bearers. The work of the regimental medical officer might be regarded as advanced first aid, but what he did and how he did it was considered to have far more influence on the final outcome than any subsequent treatment[31]. One of his responsibilities was to initiate the 'tally' or label on which was noted the nature of the injury, the treatment and, if morphine had been given, the time, dose and route; the results of the examination of wound smears was also included. This accompanied the casualty down the line, being updated as necessary.

At the next stop, the advanced dressing station, what we now call triage was begun. When an action was in progress the important task was the rapid evacuation of the casualties, either to the field ambulance or a clearing station[31]. The lightly wounded were inspected first, their dressings checked, fractured arms immobilized (not reduced) and put in a sling, tourniquets removed and bleeding points clamped and ligatured. They were sent on their way in batches. Next came those with more severe wounds, for instance of the head, chest or abdomen, and compound fractures of the leg (sometimes a badly shattered leg was amputated through the injury often with a more beneficial outcome than if delayed until the casualty clearing station). These men were evacuated by motor ambulance. Last to be evacuated were the moribund. Triage may on the surface seem a callous policy but it is essential if the system is not to become clogged up and fall apart at the seams.

The field ambulance was a mobile unit whose role was to provide earlier surgery than the casualty clearing station, particularly for those casualties who would travel badly. The casualty clearing station was sited some six to ten miles behind the front line and was the first place where facilities were available for thorough surgical treatment. Here, the wounded were segregated according to their injuries and all necessary surgery undertaken[31]. However, if a battle was in progress a number of casualties would have to be evacuated to the base hospital – unavoidable even though the time taken on the train journey might allow infection to progress to the extent of loss of limb or even life.

In the later stages of the war an American, Hiram Winnett Orr, noticed that soldiers who had merely had their wounded limbs put in plaster to enable them to be sent to America were often in far better shape than those who had received the usual treatment. This was startling since, despite the fact that the wounds were almost certainly infected, healing had proceeded quite satisfactorily under the plaster. The wound itself was loosely packed with vaseline gauze and the surrounding skin protected from the pus by vaseline and more vaseline gauze. Orr realized that the complete immobilization provided by the plaster cast enabled the natural healing processes of the body to do their job without interference[32]. Although he advocated simple plaster immobilization as a treatment of choice, Orr was unable to make any headway until some years later, when the method became accepted by a number of surgeons as the best treatment available for chronic bone infections and certain wounds. Before the plaster was applied in these cases, an incision was made to allow drainage from the site of infection. This form of plaster treatment of war wounds was really brought to the fore in the Spanish Civil War, where conditions were ideal for its use. To Orr's original technique was added the important preliminary of debridement.

In the years leading up to World War I, a great deal of work had been done in physiology, and this science of the normal functioning of the body found its way into surgery. It gave the answer to some of the problems connected with shock, the most important of which was the realization that the blood volume and blood pressure must be maintained. In war, shock assumed greater importance than in peacetime; in the immediate period after wounding it was more important even than sepsis, for unless it was treated, the casualty might never live to present the surgeon with a problem in sepsis. Over a million soldiers were killed outright on the battlefields of World War I, and of these, 10 percent died from shock and haemorrhage consequent upon penetrating abdominal wounds. The nature of shock itself was as yet inadequately understood and its treatment consisted mainly of first-aid measures. The casualty was given hot sweet tea to drink (unless wounded in the abdomen), he was wrapped up and, in an effort to keep him warm during hours of waiting, stoves were placed under the stretchers. Ambulance journeys across country and along shell-pitted roads aggravated the shock by creating anxiety, increased haemorrhage and pain; in the case of fractures where the bone ends would grate together, the outcome was sometimes lethal. Injured limbs had to be adequately splinted, and without doubt the simple but eminently practical Thomas splint saved many lives and contributed greatly to the comfort of men wounded in the legs. It was introduced by Robert Jones and other consultant surgeons, but much campaigning and education in its use were required and it was not generally employed until the second half of the war. The technique was adapted to the exigencies of war: the splint was put on over the trouser leg and boot and, to obtain extension on the limb, the boot was bandaged to the end of the splint in such a way that winding on the bandage with a stick or pencil would increase the amount of traction.

Occasionally more active measures were undertaken to combat shock, such as early attempts at blood transfusion. However, the development of blood transfusion as a practical proposition rightfully belongs to the inter-war period, for although blood was transfused in World War I, matters did not always go smoothly. The transfusion was given by some form of syringe technique directly from donor to recipient, which necessitated operating-theatre conditions. The problem of keeping the blood from clotting was solved at the beginning of the war but difficulties still had to be overcome. Blood groups were known but troubles from incompatibility were frequently encountered. By 1917 advances had been made in technique and blood was transfused more often, especially in cases of severe haemorrhage, though in grossly insufficient quantities; three-quarters of a pint was considered a large transfusion. Should the patient not recover, a condition of 'irreversible shock' was invoked, other things being equal, rather than inadequacies of the transfusion technique.

One important surgical outcome of the war was that attention became focused on the chest. As far as the heart was concerned, it was chiefly French surgeons who reported recovery after the removal of missiles, but this was without immediate impact on progress. Significant interest, however, centred around the surgical treatment of empyema – the collection of pus in the pleural cavity. The civilian method, in use at the beginning of the war, consisted in the removal of a rib and allowing free drainage to take place. However, this was soon found to be inadequate for dealing with the suppuration following war wounds, and a more extensive operation had to be evolved based on debridement, as in other types of wound.

Once surgeons had overcome their initial and quite unfounded fears that handling a wounded lung would re-start the bleeding and deepen the shock, they were able to proceed. Ribs were freely removed and those remaining on each side of the surgical wound were pulled widely apart to give free access to as extensive an area as possible. All blood, pus, dirt and foreign bodies were removed, the pleural cavity was washed out and the chest closed. This form of treatment gave by far the best results, and a similar type of extensive operation was adapted later to civilian use in ordinary cases of empyema. Nevertheless this was only half the story, since empyema was a common complication of the influenza pandemic of the end of the war. So seriously was the empyema regarded by the United States Army Medical Corps, that they appointed an Empyema Commission, headed by Evarts Graham, to investigate the problem in army camps in the United States.

The course of the influenza was exceptionally virulent, attacking the lungs and often leading with alarming rapidity to death. A small abscess in the lung would produce the empyema by rupturing into the pleural cavity, causing first a wet pleurisy and then pus formation. As soon as it became evident that there was fluid in the pleural cavity, the accepted practice was promptly to institute surgical drainage. Death then followed in from 30–80 percent of cases, varying from camp to camp. Animal experiments and post-mortem examinations showed that these patients still had an active pneumonia and that there were no pleural adhesions. The patient was thus in a bad state to withstand operation anyway and when the chest was opened, air got in which seriously disturbed the action of the heart and reduced the already parlous functioning of the lungs. The Commission reported that, at this early stage of the disease, the best procedure was to draw the fluid off as often as necessary, using a needle and syringe. Together with a good diet, this occasionally produced a cure, but in most cases operation was required later when the pus had formed and pleural adhesions kept it localized. Under these circumstances, the surgeon waited until the patient was fit and until the empyema was well surrounded by stuck-down pleura, so that when the chest was opened, drainage could take place without embarrassment to heart or lung function. After operation, irrigation of the empyema cavity by the Carrel-Dakin technique was instituted. The mortality rate fell to 9 percent: not ideal, but a creditable performance considering that anaesthetic techniques, which play an important part in chest surgery, were still undeveloped.

Once the first shock of war with its flood of casualties had been met, surgeons turned their attention to dealing with the terrible deformities of limb and face that resulted, and to seeking ways of minimizing these by adequate treatment from as early a stage as possible. Casualties with fractures or other orthopaedic problems were high on the list of priority, since no special facilities were available and many men were discharged from the army completely unfitted for civilian life. In 1915 Robert Jones persuaded the British War Office to set aside a number of beds at the Alder Hey military hospital solely for orthopaedic cases. In the following months military orthopaedic hospitals were established in other parts of the country, and Robert Jones was appointed Inspector of Military Orthopaedics. By this means the services of the orthopaedic surgeons were concentrated and the casualties benefited by receiving the best treatment. This continued uninterruptedly, through purely surgical measures, to retraining for military service or completely fresh training for a job in civilian life suited to the limitations imposed by their particular incapacity. The wide geographical distribution of the hospitals also meant that the casualty could be nursed and receive his training near his home. This marked the beginning of an extremely important branch of medicine – rehabilitation. In some instances, for example the loss of a limb or blindness, the mental rehabilitation was just as important as the physical. When the war was over the military orthopaedic hospitals disappeared, to be replaced by civilian hospitals dealing with the whole range of orthopaedic illness, whether due to injury or disease.

In addition to his achievements in the administrative field, Robert Jones also found time to advance the art of orthopaedic surgery. One of his notable successes was in transplanting muscle tendons to overcome the disability caused by injury to the radial nerve in the arm. Interest in an alternative method of dealing with injured nerves, namely by stitching the cut ends together, was also revived during the war. For some time efforts had been made to achieve success in this direction. Eduard Albert, of Vienna, in 1876 had attempted to mend a gap in the median nerve in the arm by grafting in a piece of tibial nerve from an amputated leg[33]. In 1888 Arthur William Mayo Robson achieved success with a similarly planned operation[34]. Then, in 1895, at St Thomas's Hospital, London, Charles Alfred Ballance approached the problem in a different way by attaching a nerve that served a nearby but less important part of the body (the spinal accessory root of the eleventh cranial nerve), to a paralysed nerve of greater importance (the facial nerve)[35]. However, before the war, the results of operations on nerves were extremely bad, even when it was only a case of stitching together the cut ends (the necessary technique was yet to be developed). In 1923 Harry Platt and Walter Rowley Bristow together studied the way by which a nerve regenerates and reported on the outcome in a series of patients who had had nerves sutured. Nearly a quarter of the cases were failures, and in the remainder the degree of functional recovery depended on the nerve affected and the site of injury[36].

The rehabilitation of wounded men does not stop at those with orthopaedic or peripheral nerve injuries in which purely physical capabilities are of primary importance. The psychological effect of facial wounds can be profound. The whole outlook on life of a man who has lost his nose or had his lower jaw shot away is profoundly altered, and with the large number of these and other facial injuries of World War I it became imperative to make good the damage and fit the casualties for normal life. It was not sufficient to get good wound healing, the permanent disfigurement had to be socially acceptable.

Plastic surgery is of great antiquity. Five hundred or more years before Christ the Hindus were adepts in a specialized branch of the art, since a common punishment for adultery was to cut off the nose, and the miscreants, not wishing to have their future chances nipped in the bud, resorted to surgical aid to restore their profiles. Sushruta built up new noses by using skin flaps lifted from the cheeks, while later surgeons, mainly itinerant practitioners, used triangular flaps turned down from the forehead. In the 16th century AD, Gaspare Tagliacozzi was famous for his operation in which he built up the nose from the skin of the upper arm, the patient being immobilized with his face stitched to his arm until the skin had grown onto its new site[37]. Antiseptic methods in surgery gave fresh impetus to the problems of skin grafting and led to the use of skin cut from one part of the body being implanted on another part. This is known as free skin grafting as opposed to the flap or pedicle methods in which continuity of tissue is maintained until the graft has healed in its new place.

A type of free skin graft was introduced in 1869 by Jacques-Louis Reverdin[38], and in 1872 Louis Ollier described grafts composed either of full skin thickness or of partial thickness[39]. Two years later Carl Thiersch devised a method whereby the partial thickness grafts could be cut to extreme thinness so as not to disturb the regeneration of skin in the donor area[40]. These grafts became known as Thiersch grafts and though they enjoyed considerable popularity, they were unsuited to covering large or badly damaged areas, and taken by and large the results obtained were poor, since the grafts often failed to survive and those that did became unsightly. In certain circumstances better results could be obtained by free grafts which made use of the full thickness of skin. This method was introduced to general surgery in 1893 by Fedor Krause[41] and was an idea based on the earlier work of John Wolfe, a Hungarian working in Glasgow[42], which had only found application in surgery around the eyes.

Once again World War I provided a stimulus to the advance of surgery. In Britain, William Arbuthnot Lane was active in organizing specialist services for the wounded and one of his undertakings centred round a hutted site in Sidcup. Here, wounds of the face were to be treated and the surgeon in charge was Harold Delf Gillies. Gillies had started his career with an interest in otology, but with the outbreak of war he turned his attention to plastic surgery. After a visit to France he persuaded the War Office to send all casualties with facial wounds to Aldershot. So numerous were these men that Gillies searched Southern England for a special hospital site and finally settled on Sidcup. From this beginning the whole of British plastic surgery developed; the bedded huts eventually expanded to become Queen Mary's Hospital, and along with facial injuries, other conditions demanding a plastic approach were treated. Important among these were burns which were highly liable to become infected and which healed with terribly deforming and often incapacitating scars. Free skin grafts were hardly used at all during the war, instead defects were repaired by raising flaps from neighbouring parts and moulding these to cover the injured area. From about 1917 onwards Gillies popularized the pedicle graft, which was far more satisfactory and enabled skin to be brought from distant parts. In this method, folds of skin are raised, for example, from the abdomen, and cut and stitched so that they form a tube attached at both ends. Then, in easy stages, the tube can be swung to wherever it is needed, with the proviso that one end is always firmly attached with a good blood supply[43].

After the war plastic surgery progressed rather slowly, although valuable work was being done, and the principles of the specialty, such as gentle handling of the tissues, careful apposition of wound edges, fine suture material, delicate instruments and insistence on perfect haemostasis, found acceptance in general surgery. Before World War II there existed only a handful of surgeons devoted to plastic surgery; it needed the urgency of that second war to bring the specialty into its own.

20

Consolidation

World War I marked a turning point in the history of surgery. Since the discovery of anaesthesia, and more particularly of antisepsis and asepsis, the surgical years had been full of discovery and adventure; entirely fresh avenues had been opened up and surgery had advanced in scope and success more than in all the thousands of years since Man first tried his hand at the healing art. The need for specialization had been realized and the results obtained by men who devoted their energies to one particular branch of the subject had proved its worth. Societies had been formed and many journals published to aid in the dissemination of knowledge. By the end of the first decade of the 20th century, many new operations had been worked out, in theory if not in practice. The time had come to call a pause, to review the situation, to see how techniques could be improved and surgery made safer for the patient, and, perhaps most significantly, to make the patient safe for surgery. The war had shown that there was still a great deal to be learned in this respect.

When there was need for the rugged individualistic pioneer the call had been answered by men of the right calibre, with their own particular brand of courage. They had raised surgery to heights undreamed of and invested the surgeon with a romantic aura. But times were changing and the day of the individualist had passed; the surgeon was becoming the leader of a team. At this time Lord Moynihan remarked that 'Surgery of the brilliant kind is a desecration. Such art finds its proper scope in tricks with cards, in juggling with billiard balls, and nimble encounters with bowls of vanishing goldfish.' Berkeley George Andrew Moynihan was an exceptional surgeon for any period; a skilful and beautiful operator, he lived in an era when his gifts could be put to best use. He is remembered most for his work on the abdomen and especially on duodenal ulcers, yet, unlike the men who preceded him, his name is not associated with any startling advance. By his superb operating methods and by his gentleness and care, he provided the standard for surgical technique and placed British abdominal surgery in a leading position in the world. In 1922 he was created a baronet and in 1929 he became Lord Moynihan of Leeds, the first surgeon after Lister to be raised to the peerage.

The importance of physiology to the surgeon was one of the aspects of Moynihan's teaching, and in this he showed the way for the developments that took place during the inter-war years. The relative importance of the basic sciences as applied to surgery had been undergoing considerable change. In the days when speed was all-important, a knowledge of anatomy was the prime essential. The surgeon had to know precisely where to find structures within the body. He had no time to think what the anatomical relations of various organs might be to one another; he knew instinctively. Next, in the middle of the 19th century, the science of pathology came to the fore and the surgeon had to know the behaviour and extent of disease processes so that he could design his operations accordingly. The circumstances of World War I then proceeded to show, in no uncertain manner, that there was far more to successful surgery than simply a knowledge of anatomy and pathology and of the correct surgical technique for dealing with disease. Scientists had been working on the problems of bodily function for a considerable time, but it took the war to bring home to surgeons the real importance of their researches. The factor that stimulated this interest was shock.

The reaction of the body known as shock is exceedingly complex and, depending on the type of insult to the body, it can be composed of one or more different elements. Shock itself is rather a vague term, but whatever the cause the common feature is a state of collapse. Loss of blood and nervous stimulation, which may be purely psychological, are the two main conditions producing shock, although anaesthesia, infection and hormonal changes are among other causes. In general terms, the volume of blood in effective circulation becomes reduced owing to a widespread dilatation of the capillaries which also become more permeable, so that the fluid part of the blood, as opposed to the blood cells, tends to leak into the tissues. Besides reducing the blood volume, this also makes the blood thicker. In an effort to maintain the blood pressure the small arterioles constrict, which, in the skin, leads to the pale, clammy appearance, and the heart rate increases; but as the blood pressure falls to dangerous limits, the beat becomes weaker and finally stops when the heart cannot get enough oxygen from the blood. When there has been no blood loss, or this has only been minimal, the transfusion of a suitable physiological solution is sufficient to put matters to rights; but if a lot of blood has been lost this method is inadequate as the solution leaks out of the blood stream into the tissues. It is then necessary to transfuse something that stays in the blood to restore its volume. The obvious substance is blood itself, and one of the major contributions of the 20th century to surgery was blood transfusion.

The association of blood with life dates back to primitive times and bloodletting has its origins in the Ancient Greek doctrine of the four humours (if not earlier). But whether the intention was to remove diseased material or evil spirits from the body, the practice was pursued with enthusiasm until comparatively recently. The problem of replacing it with blood containing good spirits was, however, far more difficult, although many early prescriptions had blood as a main ingredient. The theoretical possibility of giving blood directly into the blood stream was discussed as early as the 15th century, and in 1613 Andreas Libavius actually described a technique whereby silver tubes were inserted into the arteries[1]. Fifteen years later a considerable obstacle was removed from the path of experimentation when William Harvey showed that the blood circulated in the body and that the heart acted as the pump[2]. Before that time a motley array of theories, such as the blood's surging and ebbing, with the liver as an important organ, had held the field. Following Harvey's magnificent description, interest in blood transfusion achieved greater significance, and in the 1660s a number of experiments were carried out in England by Christopher Wren, Robert Boyle and Richard Lower; the first two of these gentlemen being better known as, respectively, architect and physicist. Most of their experiments were between animals[3], but on occasion they did transfuse animal blood into a human being[4]. Since they believed the blood might imbue the patient with the characteristics of the animal, considerable controversy raged over the use of lamb's or sheep's blood, which were the popular varieties. If the blood of a lion could be obtained, that was a different matter, but unfortunately no one seems to have attempted this courageous experiment. In France, Jean Baptiste Denis had some initial success in treating sick patients with transfusions of lamb's blood[5], but on the fourth occasion the patient died and the widow started a prolonged litigation. Denis was eventually absolved, although as a result of the case the practical possibilities of blood transfusion were forgotten for nearly two hundred years.

During the 1820s the practice was revived by James Blundell who employed blood transfusion for the treatment of severe bleeding after childbirth[6]. His first four cases were failures, yet he persisted in his belief and did finally obtain a few successes. The importance of his work was in his use of human donors and in drawing attention, for the first time, to the fact that animal blood was utterly unsuited for transfusion into human beings. This point was further brought out, in 1874, by Leonard Landois, a German physiologist, who showed that the serum (the clear fluid part of blood) of one animal would cause the red cells of another species of animal to clump together and dissolve[7]. Yet, in spite of this, a number of transfusions employing sheep's blood were reported at a German surgical conference in the same year. Owing to the alarming reactions, which were often lethal, and the lack of knowledge regarding their nature, blood was not often used in the latter part of the 19th century; saline solution was safer and preferred. Then, in 1901, Karl Landsteiner discovered that human blood could be divided into distinct groups[8], which have since become known as the ABO system. The blood of one group is incompatible with that of another, and this explained why reactions occurred and how they could be prevented. All modern transfusion dates from this beautifully executed work of Landsteiner.

Blood of the correct group could now be transfused, but it had to be given directly from the donor, since clotting was a serious problem. In the early 1900s the blood vessels of the donor and recipient were either stitched together or joined by a metal tube. Such methods took time and needed great skill, and any measurement of the quantity of blood transfused was impossible. The next step had actually taken place in the same year (1901) as Landsteiner's discovery, when Jules Bordet and Octave Gengou coated the inside of the syringes, tubing and other apparatus with paraffin wax and so were able to prevent clotting for a limited time[9]. This was a marked improvement, although it was still necessary to undertake the procedure as a carefully planned operation, under ideal conditions, with the patient and donor in the same room. The next few years saw scientists searching for some way of preserving blood for prolonged periods. The answer came in 1914, when three different workers discovered the same method quite independently. Albert Hustin[10], of Brussels, prevented clot formation by adding sodium citrate and dextrose solution to freshly drawn blood, and the first transfusions of this citrated blood were given by Richard Lewisohn, of New York[11], and by Luis Agote, of Buenos Aires[12]. So, at the beginning of World War I, all the necessary requirements for a satisfactory blood transfusion service were available; yet, because of failure to appreciate how large was the volume of blood lost in serious trauma, nearly a quarter of a century was to pass before blood transfusion became a routine procedure in medicine and surgery.

Two physicians at the Middlesex Hospital, London, in 1935 provided an outstanding contribution to the method of administration. Hugh Leslie Marriott and Alan Kekwick treated a patient who was bleeding severely from a peptic ulcer, with a continuous blood transfusion by a blood drip[13]. In this the blood drips from the reservoir bottle through rubber tubing and into the needle in the patient's vein. In the dependent part of the tubing is a glass cylinder where the blood can be seen dripping through. It is thus possible to regulate the rate of flow with a clamp on the tube. The whole transfusion kit now comes in disposable plastic form.

The second great contribution of the 1930s was the tentative steps taken towards the foundation of blood banks. In 1933 Sergei Sergeivitch Yudin, of Moscow, organized stores of blood that had been removed from fresh corpses[14]. There is nothing medically wrong about this and it was used in Yudin's hospital where blood was withdrawn up to six hours after death and stored for a month, but most people find something rather unethical in the practice. In 1937 Bernard Fantus, of Chicago, introduced blood banks that made use of living donors as the source of supply[15]; but the real development of these banks had to wait until the urgent crisis of World War II forced surgeons to acknowledge their extreme value.

Landsteiner, meanwhile, had emigrated to America and was working at the Rockefeller Institute where in 1940, together with Alexander Wiener, he discovered another important blood group called the Rhesus or Rh group, so named after the rhesus monkeys used in the experiments[16]. About 85 percent of human beings are Rhesus positive, the other 15 percent being Rhesus negative. In more recent years many other subgroups and new group systems have been discovered; since they may occasionally have importance in transfusion, their appearance has led to refinements in the technique of cross-matching blood.

The fluid part of citrated blood, after the red cells have settled, is known as plasma, and this holds a prominent place among the substances used for transfusion. It is not a substitute for whole blood, but it has the great advantage that it can be dried and stored for a much longer period. Hence it is more portable than blood and also does not require cross-matching; before use it is reconstituted to a fluid. Its value is greatest in cases of burns and shock and other emergencies, when it will restore the blood volume and maintain a satisfactory situation until blood becomes available.

The body chemistry and fluid balance are also of great importance, as these can be seriously disturbed in a number of surgical diseases and as a result of operation. Water is easily lost from the body tissues and in the 1820s, in a cholera epidemic, the infusion of saline solution into the veins had been used to combat the severe dehydration occurring in this disease. At the end of the century Arbuthnot Lane was one of the first to employ saline solution, given by a syringe into the veins, to counteract shock and dehydration following surgery[17]. The most practical method in use at this time was a drip, invented by John Benjamin Murphy, through which a regulated amount of saline solution could be run into the rectum[18]. Rudolph Matas, of New Orleans, was also interested in the possibilities of intravenous infusions[19], but when large quantities were given toxic reactions were prone to occur, probably due to the presence of pyrogens (fever-inducing contaminants). In 1924 he overcame the problem by giving the saline solution slowly through a continuous intravenous drip, though contact of the solution with the rubber of the tubes could still be responsible for reactions.

Intestinal obstruction is a condition presenting a problem intimately connected with the fluid balance of the body. In addition to actual disease, a form of obstruction may occur after operation (especially abdominal) in which the gut is paralysed. This is known as paralytic ileus. When the stomach is affected, the condition of acute dilatation of the stomach occurs. These postoperative effects were often the cause of death in the past and they excited much interest. When it was found that large quantities of water and salt poured into the

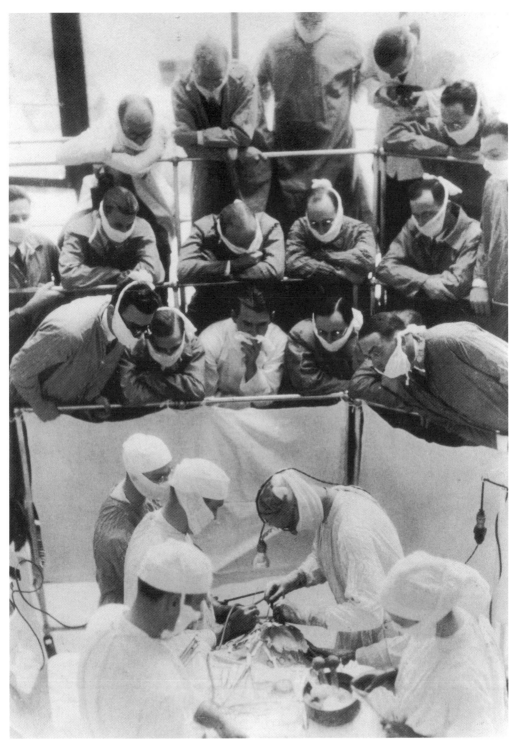

Harvey Cushing operating before the Harvey Cushing Society in 1932. (By courtesy of the Harvard Medical Library in the Frances A. Countway Library of Medicine.)

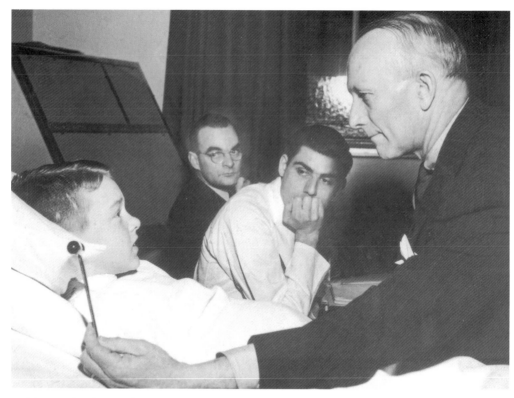

Wilder Penfield in 1947 examining a patient at the Montreal Neurological Institute. (By courtesy of Dr Wilder Penfield and Canada Wide Features.)

X-ray of a total hip replacement.

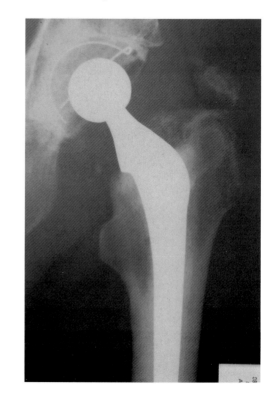

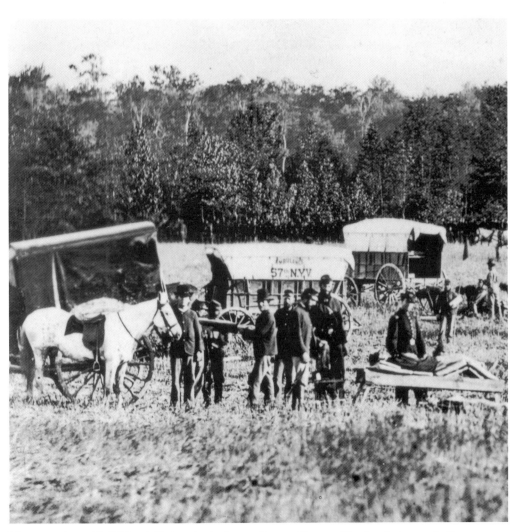

The American Civil War: A Union Ambulance Corps. (From a Brady photograph. By courtesy of the National Library of Medicine, Bethesda, Maryland.)

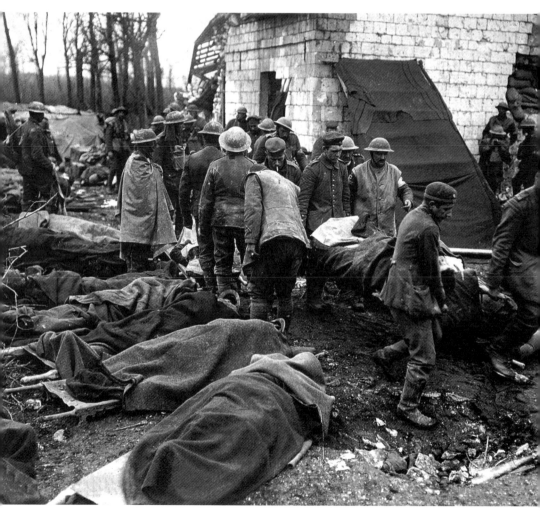

World War I: Collecting the wounded. (By courtesy of the Wellcome Library, London.)

Opposite page: The Carrel-Dakin treatment of wounds. Case 606: A large wound of the forearm showing the irrigating tubes in place (a); wound closed on the sixth day (b). Case 577: Wound of the knee with irrigating tubes in place (c); wound sutured on the four-teenth day (d). (From: Carrel A, Dehelly G. (1917). Reference 30, chapter 19.)

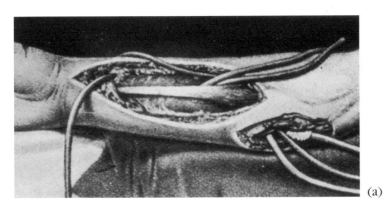

(a)

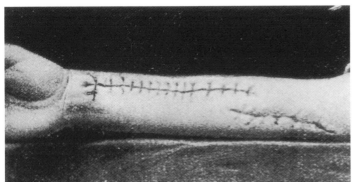

(b)

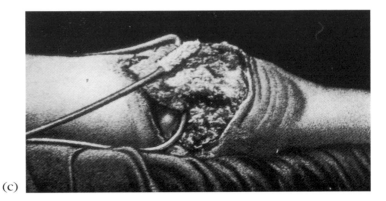

(c)

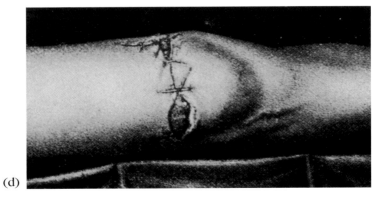

(d)

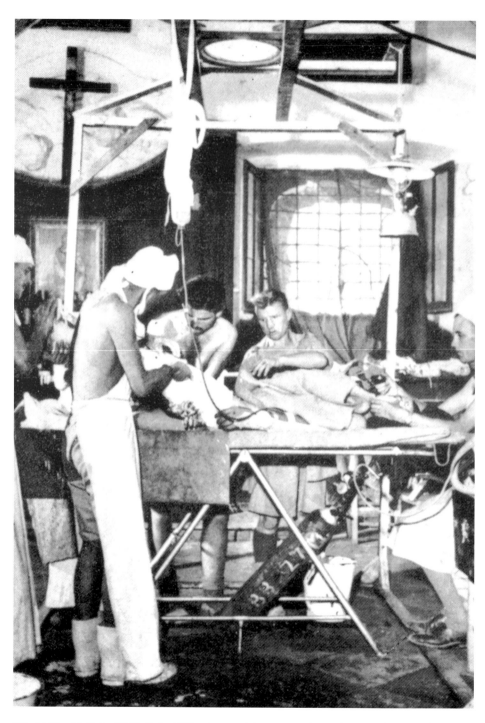

World War II: Italy, 1943. It is difficult to achieve asepsis under conditions of war. In a temporary operating theatre in a church, a British surgical team treats a soldier with a wounded leg. Note the plasma drip.

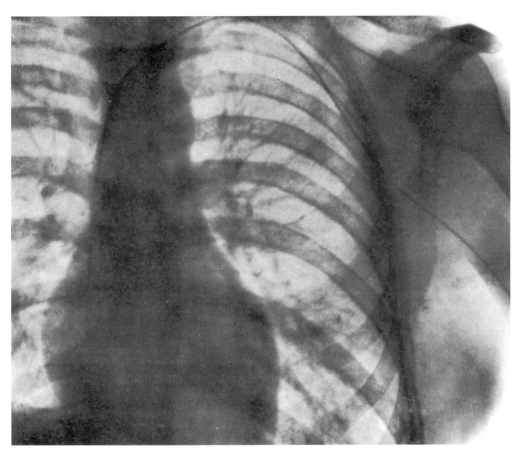

The x-ray taken by Werner Forssmann after he had passed a ureteric catheter up a vein in his arm into the right side of his heart. (From: Forssmann W. (1929). Reference 36, chapter 23.)

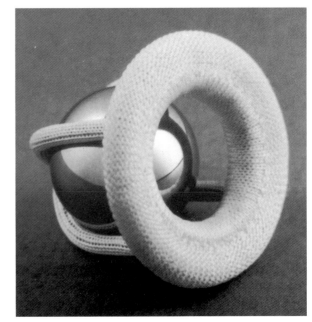

A cloth-covered Starr-Edwards mitral valve. (Photograph kindly lent by Dr Albert Starr.)

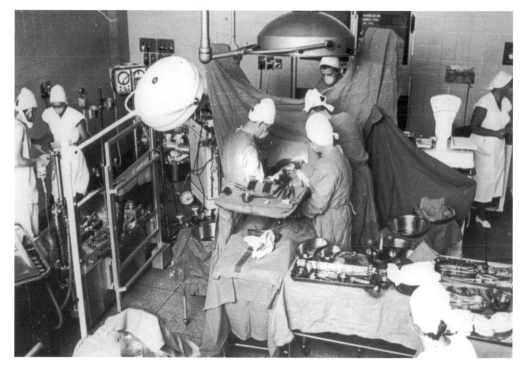

The operating theatre at Groote Schuur Hospital, Cape Town, in which the world's first human cardiac homotransplantation was carried out on December 3, 1967. (This photograph of an open-heart operation was taken the following day.) (Photo: Associated Press.)

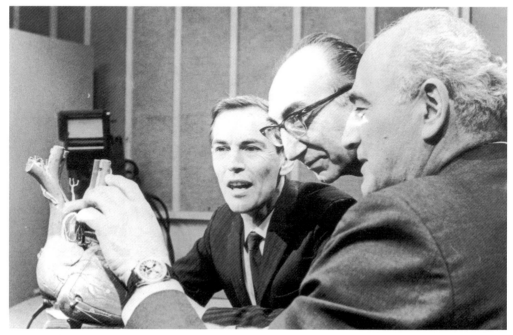

Christiaan Barnard (*left*), Michael De Bakey (*centre*) and Adrian Kantrowitz (*right*) discussing a model of the heart before giving a television interview in the USA on December 27, 1967. (Photo: United Press International (U.K.) Ltd.)

distended and paralysed gut, it became evident that this state of affairs must be set to rights if the patient was to recover. In 1920 John Ryle had been working on methods of passing tubes into the stomach[20], and the little rubber tube that bears his name is familiar to many who have had their stomach contents removed in this way. However, it was not until 1932 that Owen Hardy Wangensteen advocated intestinal decompression in cases of intestinal obstruction[21], and in 1934 Thomas Grier Miller and William Osler Abbott invented a tube with an inflatable balloon on the end that could be passed (with a fair degree of luck) through the stomach and into the small intestine[22]. The principle of treatment was to pass such a tube into the gut and apply continuous suction, by means of a suction pump, so that all the fluid would be withdrawn and the intestines thus left at rest until their normal function returned. The second half of the treatment was to replace the fluid lost, together with the normal requirement of the body, by intravenous saline infusion. At the end of the 1930s this method of suction and transfusion had dramatically improved the outcome for patients with intestinal obstruction.

Improvements in technique were hammered home to the surgical profession in the fight to prevent shock and infection; anaesthesia was improving out of all recognition and at the end of the inter-war period the discovery of the sulphonamides heralded a completely new era in the control of disease[23, 24, 25]. The progress achieved between the two world wars may not have been so spectacular as the extensive advances of the preceding half-century, but it was no less dramatic in the results obtained. Surgery had now become a safer undertaking, and the care of the patient before, during and after operation enabled more extensive operations to be withstood. The surgeon was having to call upon more and more specialized and technical assistants, and his position had become that of a leader of a highly integrated team. The flood of operative advances had been stemmed and this allowed the implications of disease and of surgical operation to be further appreciated. The pause was of vital necessity to the welfare of the patient and to the future success of surgery. The position had now been consolidated and all was ready for further progress towards the achievement that is modern surgery.

21

The last frontier

Chest surgery is dependent upon so many important considerations other than pure operative skill that successful intrusion into this body cavity lagged far behind achievements elsewhere. The physiology of respiration is extremely complex and had to be understood before any serious advance could be contemplated. The effect of opening the chest and letting air into the pleural cavity profoundly alters the mechanics of respiration, the immediate effect causing the lung on that side to collapse; there is also a variable degree of collapse of the opposite lung. If the hole is immediately closed, the lung will gradually re-expand as the air is absorbed by the body or removed by the surgeon. If the hole is big enough and remains open, air moves backwards and forwards from one lung to the other (paradoxical respiration) instead of from lungs to outside atmosphere; and the heart, great vessels, and other structures lying between the two lungs and known as the mediastinum, will flutter with the movements of breathing. The patient rapidly dies unless steps are taken to close the hole and remove the air. Should the hole into the pleural cavity act as a valve letting air in, but not out, the pressure inside the chest increases until respiration becomes impossible. When air is present in the pleural cavity, the state is known as pneumothorax and the two dangerous varieties are called open pneumothorax and tension pneumothorax, respectively.

These brief descriptions are necessary because a closed pneumothorax is used to collapse the lung in the treatment of tuberculosis; an open pneumothorax is created when the surgeon operates, and a tension pneumothorax develops if the ligature slips off the cut end of a bronchus (branch of the windpipe to the lung) after removal of a lung; it also occurs in certain wounds. The way in which these problems, and other difficulties facing the surgeon, were overcome will be considered as the development of chest surgery is unfolded.

Before doing so, however, it is advisable to digress for a moment and describe the anatomical arrangements of the lungs and pleura, otherwise an appreciation of the evolution of thoracic surgery will be rather difficult. First of all, imagine a deflated balloon that has no outlet, then make a fist of the left hand and push this into the outside of the balloon so that the fist is completely surrounded by two layers of balloon except at the wrist. Over the fist and two layers of balloon lay the open right hand. The left fist now represents the lung; and the wrist, the bronchus and blood vessels entering the lung. The two layers of balloon are the pleura; the space between them, which is potential not real, is the pleural cavity; these two layers are lubricated and enable the lung to move smoothly during respiration. The open right hand is the chest wall. If a hole is made through the chest wall and into the pleura, the pressures inside the chest are such that the pleural cavity inflates and becomes a real cavity, and the lung collapses. If, first of all, the two layers of balloon can be made to stick together (pleural adhesions) and the hole made through this stuck-down area, air will not get into the rest of the cavity. At one stage in the development of chest surgery this principle was adopted, but was later rendered unnecessary by improved methods of anaesthesia which controlled the pressure within the chest.

Until 1914 chest surgery really consisted of operations on the chest wall and the drainage of empyema (pus in the pleural cavity); then attention centred on the operative treatment of bronchiectasis (suppuration within the lung) and lung abscesses. It was not until the 1930s that the problems of surgery inside the chest became better understood and marked progress could be made. Nevertheless, the first attempts to deal with lung diseases had been made long before the ideal conditions for operation were discovered. Injuries to the chest are common in war, and although the lethal nature of an open pneumothorax has been appreciated since the days of the ancient Greeks, surgeons did not attempt to close the hole until the Middle Ages. Their enthusiasm was short lived and, except for a most successful awakening of interest during the Napoleonic Wars, a mist of forgetfulness descended. It was only in World War I that surgeons really consolidated the procedure of converting an open pneumothorax into a closed one by firm bandaging or by stitching the wound edges together.

The two chest diseases causing most concern at the end of the 19th century were empyema and tuberculosis, and in both the physician had a greater interest than the surgeon; the early operative procedures were therefore of a minor degree and guided, if not actually performed, by the physicians. In 1872 Louis Jules Béhier used capillary tubes to drain off collections of fluid in the pleural cavity[1], a slow method unsuited to the removal of thick pus. A year later, Henry Ingersoll Bowditch of Boston had operated two hundred and seventy times for empyema and had had no deaths[2]. However, all he did was to make an incision low down in the back to release the pus. But between 1877 and 1879, Max Schede of Bonn resected ribs: 'In more than one case (not children) I resected as many as 9 ribs, even going back beneath the scapula; and when this failed, I resected them still further, and once again still further. When the enormously thickened pleura fails to fall in, it is, then, the pleura that you must remove: this I thought out for myself in 1878, and I have now (1890) done this operation 10 times.'[3]

In 1879 Jakob August Estlander treated old-standing empyemas also by the removal of ribs[4], but the real achievement came three years later when Arbuthnot Lane realized that the clue to success lay in the free evacuation of pus, and to achieve this he also removed some ribs[5]. He was not concerned with long-standing empyemas, and his patients were all children with early disease in whom pleural adhesions had probably formed round the pus, so enabling open operation to be performed satisfactorily. In the years that followed, Lane's method was adapted for older children and adults. Another very important contribution to the treatment of empyema and one that was to become indispensable whenever it was necessary to drain fluid from the chest, was made in 1876 by Gotthard Bülau, a physician in Hamburg, who introduced subaqueous drainage[6]. In this a drainage tube from the chest is carried below the level of water in a bottle under the bed, thus preventing air from entering the pleural cavity. Bülau was well aware of the dangers of open pneumothorax, and so much emphasis did he put upon them that for a number of years surgeons were reluctant to attempt any form of chest operation.

The underlying principle in the treatment of tuberculosis is rest, complete, uninterrupted and prolonged – the problem was how to apply this principle to the lungs, which were perpetually on the move during respiration. But the solution had already been reached. In 1821 James Carson, a Liverpool physician, had noted the favourable effect that a spontaneous pneumothorax sometimes had on the progress of pulmonary tuberculosis; he accordingly suggested that a pneumothorax should be produced to collapse the lung and so assist in the healing of tubercular cavities[7]. Another physician, William Stokes of Dublin, came up with the same idea a few years later[8]. The next time an artificial pneumothorax was suggested was in 1882 and by yet another physician, Carlo Forlanini[9]. But at last, with the confidence provided by the successful removal of ribs for empyema, the message reached the surgical world. In 1885 Edouard de Cerenville of Lausanne reported that he had removed a number of ribs to allow the chest wall to fall in and so collapse the underlying lung[10]. Nevertheless, it was not until ten years later that J. Gourdet, in his thesis, stated the principles upon which the operation was based[11].

In the opening years of the 20th century, Ludolph Brauer drew attention to the importance of leaving the periosteum of the ribs intact, thus allowing the bone to regenerate and preserve the stability of the chest wall; he also stressed the fact that the number of ribs that were removed should be adequate to ensure collapse of the diseased lung[12]. At first this extensive rib removal had unfortunate results, since patients usually fell into the surgeon's hands when their tuberculosis was widespread. Because of the number of ribs that had to be removed, the pressures within the two sides of the chest became deranged after surgery, and mediastinal flutter sometimes developed. When early diagnosis became possible it was usually sufficient to remove part of only two or three ribs and the pressures were not then disturbed. If, for any reason, a large number of ribs had to be removed, the performance of the procedure in stages enabled the body to adapt itself gradually.

Interference with the function of the phrenic nerve, the motor nerve to the diaphragm, is another form of collapse therapy. For this, a small incision is made in the neck under local anaesthesia and the phrenic nerve is either cut or gently crushed. The result of either manoeuvre is for the affected side of the diaphragm to rise into the chest and compress the lung. Cutting the nerve, which completely paralysed the diaphragm, was first used by Ferdinand Sauerbruch in 1905 for animal experiments[13], and in 1911 Carl Adolph Ernst Stürtz suggested its therapeutic value[14]. Four years later Paul Friedrich introduced the method of crushing as opposed to cutting[15]. With this the paralysis was only temporary and was useful in some cases of tubercular cavities in the lower lobe; it was also sometimes performed after removal of a lung to help fill in the space that was left behind. This simple and safe operation enjoyed enormous popularity before receding into virtual obscurity with the arrival of chemotherapy.

Operations on the lung to remove localized tuberculosis got away to a bad start. The first occasion, in 1883, was a tragedy. The surgeon was a German by the name of Block, and the patient a young female relative who was supposed to have tuberculosis in the upper part of both lungs. She died on the table and the postmortem examination showed that she had not, after all, been suffering from tuberculosis. The distraught surgeon committed suicide. In 1891 Theodore Tuffier, of Paris, successfully removed the apex of a lung for tuberculosis[16] but, as we have seen, lung surgery of any description was advancing very slowly and was only performed on isolated occasions. Such reports as did appear were poorly documented, though it is of interest that one of these came from Macewen of Glasgow[17]. He is reputed to have removed a whole lung in stages, but doubt has been cast on the exact nature of the operation.

The events that were to form the main channel of progress were beginning to take shape at the start of the 20th century. Mikulicz was interested in the surgery of the alimentary canal. He had done much pioneer work inside the abdomen and was most anxious to add to his series by devising a satisfactory operation for cancer of the oesophagus. Although in 1886 he had removed a cancer from the upper part in the neck and restored continuity with a skin flap[18], he was still searching for a method that would prevent the lungs from collapsing when the chest was opened, a necessary manoeuvre to expose the lower part of the oesophagus. He was fortunate in having as his assistant Ferdinand Sauerbruch, who was to become the leading European exponent of thoracic surgery. Sauerbruch initially tried to keep the lung inflated by the use of a close fitting anaesthetic face mask but, apart from other difficulties, the technique had the disadvantages of inflating the stomach and preventing the removal of secretions from the respiratory tract[19]. In 1904 he tried a more physiological approach and encased the patient and the operating team in a large cabinet with their heads outside. A negative pressure was maintained in the cabinet, so that the normal conditions of pressure existing in the pleural cavity were unaltered when the chest was opened. This was a marvellous conception and ideal in theory. In practice it was far too complex and unsuited to operative work, in spite of giving the surgeon a degree of confidence he might not otherwise have felt. The patient could not be moved and the heat inside was oppressive, but though it went out of fashion for surgery, it was later re-introduced in a well-known form as the iron lung for treating patients with respiratory paralysis.

Meanwhile, work was proceeding on an aspect of anaesthesia that was to have the very greatest significance. The introduction of a tube into the trachea to keep respiration going can be traced back to the 16th century, when it was used for anatomy demonstrations on animals, but its adoption into anaesthesia naturally had to wait until there was such a thing as an anaesthetic. In 1871, Friedrich Trendelenburg devised a tube that could be inserted into the trachea through an incision made in the neck. The tube had an inflatable cuff on its inner end to make it fit snugly into the trachea, and to its outer end was attached a gauze mask which enabled a satisfactory anaesthetic to be given while the surgeon was operating on the upper respiratory tract[20]. He had no fear that blood would be inhaled or that his operative procedure would temporarily block the airway. Our versatile friend Macewen was responsible for the next major advance when, in 1878, he invented a flexible brass tube that was passed into the trachea through the mouth by sense of touch[21], a feat demanding considerable dexterity in the conscious patient. The patient's splutterings were soon controlled by the chloroform.

In the last decade of the 19th century surgeons in America were working independently on methods of giving anaesthetics directly into the trachea. In 1899 Rudolph Matas adapted the Fell-O'Dwyer apparatus for the purpose[22]. This apparatus was a form of endotracheal tube, devised by Joseph O'Dwyer[23], combined with George Edward Fell's bellows[24], and had been used for artificial respiration. The positive pressure produced would keep the lungs inflated when the chest was opened. An important feature of these positive pressure methods was the inflatable cuff round the tube, which had been further developed by Tuffier in 1895[25]. In the same year Kirstein introduced the laryngoscope[26] and this enabled the endotracheal tube to be passed through the mouth under direct vision. In the first decade of the 20th century Franz Kuhn emphasized that the tube must be wide enough to allow easy expiration as well as inspiration, and in 1902 he showed how the tube could be passed through the nose[27]. He also introduced the use of cocaine as a local anaesthetic[27] prior to intubation which reduced the gagging and coughing.

The next stage in the proceedings was the introduction of insufflation intratracheal anaesthesia by Barthélemy and Dufour in 1907[28]. This differed from inhalation endotracheal anaesthesia in that a thin tube was passed down to the bifurcation of the trachea (the point where the trachea divides into the two main bronchi to the lungs). The anaesthetic gas was delivered to the lungs under pressure by squeezing a hand bulb, and expiration took place back up the trachea round the outside of the tube. Franz Volhard, in 1908, drew attention to the fact that the delivery of gas must be rhythmical to allow carbon dioxide to be eliminated from the lungs[29]. A year later a notable paper was published by Samuel James Meltzer and John Auer, of the Rockefeller Institute, in which they reported their finding that respiration could be maintained in an experimental animal breathing air under pressure, without any respiratory movements on the part of the animal[30]. The principle underlying their work was then introduced into clinical practice by Charles Elsberg in 1910[31]. Insufflation anaesthesia under pressure meant that the respiratory exchange of gases could take place without the normal respiratory movements that had previously hampered the surgeon; unfortunately, it also meant that the lungs were distended, not an ideal feature, and that the effective elimination of carbon dioxide was interfered with. This form of anaesthesia was little used before World War I, largely because there were few surgeons prepared to run the risks of chest surgery.

After World War I, Ivan Magill and E. S. Rowbotham were working at Harold Gillies's plastic-surgery hospital using the insufflation intratracheal technique[32]. After trying out various modifications, they returned to the inhalation endotracheal method as being a better and more physiological procedure, with the patient breathing in and out through a wide-bore tube. This gave rise to fewer postoperative complications in the lungs. In 1936 Magill introduced the method of intermittent suction through a catheter lying in the endotracheal tube for removing secretions in the air passages[33]. As with many innovations, patients were at first intubated to excess, but the practice settled down to be used only for certain definite indications. In 1932 Ralph Milton Waters of Wisconsin intro-duced one-lung anaesthesia in which a tube with an inflatable cuff was passed into the bronchus of the healthy lung, thus excluding the diseased lung from any responsibility in respiration[34]. This technique was particularly applicable when the diseased lung was producing a large amount of secretion that could not be controlled.

These advances still did not solve the problem of the actual administration of the anaesthetic, and it was not until 1938 that the answer was seen to lie in some form of artificial respiration. To meet the needs Clarence Crafoord introduced a machine to control the breathing[35], and in 1941 Michael Denis Nosworthy achieved the same effect by intermittent pressure with his own hand on the anaesthetic bag[36]. This permitted respiration to be assisted or controlled with greater accuracy; moreover the pressure could be adjusted to counteract possible mediastinal movement, and to meet the wishes of the surgeon more readily. Initially drugs were used that depressed the control of respiration by the patient's brain, but when the muscle-relaxant drugs were introduced it was possible to produce complete paralysis of the respiratory movements[37], so giving the anaesthetist complete control, should this be desired.

The notions about open pneumothorax had become rather confused before World War I; experiments on animals had strengthened the fear of opening the chest, as their mediastina are less stable and thus more liable to flutter. Then, during the war years, the pendulum had swung, for a short time, violently in the other direction. The necessity for operating on chest injuries had produced the belief that the human mediastinum was more rigid than in fact it is. This led to a relaxation of the precautions to prevent both lungs from collapsing when only one side of the chest was opened. The error was, fortunately, soon appreciated.

In the 1920s physicians partially overcame their horror of surgery in tuberculous patients, thanks to the advances in anaesthetic technique and in diagnostic methods. Jean Athanese Sicard and Jacques Forestier, in 1922, introduced an oily iodine substance, lipiodol, for bronchography[38], having previously used it for x-rays of the nervous system[39]. By this method the outline of the air passages in the lungs could be seen on the x-ray.

Collapse therapy for tuberculosis now became popular again with an alternative procedure being devised to overcome the dangers of excessive rib removal and also to reduce the consequent deformity. The chest was opened and the upper part of the lung and pleura mobilized by dissection to allow the lung to collapse right away from the chest wall. This left a cavity in the top of one side of the chest which was filled with substances such as fatty tissue or paraffin and the chest then closed. The operation was performed with varying degrees of success and safety up to 1932, but with the arrival of antibiotics the operation was reintroduced using plastic substances, such as lucite balls which are like ping-pong balls, to fill the cavity. The antibiotic cover meant that the surgeon was able to leave foreign material in the chest without courting disaster. However, the outcome of more extensive operations on the lungs themselves was nearly always lethal because of failure to get hold of the patient before his disease had progressed to unwelcome extremes. Also, no satisfactory method of closure of the bronchus had been developed, and frequently a fatal tension pneumothorax would result from leakage from the bronchial stump. The high mortality discouraged other doctors from sending their patients to the surgeon, or only when the disease was far advanced, thus setting in motion a vicious circle. In one or two cases in which success had been achieved it was found that the pleurae were stuck together. Surgeons therefore concluded that if they could produce artificial pleural adhesions before operating on the lung, all would be well and, in addition, if the curse of bronchial leakage did occur, the air and secretions could be removed without involving the pleural cavity.

In 1923 Evarts Graham introduced an operation along these lines. He opened the chest wall by removing several ribs and, if the pleurae were not adherent, he placed some irritant iodoform gauze over the area and left it there until adhesions had formed. Then with a red-hot soldering iron he burnt round the diseased area of lung – 'all but the first stage may be accomplished without anaesthesia of any kind'. Further cauterizations were carried out at intervals until all diseased lung had been removed[40]. Graham eventually performed this operation on fifty-four patients, thirty-six of whom were reasonably improved and six of whom died. Wyman Whittemore of Boston used a different technique in which he sutured the diseased lobe of the lung to the chest wall leaving a piece about the size of an orange protruding; in about four weeks this died and fell off[41]. He used the procedure on five patients with two making complete recoveries, a boy of four and a man of forty-eight. These operations remained popular for bronchiectasis and suppuration until 1929.

A third type of operation carried out on the lung was lobectomy, performed in stages. The first stage, which often required more than one operation, was the production of pleural adhesions. The lobe of lung was removed at a later date – a lobe is an anatomically defined part of a lung, being roughly a half or a third, depending on the side of the chest; blood vessels, nerves and a branch of the trachea constitute the pedicle which passes into a lobe. After the lobe had been thoroughly freed, the pedicle was surrounded by an elastic tube, pulled tight and the lobe left to die; or a mass ligature was applied and the lobe cut off at once. The advantage of this wholesale ligation was its speed, an essential factor when anaesthesia was imperfect and the patient might quite easily drown in his own secretions. The fear of infection also favoured the method. Lobectomies were at this time mainly carried out for bronchiectasis and lung abscess, and the mortality rate varied between 10 and 70 percent depending on the severity and extent of the disease and upon the individual surgeon. In fact so hopeless did the procedure appear that by the end of the 1920s it had been practically abandoned. But in 1929 a ray of hope emerged from San Francisco, where Harold Brunn had performed five lobectomies for bronchiectasis and one for cancer with only one death. He had not gone through the troublesome rigmarole of creating adhesions, but had removed the lobe at a single operation. His first patient, a man of twenty-six, had been operated on in January, 1918. Brunn employed local anaesthesia with pre-medication, adding gas and oxygen under positive pressure while he was testing the security of the bronchial pedicle under salt solution[42]. The secret of his success lay in the institution of suction every two hours for five days after operation to carry off any air and secretions, and so allow the remainder of the lung to expand satisfactorily and fill the space.

Brunn's paper did much to revive interest in the possibilities of chest surgery, and in 1931 surgeons were contemplating removing the whole of one lung. This was first done by Rudolf Nissen, then of Berlin, on a twelve-year-old girl who had been run over. She developed an empyema on the left side which was drained, but over the next few months signs of chronic pulmonary suppuration developed and bronchiectasis of the entire left lung was evident. Her general condition was bad, but in view of the hopeless conservative prognosis Nissen decided to remove the lung. During the operation she collapsed and so Nissen simply packed the whole operation area with gauze. Fourteen days later he removed the lung. The chief fear was over the ligation of the main branch of the pulmonary artery which carries blood from the heart to the lung. It was quite possible that this necessary procedure might be lethal. The effect of the loss of one lung upon respiratory function was not a problem, but there was some doubt as to the future of the large space that would be left. None of the feared complications developed, and the space became filled by the diaphragm rising up, the mediastinum partly moving across, and by the chest wall contracting inwards[43].

In 1932 Norman Shenstone introduced a technique for tying off the bronchus and blood vessels of the lobe. It consisted of leaving a pedicle three-quarters of an inch long which was divided between loops of heavy cord applied by means of modified tonsillar snares. The area was drained simply and then, after the first twenty-four hours, this was changed to continuous siphon drainage[44]. The technique made the operation easier and quicker and was therefore adopted quite extensively, but it had the disadvantage of leaving more tissue behind in the bronchial stump and so was unsuited to the extensive removal required for cancer. More significant still was the fact that, because of its ease of use, it delayed the advance of the dissection method that was destined to become the accepted procedure.

Cancer of the lung was not a major surgical problem at this period of history. The disease was less common than today and diagnosis was rarely made soon enough for surgery to be effective. In addition, the very nature of the operations then in use, with their prolonged preliminary stages, rendered them thoroughly unsuitable for a rapidly progressing disease. But although operations for lung cancer were few and far between, as far back as 1913 Morriston Davies had removed a lower lobe for cancer, and had actually dissected out each structure entering the lobe and ligated it separately[45]. His patient, a man of forty-four, was in a good condition for six days but then developed empyema and died on the eighth day. In 1929 Arthur Tudor Edwards, who may justly be considered the founder of British thoracic surgery, performed a similar operation[46].

The third successful operation for cancer was the occasion of the first removal of a whole lung; it was performed by Evarts Graham and Jacob Jesse Singer on April 5, 1933. A lobectomy had been planned, but at operation it was found that the disease had spread and that a pneumonectomy was therefore necessary. Graham did the operation in one stage, ligating all the hilus, except for the pulmonary artery, with catgut. The artery he ligated separately since he had no knowledge of Nissen's case and was seriously concerned about the effect of ligation. He inserted seven radon seeds into the stump (a form of local irradiation) and also transfused 500cc of blood[47]. As he was afraid of leaving so large a space, he removed the third to ninth ribs to ensure that the chest wall would fall in. The bronchus started to leak a short time later and caused a small empyema which necessitated removal of the first two ribs. The patient was a forty-eight-year-old doctor, and when told the nature of his illness and had agreed to an operation, he went home for a day or two to set his affairs in order. He had his teeth seen to, a nice gesture of confidence, but he also bought himself a plot in a cemetery. The plot was not required. He was able to carry on a busy practice and was still alive in 1957, the year that Graham himself died at the age of seventy-three, ironically a victim of lung cancer.

A few months later on July 24 of the same year (1933) William Francis Rienhoff of Johns Hopkins University performed a planned pneumonectomy on a three-and-a-half-year-old child for a benign tumour of the left primary bronchus. He was the first surgeon to enter the mediastinal pleura, carefully dissecting out all the vessels to the lung and ligating them separately. When he had removed the lung he closed the bronchus with a number of individual sutures and then covered the stump with a layer of pleura. He did not institute drainage and did not perform a thoracoplasty. There were no postoperative complications and the bronchial stump healed without trouble[48]. Although leakage from the stump was still a possible complication, Rienhoff solved this very difficult problem by his method of dissection and individual ligating. In the years that followed he improved on his technique for closing the bronchial stump[49].

Prior to 1930 the choice of anaesthetics for chest surgery had lain between ether and nitrous oxide, or both, combined with oxygen; then, in that year, Ralph Waters started work on cyclopropane which was introduced into anaesthetic practice in 1933[50]. It is a very explosive gas and liable to produce irregularities of the heartbeat, yet it was used quite extensively because it can be mixed with a high percentage of oxygen. It was particularly suited to chest surgery, since lung movements can be reduced to a minimum and the poor muscular relaxation it produces is not of great moment. In 1934 John Lundy of the Mayo Clinic initiated the use of Pentothal (a barbiturate drug) for intravenous anaesthesia[51], thus bringing to a climax a long series of trials by many workers to find a suitable intravenous drug. This makes the anaesthetist's task much easier and, from the patient's point of view, it does away with the need for starting the anaesthetic under a mask, although inhalation anaesthesia is used once he is unconscious.

For many centuries curare has been used by South American Indians to tip their arrowheads; the victim dies from paralysis of the muscles of respiration. In 1595 Sir Walter Raleigh brought the drug to Europe, but it was not until the 19th century that the great French physiologist Claude Bernard studied its properties[52]. Then, in 1942, Harold Griffith and Enid Johnson of Montreal produced muscular paralysis by the injection of a purified preparation of the drug[37]. Curare proved to be of great benefit to both surgeon and anaesthetist, since profound relaxation could be produced by its injection while the patient was under the anaesthetic. Since 1942 a number of preparations, with two main differing modes of action, have been introduced for this purpose.

The progress of anaesthesia and the advance in chest surgery came at an appropriate time since in the 1930s the incidence of cancer of the lung increased. (In the 1970s it began to decline in men, though not in women.) As if to compensate, bronchiectasis and lung abscesses are less common and no longer occur in the severe form of earlier years. The same was true of tuberculosis, with campaigns like mass radiography bringing the patients under medical care at an early stage. In 1943 Richard H. Overholt revived interest in the possibilities of lobectomy for tuberculosis by an improved technique and by using nerve block with local anaesthetic infiltration rather than general anaesthesia[53] – and, as it happened, the timing could not have been more opportune, since shortly afterwards the antibiotics came into their own. The first of value for tuberculosis was streptomycin, to be followed by para-aminosalicylic acid (PAS) and isoniazid. By using these drugs in planned combinations tuberculosis could be brought under control and the bronchi rendered reasonably healthy before operation. After operation they prevented the complications of spread or flare-up of the disease. In 1939 E. D. Churchill had drawn attention to the important fact that the segment, and not the lobe, was the anatomical unit within the lungs[54]. This meant that the smaller segment could be removed if the particular disease was limited in extent, thus saving the patient from a bigger operation and preserving healthy lung tissue. Regrettably, for various reasons such as poverty, malnutrition, HIV/AIDS and drug resistance, tuberculosis is once again becoming a problem.

Operations on the upper part of the stomach or the lower oesophagus demand a wide exposure in which both chest and abdomen are opened – the thoraco-abdominal approach. This was used by Martin Kirschner in 1920[55] but, because he was in the right place at the right time, credit for its introduction into modern surgery goes to a Japanese surgeon, T. Ohsawa who, in the early 1930s, reported his results of operating on cancer of the oesophagus and upper stomach by this route[56, 57]. The first successful removal of the oesophagus for cancer had, however, been performed by Arthur Evans in 1909 on a woman with a growth involving the cervical and upper part of the thoracic oesophagus, a stubborn site[58]. The patient was known to be still alive twenty-three years later[59]. This achievement, by another of those strange quirks of history, has been overshadowed by the operation of Franz Torek, an American, on a woman of sixty-seven on March 14, 1913. (He even entitled his paper 'The first successful case....') He had created a gastrostomy some time previous to the main operation at which he removed most of the thoracic oesophagus, leaving the upper end in a hole in the neck connected by a rubber tube to the gastrostomy. A hot coffee enema with whisky and strychnine was given at the end of the operation, which had lasted one hour and forty-five minutes[60]. The patient survived for eleven years. Torek certainly had the courage of his convictions as, at this time, Sauerbruch had been advising that cancer of the mid-thoracic region should be left untouched owing to its inaccessibility behind the arch of the aorta and to the danger of damage to the vagus nerves. The method was later modified by the use of grafts of small intestine running beneath the skin of the chest wall, but the procedure temporarily went out of fashion when an extensive operation carried out through the thoraco-abdominal approach was introduced. In this the stomach is mobilized and carried up through the chest to be joined to the pharynx or to the upper end of the oesophagus in the neck. The feat was shown to be possible on May 8, 1943, by John Garlock of New York[61].

The last anatomical frontier had thus been crossed and the surgeon was now able to operate successfully on structures lying within the chest. There remains, however, one most important organ still to be mentioned. Surgery of the heart has a surprisingly long history which was gathering momentum in the late 1930s but, owing to a second world conflict, its further progress was delayed for six years.

22

More in a military vein

The curtain raiser to World War II was the Spanish Civil War. If the years of peace had led to considerable advance in the practice of surgery, so also had they produced vastly improved methods of destruction. The internal strife in Spain provided a suitable opportunity for countries with militaristic aspirations to experiment without fear of national failure or repercussion, and the consequent bloody slaughter provided surgeons with plenty of material upon which to exercise their skill. At the beginning of the war the Carrel-Dakin system of wound irrigation was used, but was not attended by the same degree of success as in World War I. Conditions were different and those peculiar to this civil war made possible a simpler line of treatment.

Generally speaking, the casualties were picked off the streets and hurried to hospital without the delay that was unavoidable in a full-scale war. This gave surgeons a chance to operate before infection had got a serious hold on the wounded tissues, and so Joseph Trueta, of Barcelona, applied his peacetime researches to meet the emergency of all limb wounds, whether fractured or not. His treatment was based on that of Winnett Orr in World War I and that of Lorenz Böhler at Vienna in the postwar years. Orr had appreciated the great value of rest and immobilization and had returned wounded men home to America in plaster casts. And Böhler, with a large experience of fractures in his clinic, had introduced many innovations including a number of valuable splints and skintight plasters[1]. However, the idea of applying plaster of Paris without padding filled his contemporaries with horror, but as the anticipated pressure sores and skin reactions did not develop, his method was eventually accepted.

Before the Spanish Civil War broke out Trueta had been experimenting on the use of Orr's technique and had modified it considerably. As far as war injuries were concerned, he first performed a thorough debridement (in the modern sense), if necessary extending the wound by longitudinal incisions at its ends. To prevent gaping, he stitched these extended surgical incisions by primary suture, thus leaving only the original wound cavity open. This he covered with a special close-meshed gauze (not vaseline gauze as Orr had used) and lightly packed the cavity with more gauze. If a fracture was present, it was accurately set. The plaster cast was then applied with padding only over the bony prominences, and left for four to six weeks; elevation of the limb was necessary during the first seven to ten days to prevent the collection of fluid within the tissues. The gauze and the plaster itself absorbed the secretions from the wound and only in severe cases that had come late to surgery was the smell troublesome; but provided the patient's condition did not deteriorate, usually shown by a rise in temperature, all was well and the wound could safely be left alone. Thereafter the plaster was changed every two months until healing was complete[2].

Trueta's results were magnificent; among his first 1073 cases there were only six deaths. At the end of the war he had treated some 20 000 casualties with only four patients coming to amputation and with just under a hundred unsatisfactory results. Other surgeons, who could not equal this achievement, failed either because their debridement was not thorough enough or because their immobilization was inadequate. It was in these improperly treated cases that infection got a hold and pus oozed from the plaster cast with an overpowering stench.

When World War II broke out surgeons were once more uprooted from the organized routine of hospital life to find that civilian surgery could not be applied directly to conditions of war; many of the lessons of World War I were forgotten and had to be learned all over again, but as the second war progressed, the surgical achievements reached an extremely high standard. This war was truly global and the methods for dealing with casualties had to be modified according to the particular climatic and geographic conditions. The nature of the military campaign also governed the choice of surgical procedure. Since 1918 the technique of waging war had changed; no longer was it a relatively static affair in trenches. The internal-combustion engine had brought about a profound alteration in military strategy and enabled armies to move with hitherto unexpected swiftness. German mechanized divisions thundered across Europe ignoring the 'barrier' of frontiers. A mockery was made of outdated modes of defence. The casualty evacuation system that accompanied the British Expeditionary Force to France was still geared to the past. Its immobile base hospitals were not organized to cope with the situation, more especially as the BEF was retiring. However, mechanization was not without its benefits. The long, tiring forced marches, often at night, that had sapped the strength of troops in

World War I were replaced by transportation in vehicles, so that on the whole men were in a fitter state at the time of wounding. Casualty evacuation was quicker, and when air evacuation came into being the wounded could be got back to receive early surgery with notably beneficial results.

The character of the wounds also changed. Virtually all weapons were fired from a distance and their design had changed dramatically. The missiles, whether bullets from rifles and machine guns or shell and bomb fragments, travelled at much higher velocities. A missile may pass straight through and cause little damage, but if it is slowed either by tumbling or by hitting bone, the kinetic energy expended on the tissues causes them to expand. This phenomenon is known as cavitation and the negative pressure within the cavity sucks in foreign material and dirt. In World War I cavitation was recognized but was thought to be due to the missile exploding or expanding (as happened with the soft-nosed dumdum bullet); its real nature was not understood. [The kinetic energy expended on the wounded tissues is proportional to the mass of the missile and the velocity of the fragment.]

Nevertheless, the wounded man, especially the seriously wounded man, now had a far better prospect of recovery thanks to advances in surgical techniques. Pre-operative and postoperative care had improved, particularly in the attention paid to maintaining fluid balance by intravenous transfusion of saline solution, plasma or blood – in the tropics dehydration was an ever-present risk. In casualties with abdominal wounds the gut could be adequately rested by removal of the intestinal juices by stomach suction through a Ryle's tube; intestinal suction with the Miller-Abbott tube was usually unnecessary under war conditions.

Anaesthesia came into its own as a specialty. Anaesthetists had gained recognition in the immediate prewar years, yet it required the emergency of war to show the immense benefit of good anaesthesia administered by specially trained doctors. Where there was a military surgical unit, there was also found at least one anaesthetist. Intravenous anaesthesia with Pentothal was a tremendous boon, and was used in 80–90 percent of all operations, either for the whole operation or just to get the patient under. One lesson that was quickly learned was that a severely shocked casualty would tolerate less Pentothal than a fit, unshocked person. Cyclopropane was a popular anaesthetic agent, since it could be used in a closed-circuit system. This means that the expired air from the patient's lungs is not breathed into the atmosphere, but passes back into the anaesthetic machine where carbon dioxide is absorbed by soda lime and the gaseous mixture is then rebreathed. The use of this system conserved the cyclopropane and was particularly useful when supplies were short.

Another important advance was the development of the Oxford vaporiser. Just before the war the need had been realized for a suitable and portable means of giving a simple anaesthetic, and as a result of work carried out at the Nuffield Department of Anaesthetics at Oxford, the Oxford ether vaporiser was invented.

Hot water supplied heat to calcium chloride contained in the apparatus and, owing to the properties of this chemical, it kept the ether at a constant temperature of 30°C; the liquid, therefore, vaporised at a constant and measurable rate[3, 4, 5, 6]. The apparatus could be used with an endotracheal tube when necessary, and thus proved itself a valuable and adaptable addition to the anaesthetist's armamentarium.

In the inter-war years a discovery had been made which prepared the way for a revolution of such magnitude as to take its place beside the discoveries of anaesthesia and antisepsis in its benefit to mankind. The modern chemotherapeutic era had been ushered in by Paul Ehrlich's discovery of his 'magic bullet', a drug known as salvarsan which was used in the treatment of syphilis[7]. This was followed by the production of other chemicals of value in certain diseases, but nothing was found that was active against the common bacterial diseases. Until, that is, 1932 when a German doctor, Gerhard Domagk, working for the big dye industry, I. G. Farbenindustrie, came across a dye, prontosil red, which cured mice infected with streptococci[8]. Thinking that they were on to a good thing, the Germans continued their research into the therapeutic possibilities of other dyes, patenting those that seemed most hopeful.

In 1935 knowledge of what was going on leaked out and M. and Mme J. Tréfouël and their French colleagues skilfully outplayed the commercial ambitions of the Germans by showing that the active constituent of prontosil was sulphanilamide[9]. This had not been patented. Results of the clinical use of prontosil and sulphanilamide did not at first stand up to statistical analysis, so Leonard Colebrook and Méave Kenny carried out controlled trials of the drugs in patients with puerperal sepsis and proved clearly that both, but especially sulphanilamide, were of marked value in the treatment of the disease[10]. After this trial doctors proved the benefit of sulphanilamide in such diseases as gonorrhoea, pneumonia, peritonitis, cellulitis and certain other bacterial infections. The results were dramatic. So dramatic, in fact, that the drug was used without due care, and before long reports appeared of the toxic effects which included rashes, fevers and sometimes a lethal allergic reaction. During the next few years new sulphonamide compounds were brought out, largely in Great Britain. Some of these were liable to form crystals in the kidney unless large amounts of water were taken. Eventually, in America, the compound sulphadiazine was discovered, which had the least harmful effects[11]. Since then more varieties of the sulphonamide group have been developed, suitable for different diseases.

Great hopes were held out for the sulphonamides in the prevention of infection in war wounds, but unfortunately they did not live up to expectations. They were not active locally in the wound and their possible toxic effects limited their use by mouth. At first too much reliance was placed on their powers and their use did not replace the need for adequate surgery.

In World War II, as in World War I, about 70 percent of the wounds were open wounds of the limbs and since the principles of wound surgery are basically the same regardless of the part of the body injured, the lessons learned from treating these wounds were applied to other injuries, modified as circumstances demanded. Amputation was indicated only occasionally, as the limb could usually be saved even in severe, extensive injuries. The chief reason for amputation was damage to the main blood vessels, which was in marked contrast to the state of affairs in World War I, when amputations were often performed in serious injuries because of the fear of infection.

The treatment of wounds in World War II went through three phases, roughly corresponding to the opening years, the campaign in North Africa and the final Italian and European campaigns[12]. Each was fought under different conditions and to each surgery adapted itself. Primary suture of wounds was again attempted at first, but to all intents and purposes it failed miserably. Under conditions of war, wounds just could not be sewn up immediately. There were, however, certain exceptions to this generalization as, for example, wounds of the face. The extension of war to involve the civilian population also provided other exceptions, since civilian casualties would find themselves rapidly transported to a hospital where they would stay under the care of one surgeon until their wounds were healed. But in the field, where the casualty had to pass through the hands of many surgeons along a long route of evacuation, primary suture was impossible.

Trueta's method of debridement and immobilization in plaster was the standard method of treating wounds in the early years. It was of great value when organization was not fully developed and when there were large numbers of casualties with insufficient personnel to meet their needs. Although Trueta's method, as described by himself in all its details, was finally vindicated, there was considerable controversy and confusion regarding its application. Different surgeons placed different emphasis on different details. Results therefore varied, and faith in the technique was lost in some quarters. Trueta's reasons for lightly packing the wound with absorbent material were not always appreciated. The plaster cast had to include the joints above and below the wound and the plaster had to exert a uniform pressure over the wound area. The debridement performed was not always sufficient. On the other hand, for some time there was an incorrect idea prevalent that the wound area had to be excised en bloc, and this led to the sacrifice of too much skin with unnecessary mutilation. Nevertheless, despite a certain amount of failure in appreciating the underlying principles of the technique, Trueta's method played an extremely valuable role in the early years.

By the time the main scene of military operations had been transferred to North Africa, surgeons had had the opportunity to gather themselves and to assess the problems of war. The effect was soon apparent. In this particular phase, treatment was governed by the many hundreds of miles of desert between the front line and the base hospitals in Cairo and the Sudan, and penicillin, which became available about this time, contributed in no small manner to success. Wounds were excised, drainage was instituted, and the limb put in a padded plaster cast. Before evacuation all circumferential plasters were split to allow for swelling of the limb. At base, closure of the wounds was performed by secondary suture or skin grafting as soon as the wound surface was healthy. This routine was ideal for the great distances to be covered and for the rapidly moving nature of the battles. Besides ensuring immobilization and relative comfort, the plaster casts had the added advantage of discouraging interference unless the patient's condition was obviously deteriorating. It was a sore temptation for a medical officer on the long route of evacuation to take a peep at the wound and to satisfy himself that all was well, but to do so was tantamount to asking for infection.

Wounds of the thigh posed a tricky problem in plaster technique in desert conditions, and to overcome the difficulties the Australians introduced the Tobruk splint. The leg was placed in a Thomas splint with traction exerted through sticking plaster stuck to the sides of the calf. The leg was well padded and the plaster-of-Paris bandages were then applied from the top to just above the ankle. From time to time during evacuation the traction was tightened by means of a Spanish windlass sited between the foot and the end of the splint. So effective was the Tobruk splint that it became the routine method of splinting thigh and knee wounds throughout the rest of the war. Wounds of the buttock were treated similarly, but with considerable modification to the upper part of the splint.

Penicillin is one of the finest discoveries of all time. Together with the other antibiotics that have followed, it has transformed the whole pattern of infective disease (though it may be argued that the natural pattern was changing anyway). Surgery was no longer required for chronic complications of many acute infections for the simple reason that antibiotics had prevented the complications from developing. The mortality rates from the acute diseases themselves were greatly reduced. The gains, however, were not achieved without certain unwelcome disadvantages, chief among which was the emergence of strains of bacteria (notably staphylococci) that were resistant to the charms of the drugs, and the problematical effect on the gut of some of the later antibiotics. Had Joseph Lister been granted greater good fortune than was already his share, penicillin might have been discovered more than half a century earlier. In 1871 he had noticed that the activity of certain bacteria in a urine specimen was inhibited by contamination of the urine with a mould, *Penicillium glaucum*[13]. He pursued his observations and was obviously knocking on the right door, but his reports failed to attract any attention. Strangely enough, in the same decade two other scientists, quite independently, made similar observations. William Roberts, a physician in Manchester, in 1872[14] and John Tyndall (better known as a physicist) in 1876[15] both observed the antibacterial activity of *Penicillium glaucum*. As Tyndall wrote 'In every case where the mould was thick and coherent the *Bacteria* died, or became dormant, and fell to the bottom as a sediment.' This particular variety of the mould, unfortunately, does not yield penicillin and only produces substances toxic to human beings.

Continued research might have led towards penicillin, but when one considers the circumstances of Fleming's discovery, it seems an almost inescapable conclusion that the Fates had decided to take a hand. Fleming recorded that he set aside a number of plates which he examined from time to time. In 1928 he found that a culture of staphylococcal bacteria had been contaminated by *Penicillium notatum*, a variety uncommon in Great Britain, but one that produces penicillin. Yet, despite the unfavourable odds, a stray spore had drifted through the window and settled on the culture plate. Fleming noted the antibacterial effect and gave the name 'penicillin' to the active substance. He wrote: 'It is suggested that it may be an efficient antiseptic for application to, or injection into, areas infected with penicillin-sensitive microbes.'[16] Nine years of near-forgetfulness were to pass before interest in penicillin was revived.

During these years the sulphonamides had put doctors in the right frame of mind for discovering new modes of attack on bacteria and, recalling Fleming's observations, Howard Florey and Ernst Chain in Oxford set about extracting penicillin from the mould. The task was slow and laborious, but by 1941 they had produced enough of the drug to give it a small clinical trial on human patients[17]. In all their cases the results were excellent. Florey was then faced with the problem of providing sufficient penicillin for large-scale use, and since British firms were too hard-pressed by other commitments of war, he went to the United States. The Americans responded nobly, and in a very short while the production of penicillin on a commercial scale was proceeding apace. In North Africa penicillin received its first major trial and showed its great value. It could also be applied topically to wounds with the great benefit of allowing earlier closure by skin grafts. There are, however, certain types of bacteria that inactivate the drug and it was soon found that, despite its almost miraculous powers, adequate surgery was still required if penicillin was to work properly and the best results to be obtained.

Blood-transfusion services reached a high standard during the North African campaign. About 10 percent of those wounded, both military and civilian, required blood transfusion and their needs could only be met by an organized blood-bank system. Blood was but one part of the comprehensive service that provided plasma, serum, saline and synthetic fluids that could stand in for plasma. At the beginning of the war it had been calculated that a hundred pints a day would be needed, but as the war progressed donors in Great Britain were giving over 1250 pints of blood a day. The main blood-transfusion centre for the Army was at Bristol under Lionel Whitby and from here blood and the other fluids were sent to any part of the world where British troops were in need. Initially the blood could only be stored for ten to fourteen days, but later improved methods enabled this to be lengthened. During the desert battles, G.A. Buttle made it clear that blood should be transfused in adequate quantities and at a rate sufficient to replace that lost. Blood transfusion was first used on a grand scale at El Alamein, and the practice of giving the transfusion while the casualty was being transported in the ambulance came to the fore. In theory this is ideal, but in practice the patient would often arrive at his destination with the transfusion needle adrift from the vein or with the bottle empty. The great importance of transfusion and resuscitation led to the recognition of transfusion officers as specialists. Their clinical acumen and accurate judgment were of the greatest value to the surgeon in determining the best time for operation.

Evacuation of casualties by air started in North Africa; most wounded men are suitable for transportation by this method and in those cases in which the air was not ideal it was usually preferable to a long and rugged ground journey. In furtherance of the objective of getting major surgery to the casualty as soon as possible, mobile surgical teams also made their first effective appearance in this campaign. They got away to a slow start owing to a lack of vehicles, and initially they were sometimes placed too far forward. This meant that the surgeons were covering too narrow a front and full use could not be made of their particular talent; in addition, under the circumstances of the fighting, they were often unable to hold their casualties after operating. This necessitated the evacuation of men who had recently undergone major surgery: not a desirable thing under the best of conditions, but positively dangerous for abdominal cases when the road was a bumpy desert track. However, the psychological effect of the surgeon's presence was immense. In the chapter on Field Conditions in *The History of the Second World War (Surgery)* Sir Gordon Gordon-Taylor recorded the following authentic incident: 'Seeing a pal passing him with his battalion which was marching up to the line, a stretcher case was heard to say "Watcher, Bill – good luck and watch yourself – and don't worry mate – 'alf 'Arley Street is just in front of us."'[12]

In 1942 field surgical units replaced the mobile surgical teams – if only in name. These units were self-contained and mobile, but had to be attached for operation to some parent unit such as a field ambulance or casualty clearing station. Their job was to provide surgery where the need was greatest, but they were not responsible for the after-care and nursing of the casualties; this was done by the parent unit.

The third phase of surgical treatment coincided with the fighting in Italy and later in Europe. Conditions were favourable, there was little or no fear of retreat, and the Allies had air superiority. Wounds were, therefore, excised at forward units, the casualty was evacuated, often by air, and delayed primary suture could take place at base within three or four days. Combining the lessons learned in the later years of the war, certain basic principles of wound treatment emerge. An x-ray taken before an operation was of great help to the surgeon in coming to an accurate diagnosis and in locating foreign bodies; however, the benefit of radiography in advanced surgical units was not finally settled. As far as forward surgery was concerned, asepsis was always practised as much as conditions would allow. The patient was partially prepared before coming onto the table, but his wound was left undisturbed with the first-aid dressings still in place. On the table the dressings were removed, the nature of the wound assessed and the wound area prepared by shaving, scrubbing with soap and water and painting with an antiseptic. Debridement was then carried out, although the procedure was limited in wounds more than twelve hours old because of the danger of spreading sepsis. Bleeding was controlled by the application of hot wet packs; ligatures were only used if absolutely necessary and thread was preferred to catgut. In the early years of the war bone fragments were removed to avoid possible infection, but the arrival of penicillin made it quite safe to leave fragments, particularly if attached, behind when they could act as chip grafts and aid bony union. After debridement, penicillin and sulphonamide powder was carefully dusted into all corners of the wound.

At base hospitals soft tissue wounds were inspected only in theatre, thus avoiding excess interference that could so easily lead to infection. The wound was again assessed and the form of treatment decided. At the earliest possible moment after his arrival, the physical and mental rehabilitation of the casualty was begun and after discharge was concluded at special rehabilitation units. Further evacuation, if necessary, only took place after the patient had had his stitches removed.

Segregation of the casualties was essential when specialist treatment was required and was partially achieved by having specialist surgical units operating in conjunction with casualty clearing stations; however, complete segregation was not really practicable further forward than base. A great advance in the treatment of wounds of the large bowel was made by Heneage Ogilvie who, in the East African campaign, first used a method of exteriorization of the wounded colon[18]. The abdomen was explored through a surgical incision to determine the site and extent of injury and then, through another incision, the wounded part of the bowel was brought out to the surface of the abdomen and the wound allowed to act as the colostomy through which the bowel motions were evacuated. This was later closed. Although it was decreed that all wounds of the large bowel should be treated in this manner, wounds of the caecum and right side of the colon often led to dehydration and other troubles, since in this site the bowel contents are fluid. Because of this, many surgeons sutured the wound in the bowel and joined the small intestine to the transverse colon so as to by-pass the wounded area. The aids to modern surgery also contributed to the success of abdominal operations and at the end of the war the magnificent achievement of 70–80 per cent recovery rate in abdominal wounds was recorded.

Surgery of the chest was unsatisfactory at the start, since wounds were stitched without excision and collections of blood in the pleural cavity were not evacuated with anything like the urgency that they demanded. Both these factors led to a very high rate of sepsis. By the time the North African campaign was under way the situation was rectified and the treatment of chest wounds divided into two stages. In the first the wound was excised and the physiological derangements were corrected by the closure of a dangerous pneumothorax and the removal of air and blood from the pleural cavity. The second stage consisted of getting the lungs back to normal function. Foreign bodies were removed, and sometimes it was necessary to excise a number of ribs and decorticate the lungs. Decortication consists in the removal of thickened pleura or scar tissue surrounding the lungs that was preventing their expansion. The scar tissue may be formed from the organization of pus or blood. There was also an interesting change of approach to the problem of empyema. Evarts Graham and his Empyema Commission of World War I had shown how disastrous it was to operate in the early stages of the disease. But times had changed and penicillin had been discovered. Even in the presence of active infection it was now the policy to operate on empyemas caused by war injuries, since the best way to cure the empyema was to get the lung to expand. As far as the heart was concerned there were no occasions on which British surgeons actually entered the organ, but an American surgeon, Dwight E. Harken, successfully removed missiles from inside the heart on thirteen occasions[19], and another American, Laurence Miscall, at his centre in northern England, had removed thirty-nine foreign bodies from the heart, again with no deaths[20].

Plastic surgery had undergone great development in the inter-war years and the work carried out in the reconstruction of noses, ears, faces and deformities and injuries of other parts of the body was applied with great success to the wounds of war. In Great Britain in 1939, the number of plastic surgery specialists was few and only a handful of hospitals had plastic surgery units; but under the leadership of Sir Harold Gillies, the formation of new units and the training of surgeons was very soon accomplished. One of the main advances was in treatment of burns. Since 1925 tannic acid had been used; this produced a hard coagulum and left a firm contracted scar requiring subsequent removal and grafting. The tannic acid itself was sometimes toxic, as also was the local use of sulphonamides that succeeded it. This in turn gave way to penicillin powder, which completely transformed the issue. With extensive burns it was necessary to pay particular attention to the fluid balance, transfusing blood and plasma as required.

Skin grafting was vital when skin loss had been extensive, as for instance with burns, and the introduction of penicillin enabled the grafting to take place earlier and with more certainty of a take. Sulphonamides and, later, penicillin both reduced the long delay that previously had been necessary between the stages of plastic operations. In 1939 Earl Padgett had introduced the dermatome[21], which enabled shavings of skin to be cut from areas such as the abdomen and back, and thus allowed a large area of the body to be available for grafts. The use of multiple small grafts to cover a large area had been known for some time, but was brought into prominence in 1943 by P. Gabarro[22], of Barcelona, and Denis Bodenham[23], working independently. In the same year Archibald McIndoe employed what he called postage-stamp grafts of about one half to one inch square[24]. These were laid over the area with gaps between to allow for discharge from the wound. Firm pressure was applied and the grafts had 'taken' when capillaries had grown into them. They then spread with great rapidity from all four sides.

Wounds and burns of the hand also benefited greatly from plastic surgery. Again early coverage with skin was important, as it helped to prevent infection and enabled movement to take place, maintaining function. When tendons on the back of the hand had been lost, replacements could be grafted and made to run through the fat of an abdominal skin graft. When that most valuable digit, the thumb, was lost, tendons could be so rearranged that the index finger acted as a substitute. By the 1960s toes were successfully grafted to replace missing fingers.

Plastic surgery also achieved almost miraculous results in the reconstitution of injured faces. What with flap grafts and pedicle grafts, bone grafts and cartilage grafts, and with superbly skilful surgery, there was no face so severely injured that it could not be restored to give its owner self-confidence and a semblance of expression.

Before the memory of World War II had begun to fade, surgeons were once again faced with the problems of wartime surgery, on this occasion in Korea. A most striking contrast was provided by the methods of dealing with casualties in the opposing forces. The North Koreans and Chinese gave treatment that was little better than crude first aid; the seriously wounded they usually shot, a fate that befell a number of Americans in the early stages. The United Nations strove for and attained an extremely high standard. Evacuation by helicopter to early surgery, and superb international co-operation were the outstanding features of the war. Forward surgery was carried out by the Americans and Norwegians; at Seoul there was a small Commonwealth hospital acting as a relay station to the base hospital in Japan, where Commonwealth surgeons were responsible for the definitive treatment[25]. This cosmopolitan organization demanded a routine to which all surgeons had to adhere, and instructions for early surgical technique, which agreed closely with accepted British practice, were laid down by the Americans. However, the Tobruk splint for wounds of thigh and knee was not adopted. Instead, a padded plaster was applied round the hips and affected leg: a procedure which, in the British opinion, predisposed to pressure sores and infection.

At the regimental aid post or the casualty clearing station, the casualty received first aid, penicillin, anti-tetanus serum and, when necessary, his blood pressure was restored by transfusion of dextran, a plasma substitute. In view of the fact that surgery and anaesthesia were going to take place very shortly after, the time-honoured custom of giving the casualty a cup of hot, sweet tea became a thing of the past. The wounded man was next evacuated to a Mobile Army Surgical Hospital (MASH) by helicopter which proved to be an easy matter owing to the air superiority enjoyed by the United Nations. The MASH was staffed by Americans or Norwegians and was geared to provide constant surgery on four or more tables. These units were sited within a few miles of the front line, ensuring early surgery in almost every case, and it was there that debridement was performed after x-ray and further transfusion, if required. Blood in adequate quantities was available, and a new departure was the disposable transfusion sets which were used once only. This eliminated the possibility of infection from contaminated apparatus even after re-sterilization, although this was admittedly a rare occurrence. In casualties almost moribund, transfusion was sometimes and successfully given under pressure into an artery in the leg. Attached to the MASH was a small ward where those casualties not fit for evacuation on the next day were held. Evacuation then took place by hospital train to Seoul where, after a variable delay, the patient was transferred to a plane for Japan.

Most casualties reached Japan within six days and could have their wounds closed by delayed primary suture. This meant that the skin edges of the unclosed debrided wound were freshened up and the gap stitched together. If the stitching could not be done without tension, there were various manoeuvres that might be adopted, but if these were impracticable, skin grafting was necessary. A number of casualties took more than six days to reach Japan and their wounds had to be excised again and closed by secondary suture. When infection had developed, as was more prone to occur in the late arrivals, it was necessary to be more ruthless in the second debridement and not to close the wound for a further four days, during which time penicillin and other antibiotics were given.

A major advance in surgical technique since the end of the world war had been the repair of arteries. It will be remembered that damage to the main blood vessels was one of the major reasons for amputation in World War II, accounting for nearly a quarter of those performed. In World War I, attempts had been made to preserve continuity of blood flow by using silver tubes, but they became blocked by clot-formation within a few hours. Glass and plastic tubes and, with more success, vitallium metal tubes lined with a vein graft, were used occasionally in World War II, but they were by no means general procedures. In

Korea, the Americans devoted one MASH to the treatment of arterial injuries. Spasm of the artery, one of the troubles of this sort of surgery, was overcome by the local use of the drug, papaverine. When possible, the severed artery was treated by direct anastomosis, but more extensive damage required replacement either with a length of vein taken from elsewhere in the patient himself or with a stored arterial graft; in the latter case the subsequent amputation rate was 33 percent. If the artery had to be ligated, the amputation rate was 51 percent, but the overall rate for the 304 major vessels repaired was 13 percent – compared to 36 percent in World War II[26].

In both World War II and the Korean War adequate surgery was achieved ever earlier; evacuation of the casualty was speeded by air transport and was made more comfortable. All the miracles of contemporary surgery had been brought to the aid of the wounded man, and death, deformity and loss of limb were reduced to a minimum. Nevertheless, many questions remain unanswered, not the least of which is the apparently insoluble problem of mass casualties overwhelming the system. Just remember, for instance, that the atomic bomb dropped on Hiroshima killed some 80 000 people and injured more than 70 000; a vast area of the city was burnt out or reduced to rubble. All this was achieved by a single bomber and its crew.

23

Surgery of the heart

H aving traced the stories of other branches of modern surgery, it will surely come as no surprise to learn that heart surgery has a history extending back considerably further than the past fifty or so years. The early operations were sporadic and rarely successful. A few visionaries, seeing the possibilities, worked out theoretical procedures; very, very occasionally, a surgeon managed to put theory into practice. On the whole the attitude of the profession was overshadowed by doubt and disbelief; wounds might be sewn up, as they would be fatal anyway, but beyond this hearts belonged to the physician and he was reluctant to part with his patients.

Like the lungs, the heart is surrounded by two layers of lubricating membrane (the pericardium) forming the pericardial cavity, which again is a potential and not a real space. Fluid can collect in this cavity as a result of disease, and in the past this quite often became infected and turned to pus. In the 19th century one or two attempts were made to incise the pericardium and drain away the pus; notable among these were the operations of Dominique Jean Larrey in 1810[1], of Friedrich Joseph Hilsmann in 1844[2], and of Bernhard Langenbeck in 1850[3], all of which were successful. Nevertheless, feelings ran high over the respective merits of aspiration and open operation until a Toulouse surgeon, Georges Dieulafoy, in 1873[4], brought the weight of his opinion to bear in favour of aspiration. A few years later, however, the accepted practice was to aspirate if only fluid was present and to perform an open operation for pus.

The first operations on the heart itself were on patients with stab wounds; in 1895 Axel Cappelen[5], a Norwegian, and in 1896, Guido Farina[6], an Italian, attempted to stitch a heart wound, but success eluded them, only to come a few months later to Ludwig Rehn[7] of Frankfurt. At the end of the same decade

Herbert Milton[8] and Daniel Samways[9] quietly mentioned that a surgical approach to the mitral valve might one day be possible – so quietly, in fact, that no one paid any attention – and Arbuthnot Lane had worked out, on cadavers, a method for the surgical treatment of mitral stenosis, an acquired disease almost invariably due to rheumatic fever, but was unable to induce his colleagues to give him a living patient[10]. But when, in 1902, a physician, Lauder Brunton, again suggested the operation[11] and the message this time was heard, the outcry was such that it thoroughly prevented any further consideration.

It is now common knowledge that occasionally the heart may stop beating during the course of an operation, even quite a minor one, and when this occurs all other surgical considerations are thrown to the winds while the surgeon attempts to massage the heart back to life. Tuffier first tried the manoeuvre in 1898, but was unsuccessful[12]. In 1901, Kristian Igelsrud, after removing the ribs over the heart, was rewarded for his initiative[13]. A year later, when Lane was removing an appendix, the same catastrophe occurred. He at once plunged his hand through an abdominal incision and successfully massaged the heart through the diaphragm[14]. Some fifty years later came the recognition of two forms of cardiac arrest and the introduction of external methods of resuscitation. When the heart stops it may just stop or it may go into what is known as ventricular fibrillation. In the latter case it twitches uselessly for about twenty minutes before finally stopping; these twitches are very faint and can only be appreciated when the chest and pericardium are opened. But the important point is that a normal beat can only be restored by an electric shock – massage is only of use to keep the circulation going until the electric defibrillator can be obtained. The first successful defibrillation was performed by Claude Beck of Cleveland in 1947[15]. Since, in about half of all cardiac arrests the heart is in ventricular fibrillation, the importance of differentiating the condition from cardiac asystole (complete stopping) can be readily appreciated; it also helps us to understand why many of the early attempts at massage failed.

Restoration of the heartbeat by external massage, without opening the chest, was a most significant step forward. No longer did the agonizing decision to open the chest have to be made – a decision that might well waste valuable minutes or seconds. The doctor, or a trained person, can act at once and then think while he is acting. The idea came accidentally in 1960 to William Kouwenhoven of Johns Hopkins University[16]. He was working on the effect of electricity on the heart when he noticed that the pressure of the heavy electrodes on a dog's chest caused its blood pressure to rise slightly. By pressing regularly on the chest he then found he could keep an adequate circulation going in the dog, whose heart was fibrillating. From this observation developed the technique of using rhythmic pressure with the hands on the bottom end of the sternum (breast bone) as an effective means of cardiac massage. Kouwenhoven also drew attention to the importance of having a second person give mouth-to-mouth artificial respiration in cases of cardiac arrest, since it was no good keeping the circulation going if the blood was not being oxygenated. Mouth-to-mouth respiration has had a very long history, in fact it is sometimes known as the biblical method on the grounds that this was how Elisha revived the Shunammite's son (II Kings, 4,verses 18–37); but these grounds are tenuous in the extreme. In the 18th and 19th centuries it was sometimes used, mainly on newborn babies, yet it failed to make an impression until the 1950s, since when it has been linked with external cardiac massage as the definitive form of resuscitation.

But we have wandered ahead of our subject and must return to 1902 when Ludolph Brauer, a physician, devised an operation for chronic adhesive mediastino-pericarditis (the pericardium gets stuck to the chest wall and hampers the heart's action). Brauer's surgical colleague simply removed the ribs overlying the adherent area and released the heart[17]. In 1908 Alexander Morison advised the same operation for an enlarged heart, but it only allowed the heart to enlarge still further[18]. The procedure was also considered for constrictive pericarditis, a condition in which the pericardium becomes thickened or calcified and slowly strangles the heart. The operation was simple and was performed fairly frequently until its inadequacies became apparent and surgeons realized that any effective operation would have to remove the constricting pericardial membrane. This had originally been suggested by Edmond Delorme in 1895[19] but was not carried out until 1913, when Rehn[20] and Sauerbruch[21] both were successful. In spite of their achievements, the operation was only occasionally performed in the following years.

In 1908 Friedrich Trendelenburg of Leipzig twice attempted to rescue a patient from the very jaws of death[22]. In each case, a healthy young person had undergone a surgical operation and was progressing quite favourably until a clot of blood formed in a vein and was carried into the pulmonary artery, where it blocked the circulation. To all intents and purposes the patients were dead. However, they were immediately rushed to the operating theatre, where Trendelenburg was waiting. The chest was opened, the ribs removed, the pericardium opened, the heart exposed, the pulmonary artery located and explored and the clot withdrawn: all in a matter of minutes. Regrettably the patients only lived for a few hours after these heroic operations and, despite occasional attempts by other surgeons, not until 1924 was success attained by Martin Kirschner of Konigsberg[23].

A few years later Clarence Crafoord was also successful[24]; but despite a handful of other successes the operation was considered of doubtful value and was virtually abandoned until 1958 when Richard Steenburg at the Peter Bent Brigham Hospital in Boston achieved the first American success[25]. This aroused surgeons from their despondency and when Denton Cooley of Houston, Texas, in 1961 carried out an embolectomy for the first time using a heart-lung machine[26], the operation took its place as a worthwhile lifesaving measure.

Before we move inside the heart there is one more notable observation worthy of record. In 1907 John Cummings Munro, of Boston, suggested that a persistent ductus arteriosus, a congenital defect, might be tied with a ligature in an attempt to prevent the bacterial infection that was so likely to develop[27]. Besides the suggestion, he also devised a practicable technique, but alas he was ahead of his time and more than thirty years had to pass before the operation was performed. His idea was all the more remarkable since the nature of congenital heart deformities was then very poorly understood.

The first surgical offensive inside the heart took place in 1912 when Tuffier made an ingenious attack on a stenosed aortic valve. He did not incise the heart or the aorta, but simply invaginated the wall of the aorta just above the valve with his finger and so dilated the valve from outside[28]. Although the twenty-six-year-old patient survived, somewhat improved, Tuffier did not repeat the procedure. The next year Eugene Doyen divided a stenotic pulmonary valve, making his approach through the right ventricle. The patient, a young woman of twenty, died and at the post-mortem examination the condition of the heart was seen to be such that the operation could never have succeeded[29].

After World War I surgeons returned to the problems of heart surgery with renewed vigour. Evarts Graham and Duff Allen, in America, in 1922 designed an instrument they called a cardioscope, which enabled them to see the valves inside the heart. Using this instrument on dogs, they entered the heart through the left atrial appendage (a little cul-de-sac-like part of the atrium) and under direct vision were able to cut the mitral valves. They had a very low mortality among the dogs, but unfortunately when they came to try the operation on a human being, the patient died on the operating table before the cardioscope was even used[30]. The following year, 1923, Elliott Cutler operated successfully on a patient with mitral stenosis, cutting the rigid valves that had become joined together, thus allowing them once again to fulfil their normal function. Cutler used a modified cardioscope and a knife originally intended for cutting tendons[31]. The patient lived for a further four and a half years, much improved in health. Cutler and Claude Beck, of Cleveland, then performed the operation on a few more patients with mitral stenosis and designed a special knife known as a cardiovalvotome, but they had no successes[32].

Then in 1925 Henry Sessions Souttar of The London Hospital carried out the operation by a method that is essentially a modern technique. He passed his finger through a hole made in the left atrial appendage and digitally dilated the stenosed valve. The hole was then closed around the withdrawing finger[33]. Lily Hine, aged fifteen years, lived for seven more years in quite good health. Despite Souttar's success he got no more patients from the physicians who were obsessed with the idea that the essence of the disease lay in the heart muscle, rather than in the valves. Six months later a German, Bruno Oskar Pribram, removed part of a stenosed mitral valve, using a method similar to Cutler's, but the patient only survived a few days as the heart disease was extensive and had affected the aortic valve[34].

Nearly a quarter of a century now passed before interest in the surgery of the mitral valve was revived. The main reason for the hiatus was the insufficient development of the techniques essential for successful surgery of this nature. Anaesthesia, blood transfusion and the methods of accurate diagnosis were inadequate. Only the intensive research and experimentation carried out in the 1930s and during the years of World War II made the road into the heart fit for travelling. For example, cardiac catheterization is a most important tool, not only for investigation but also for treatment. In 1905 Fritz Bleichroeder, of Berlin, successfully catheterized his own inferior vena cava through a vein in his thigh[35], and in 1929 Werner Forssmann catheterized his own heart with a ureteral catheter and verified the position of the catheter by fluoroscopy[36]. But these achievements remained simply of academic interest until 1937 when George Robb and Israel Steinberg of New York developed a satisfactory method of injecting contrast medium into the circulation through an arm vein thereby obtaining good x-ray pictures of the heart chambers[37]. This diagnostic advance was further developed when André Cournand, also of New York, showed the practical value of catheterization of the heart, to both physician and surgeon[38]. Nevertheless, none of the methods for contrast radiography of the heart showed the coronary arteries in a thoroughly reliable fashion, and this was vital when direct surgery on these vessels became possible. In 1962, after a great deal of research, Mason Sones and Earl Shirey of Cleveland published their technique of selective catheterization of the coronary arteries[39] which, although a tricky undertaking demanding much technical skill, is now an essential diagnostic measure before coronary-artery surgery is performed.

The search for some way of relieving the agonizing and incapacitating pain of angina pectoris has occupied surgeons, as well as physicians, for a goodly number of years. The original surgical efforts were aimed at easing the pain rather than treating the heart. In 1916 Thomas Jonnesco[40] of Bucharest operated on the sympathetic nerves (special nerves governing involuntary functions of the body) in the neck and thus put into effect a suggestion made by C. E. François-Franck, a professor of physiology in Paris, in 1899[41]. Charles Mayo had previously performed a similar operation in 1914, but did not record it until many years later[42].

In 1932, Claude Beck started on his experiments to find a way of improving the blood supply of the heart muscle, the cause of the trouble, and for the rest of his career worked with indefatigable energy, but without finding the answer to the problem. Moreover, the results were not sufficiently convincing to lead to widespread adoption of the varied techniques. Beck in 1935[43], followed by Laurence O'Shaughnessy, an English surgeon, in 1936[44], reported on the experimental work and also on the methods they had used in human beings. These included grafting part of a pectoral muscle, lung or omentum (the fatty apron that hangs down inside the front of the abdomen) onto the heart, with the object of bringing more blood to its muscle by means of the grafts, which remained still attached to their original source. Such operations aroused considerable interest at the time but were later abandoned.

In the late 1940s Beck devised a method by which the aorta was connected by a vein graft to a vessel known as the coronary sinus in the heart muscle[45]. Another way in which the blood supply could be improved, and which had its run of popularity, was to set up a sterile inflammation over the surface of the heart; the body reacted to this by increasing the blood supply to the affected area. Beck's method was to remove the surface layer of the heart by abrasion, and then to powder it with asbestos dust (he originally used powdered beef bone). Dwight Harken favoured 95 percent carbolic acid followed by a powdering of sterile talc[46]. There was, however, evidence that these operations relieved the pain of angina pectoris by destruction of nerve fibres and not by increasing the blood supply.

The only operation for angina pectoris that seemed to have a future, and the only one for which there was objective evidence that it increased the blood supply of the heart, was implantation of the internal mammary artery. This was devised by Arthur Vineberg of McGill University. After five years of experimental work, he first performed it in 1950[47]; three years later, he wrote:'from a condition of complete disability' this man 'can now walk 10 miles through the bush.'[48] Despite widespread criticism and failure of others to reproduce his results, Vineberg stuck to his guns. His technique was to dissect out the internal mammary artery, which runs behind the side of the sternum, and bury its bleeding end directly into a tunnel he had prepared in the heart muscle. The operation might be done on both sides when both coronary arteries and their branches were diseased; in 1962 he added to the technique by removing the greater omentum from the abdomen and wrapping it round the heart as a free graft to increase the blood supply still further[49].

In the 1950–60s another group of operations for disease of the coronary arteries came into prominence owing to the recognition that the occlusion was sometimes limited in extent and might occur at the beginning of the artery. Walton Lillehei in 1956 reported on coronary endarterectomy – reboring the artery – and on a variety of anastomotic operations; for instance, bringing the subclavian artery into anastomosis with the circumflex branch of the left coronary artery[50]. Working independently, Angelo May attacked the problem by curettement of the coronary arteries; his first experiments on dogs took place in 1954[51] and in 1956 Charles Bailey, his colleague, performed the operation on a fifty-one-year-old man[52]. Åke Senning, a colleague of Crafoord in Stockholm, in 1959 introduced patch grafting of the coronary artery after the inner core had been removed by endarterectomy[53].The graft was taken from one of the patient's own veins and sewn into an incision in the artery to increase its diameter.Then, at the beginning of 1967, Philip Sawyer and his New York colleagues used jets of carbon dioxide gas sprayed in short bursts down the wall of the affected artery between the inner and outer layers[54]. This separated the diseased core, which could be withdrawn through a small incision. Before trying this technique on a human patient, these surgeons had practised on many cadavers and had also had more than a year's experience behind them of using it successfully on larger arteries in the neck, abdomen and legs.

Yet even as all this ingenuity was being expended on endarterectomy in its variety of forms, the operation that was to supersede it was taking shape at the Cleveland Clinic, Ohio, and on May 9, 1967, the Argentine, René Favaloro who was working there, performed the first coronary artery bypass on a fifty-one-year-old woman. A length of saphenous vein from her upper thigh was used for the bypass from the aorta to beyond a total blockage of the right coronary artery in its proximal third. The patient made an uneventful recovery and cineradiographic studies twenty days after operation showed 'total reconstruction of the right coronary artery.'[55] Since then multiple grafts have been inserted when more than one artery has been affected and, in selected cases, a length of internal mammary artery has been used as the graft.

Ten years later, a technique that complements coronary artery bypass appeared on the scene: percutaneous transluminal coronary angioplasty. This procedure, which is almost invariably performed by a physician, was introduced by Andreas Grüntzig of Zurich who, in 1977, reported on five patients with severe stenotic lesions associated with refractory angina[56]. He used a catheter with a sausage-shaped balloon at its tip which he inserted through the femoral artery; when the balloon was seen, radiologically, to be in position he filled it with saline solution and contrast medium under pressure and thus compressed the obstructing atheromatous lesion, leaving a smooth inner surface to the artery.

Between them these two techniques have transformed the outlook for patients with coronary artery disease and, what is important for the surgeon, their effects can be assessed objectively by a wealth of modern techniques. No longer does the value of an operation have to be judged solely on whether or not the angina is relieved.

The modern era of heart surgery began in 1938, with the now famous operation of Robert Edward Gross, of Boston, who successfully tied a persistent ductus arteriosus[57], thus putting into effect Munro's suggestion of thirty-one years earlier. (The ductus arteriosus is a vessel that during embryonic life diverts blood from the inactive lungs. It joins the pulmonary artery to the aorta and normally closes automatically after birth. Sometimes it remains patent and causes trouble later in life.) Once Gross had closed a patent ductus as a planned undertaking, other surgeons soon entered the field. The operation became extremely popular, and before long it was found that it prevented bacterial infection of the heart, as well as prolonging the lives of the patients.

The next step was more ambitious and concerned a very complicated congenital malformation known as Fallot's tetrad (or tetralogy); babies suffering from this condition are the original blue babies. The defects in the heart combine to deprive the lungs of blood. The pulmonary valve is stenosed, the aorta and pulmonary artery are muddled, there is a hole in the wall between the two ventricles, and the right ventricle is hypertrophied; the result is that blue un-oxygenated blood gets pumped around the body. It occurred to Helen Taussig that it might be possible to direct some of the blood from the aorta into the lungs and thereby ensure a more satisfactory degree of oxygenation. Accordingly she discussed the problem with Alfred Blalock, the Johns Hopkins surgeon, who had had many years of experience with blood-vessel surgery, and together they devised an operation for joining the left subclavian artery, a branch of the aorta, onto the left pulmonary artery. Blalock performed the first operation on a baby girl on November 29, 1944, with an immediate and dramatically good result; a blue, crippled girl was transformed overnight into an almost normal individual[58]. In 1946 Willis John Potts of Chicago sewed the side of the aorta directly onto the side of the pulmonary artery, which was just a different way of achieving the same result[59]. Potts's operation can only be performed on one side and is more dangerous if troubles are met; on the other hand it has a lower mortality rate than the Blalock-Taussig procedure, 9 percent as opposed to 12–18 percent. In both types early beneficial results are obtained in over two-thirds of the children. Either may still be used to tide very young patients over until they are ready for a total correction.

Surgery of heart conditions was still, however, restricted to overcoming the physiological upsets by operating on blood vessels, and it was not until 1948 that surgeons once again went inside the heart. Russell Brock of Guy's Hospital had investigated the problem closely, and on occasions, when operating on the lungs, he passed an instrument into the heart along the pulmonary vessels to study the heart valves. He then developed a method of cutting the rigid valve in pulmonary stenosis by introducing a special knife, known as a valvulotome, through the wall of the right ventricle[60]. Holmes Sellors of the Middlesex Hospital had performed a similar operation in December 1947[61] but his paper was not published until a fortnight after Brock's. As experience was gained, patients with Fallot's tetrad were treated by operating on the pulmonary stenosis part of their defect, and when open-heart surgery became possible they could also have the hole between the ventricles repaired. This complete correction was first done in 1954 by Walton Lillehei and his team from the University of Minnesota (he found that the muddled positions of the aorta and pulmonary artery created no technical problem) and they were thus able to give their nineteen-month-old boy patient a normal cardiac physiology[62].

The year 1948 also saw the first successful operations of the modern period for stenosis of the mitral valve. In January, Horace Smithy used a Cutler valvulotome[63]; in June, Charles Bailey[64], then of Philadelphia, and Dwight Harken[65] of Boston, and in September, Brock[66], all attacked the valve using the approach through the atrial appendage employed by Souttar twenty-three years earlier. Special knives, attached to metal rings on the surgeon's finger, were invented for cutting the leaves of the mitral valve when these could not be split by the finger alone. In the same year, Gordon Murray in Toronto successfully closed a hole between the two atria[67].

Thus surgery within the heart was well and truly launched and in the ensuing years many patients were operated on in centres all over the world. There was, however, one disadvantage to every technique employed up to 1953, namely that the operations were done 'blind'. Surgeons had to work by touch alone, and it speaks very highly of their superb skill and anatomical knowledge that they were able to operate inside the heart without the aid of vision. They had no choice in the matter, for they were unable to stop the heart which, during the course of an operation, was pumping gallons of blood round the body. Accordingly they devised techniques which virtually isolated one part of the heart and allowed them to work through this with a minimal loss of blood and without interfering with the heart's function. For instance, in 1951 Gross developed a rubber well that was like a bag with no bottom. It was sewn onto the right atrium and the incision made into the heart through the bottom of the well[68]. Since the pressure in the atrium is not particularly high, the blood only filled part of the well and Gross was able to feel inside the heart and repair holes between the atria with great accuracy. Other surgeons devised their own methods for getting inside the atrium, and Gross himself later found he could dispense with the well, although it continued in use in other surgical centres. However, one of the first lessons a surgeon learns is to get a good exposure, in order to see precisely what he is doing, and to achieve this end scientists of divers interests put their heads together. As the result of an immense amount of research and experimentation two important methods – hypothermia and extracorporeal circulation – were devised, both making their appearance in clinical practice in 1952/3.

Hypothermia means that the temperature of the whole body is reduced. It is used because the vital organs of the body, in particular the brain, liver and kidneys, require less oxygen at low temperatures and can therefore be deprived of their blood supply for a longer period than at normal body temperature. Normally the circulation can only be stopped for two or three minutes before irreversible damage occurs in the brain, but by reducing the body temperature to about 28°C this period is extended to ten minutes. Wilfred Bigelow[69] of Toronto and William McQuiston[70] of Chicago in 1950 were responsible for bringing hypothermia into the limelight, and the method was first used to produce a defunctioned heart for closing a hole between the atria in 1952 by F. John Lewis[71] of the University of Minnesota and in 1953 by Henry Swan[72] of the University of Colorado.

The state of hypothermia can be brought about in a variety of ways, the easiest being to plunge the anaesthetized patient into a bath of cold water as done, for instance, by Robert Virtue in Swan's clinic. In order to compensate for the continuing drop in temperature, the patient is removed from the bath when his temperature is around 31–32°C and is wrapped in a plastic rewarming blanket. The operation is performed when the temperature drops to the minimum of 28–29°C. Alternatively, the anaesthetized patient may be wrapped in a special blanket through which ice-cold water is pumped. The time taken to reduce the temperature varies from half an hour upwards.

A different method, originally described in 1951 by Ite Boerema[73], and in 1952 by Edmund Delorme[74] of Edinburgh, involved inserting a cannula into the patient's femoral artery from which plastic tubing carried the blood through an ice bath and back into the body through another cannula in the femoral vein. To overcome some of the objections to this method, Donald Ross of Guy's Hospital in 1954 introduced a technique whereby the blood from one of the great veins near the heart is withdrawn, cooled and returned through another great vein[75]. The advantages and disadvantages of the various methods for producing hypothermia are complicated and technical, but whichever method is used, once the temperature is lowered sufficiently the heart may be cut off from the circulation for a few minutes. Snares are placed on the superior and inferior venae cavae (the veins entering the heart) and the aorta and pulmonary artery are clamped. The blood inside the heart is then sucked out and the operation performed. Afterwards the snares are released first, so that the heart fills with blood, before the clamps are removed from the arteries.

An important advance was made in 1959 when Charles Drew of the Westminster Hospital introduced the technique of profound hypothermia[76]. Having overcome the difficulties associated with passing cannulae into the heart, he was able to construct a bypass and divert the blood through a heat exchanger. With this apparatus the patient's own lungs were used to oxygenate the blood and the temperature of the body could be lowered to around 15°C, so allowing about forty-five minutes of operating time. A further development was to replace the lungs with a simple extracorporeal circuit; this gave the surgeon virtually unlimited time inside a still heart and enabled complex operations to be performed without a desperate need to hurry.

Hypothermia is also a great asset for certain operations on the brain. This time the carotid arteries taking blood to the brain are clamped off. However, for whatever purpose hypothermia alone is used, the operation must be performed quickly, and this is a serious drawback when prolonged reconstructive procedures are required inside the heart. There are also problems connected with the continued drop of body temperature after active cooling has ceased, and with the speed of warming the patient after operation. The method itself is not without its complications as the heart may suddenly start beating very irregularly and death ensue. This dangerous happening can usually be overcome by electrical stimulation.

Extracorporeal circulation is the other important method that enables surgeons to work on an almost dry, slowed heart. With this technique the patient's heart and lungs are bypassed from the circulation, and the blood is led off to some external agency which takes over the job of pumping and oxygenation. The construction of a machine to oxygenate the blood without destroying its properties is an extremely difficult matter; it is easy to damage the red cells or to remove the part of the blood concerned with clotting, and if blood of this nature were to be returned to the patient the effect would be disastrous. As far back as 1937 an American, John H. Gibbon, Jr, reported on his pioneer work of making a suitable machine[77]. He continued his researches, and in 1953 his apparatus was used during the repair of a hole between the two atria of the heart[78]. Oxygenation took place because the blood was converted into a thin film which flowed over a stationary vertical screen in an atmosphere of oxygen. A variant, developed by Viking Olov Björk[79] of Stockholm, and taken up by Denis Melrose[80] of London, involved the passage of the film of blood over a moving surface. Another method, used in many clinics, was to pass bubbles of oxygen through the blood. The technique was essentially the same whichever type of pump-oxgenator was chosen: catheters, placed in the two great veins returning blood to the heart, were so arranged that all the blood flowed into them. The blood was then pumped into the oxygenating machine, oxygenated and pumped back into either a subclavian or a femoral artery. The aorta was clamped across just above the heart.

Melrose, in 1955, made an outstanding contribution by showing how the heartbeat could be stopped at will[81]. Once the machine is connected up and working, potassium citrate is injected into the aorta on the heart side of the clamp. The drug immediately gets into the coronary arteries and the heart stops in a relaxed state. The surgeon now has ideal conditions in which to perform his operation. When he has finished, the clamp on the aorta is released and blood flows back into the heart, washes out the potassium citrate from the coronary vessels, and the heart once again starts beating. In 1955, Conrad Lam, in

America, introduced acetylcholine as an alternative drug for producing elective cardiac arrest[82].

For a short time in 1954 Walton Lillehei used a human being (a parent) of suitable blood group in place of a machine, since he felt that the apparatus was not yet sufficiently developed for his requirements[83]. After a great deal of experimentation, he found that the body could survive quite satisfactorily for the duration of an operation if the amount of blood in circulation was drastically reduced. The basis for this reduced blood-flow cross-circulation technique was laid by the experimental work of Anthony Andreasen and Frank Watson at the Royal College of Surgeons, England, between 1949 and 1953[84]. Lillehei's important contribution to the technique was the fact that he improved the pump between patient and donor to control the amount of blood recirculating in the patient, and to keep its volume reduced. He had no deaths among the donors. In 1955 he used a dog lung as an oxygenator for a small series of patients[85], and later the same year he devised a simple disposable oxygenator made of plastic[86]. Variations of the latter have also been developed in other clinics. With these methods Lillehei operated under direct vision on a considerable number of serious malformations of the heart, and had exceedingly good results considering the critically ill state of many of his patients. At the Mayo Clinic, John W. Kirklin also operated on similar cases using a more orthodox, but more expensive, heart-lung machine[87].

Surgery of the aortic valve was a late arrival. In 1952 surgeons such as Brock, and Bailey, approached the valve in patients with aortic stenosis with an instrument passed 'blindly' through the wall of the left ventricle. Brock had in fact used what is known as a retrograde approach to dilate the valve in a few patients since 1947[88], but the results were bad and he abandoned it. Stenosis in this site poses far more problems than does mitral stenosis; therefore Bailey, in 1953, devised a method of approach through the aorta, which enabled the surgeon to assess the state of the valve with his finger before attempting anything further[89].

Aortic incompetence, a condition in which the blood regurgitates back into the heart, has been tackled by, among others, Charles Hufnagel of Georgetown University, Washington. In 1952, after a number of years of experimentation, he began a series of operations in which he inserted a plastic valve into the descending part of the thoracic aorta[90]. In 1955 after much experimental work on animals, Gordon Murray replaced diseased valves with ones taken from healthy human cadavers. A man of twenty-two who had his incompetent aortic valve replaced in that year was alive and free of symptoms six years later[91].

Since those early days when the heart-lung machine virtually gave surgeons the freedom of the heart, progress has been quite staggering. When function cannot be restored to the heart valves there is really only one answer, and that is to remove them and replace them with something else. Once Hufnagel and Murray had shown that either artificial or human valves could be successfully used for this purpose, research proceeded apace.

The amazing progress in cardiac surgery was achieved by doctors and scientists working as closely knit teams; years of thought and experimentation passed before the surgeon took up his scalpel to lay bare the human heart and attempt some new procedure. The pathway along which cardiac surgery nevertheless advanced so rapidly was strewn with discarded operations, some of which served their purpose for a short time. Many operations are now standard practice; for instance the congenital defects of patent ductus arteriosus, coarctation of the aorta, certain holes between the atria, and pulmonary stenosis and uncomplicated mitral stenosis can be dealt with quite safely. Operation for holes between the ventricles and the various manifestations of Fallot's tetrad are also routine but slightly more risky. Beyond this, a challenge remains.

One of these is heart failure. Admittedly the treatment of this is medical, but if the surgeon can assist in any way he is always ready to do so. For instance, the first attempt at helping a failing left ventricle to do its work was made by Adrian Kantrowitz at Maimonides Hospital, Brooklyn, on February 4, 1966. He used an auxiliary pump but his patient died after twenty hours[92]; nevertheless, he continued working on pumps of various different designs. Later that year, Michael De Bakey of Houston, Texas, had a critically ill patient in left ventricular failure who had already had a calcified, stenotic aortic valve replaced. So, on July 19, he bypassed the left ventricle with an air-driven pump. This was used continuously and efficiently during the last four days of the patient's life[93]. Then, on August 8, he inserted a squeezing type of tube pump after replacing both mitral and aortic valves in Esperanza del Valle Vasquez as her ventricle was failing. Ten days later, the pump was removed and a year afterwards Mrs Vasquez was free of symptoms and working as a beautician[94].

De Bakey had for some years been concentrating on the technique of left ventricular bypass as he considered there were too many problems to be overcome before total replacement of the heart with an artificial pump became a practical proposition. The problems are indeed immense, but progress, although slow, had been steady since artificial hearts were first constructed in the 1950s. Among those carrying out intensive research were Willem Kolff and Tetsuzo Akutsu in Cleveland, Ohio, and Kazuhiko Atsumi in Tokyo. In 1965 Kolff reported that he had kept a calf alive for more than thirty hours with a pump implanted in its pericardial cavity[95]. Atsumi, who began his work in 1958, experimented with many designs of pump and various materials; in 1967 he kept a dog alive for twenty-seven hours[96]. He also linked his devices to a computer to enable the mechanism to respond to the changing demands of the animal's body.

The survival times in these animal experiments could not compare with those achieved by the alternative method – the use of a living human heart. And when Christiaan Barnard in December 1967 and January 1968 transplanted the human heart he thrust wide the door at which surgeons had been knocking for all those years.

24

Arterial surgery

C losely allied to surgery of the heart is arterial surgery, a story that once again goes back for many years. Since the time of Galen and Antyllus, in the second century of our era, aneurysms, or bulgings of the arteries, when occurring in the limbs have been a source of interest and the objects of much dubious surgery. It was not until the closing years of the 19th century that surgeons began to move away from the traditional methods of compression, ligation and a variety of techniques designed to prevent the aneurysm from enlarging without compromising the arterial supply to the area beyond. In 1888, Rudolph Matas, of New Orleans, was faced with a man of twenty-six who had been shot with bird-shot and had developed an aneurysm of his left brachial artery involving practically all his upper arm. Initially, he intended to excise the aneurysmal sac but was thwarted as it was adherent to nerves. So, on April 23, he applied a ligature above the sac and, fifteen days later, another below it. But as the pulsations failed to disappear, Matas used an Esmarch bandage (an elastic bandage that squeezes the blood from a limb and then acts as a tourniquet) to give him a bloodless surgical field and proceeded to suture the orifices of all the entering vessels and to excise part of the sac. The patient was discharged fit on May 21[1]. Twenty years later Matas reported on his series of patients cured by this technique of endoaneurysmorrhaphy[2].

However, of far more significance would be the ability to anastomose blood vessels by end-to-end suture as this would open up a much broader field than the comparatively restricted one of aneurysms. The search was on and the first to report success was Mathieu Jaboulay of Lyon. With dogs as his experimental animals, he inserted U-shaped sutures that everted the ends of the vessels so that undamaged intimas (inner layers) were brought together. The circulation was re-

225

established without haemorrhage[3]. Jaboulay was also the first to transplant a segment of artery experimentally. Another important contribution was that of John Murphy who used a different technique in his experiments on end-to-end arterial suture and who, in 1897, repaired perforations in two leg veins of a thirty-year-old man and in the femoral artery and vein of a man of twenty-nine. Both patients recovered satisfactorily[4].

At the turn of the century, surgeons expended their energies searching for some artificial product to make sure that intima was approximated to intima (the essential requisite for successful anastomosis). For instance, T. Nitze, in 1897, demonstrated his use of rigid rings of ivory[5], and Erwin Payr tried absorbable rings and cylinders of magnesium[6]. And, to replace diseased lengths of arteries, glass, aluminium and gold tubes were all used at times, but none was suitable: the blood within them clotted with dismal regularity. Nevertheless, they were an improvement on the technique of Pierre Dionis, who in the 18th century tackled the problem by chewing a wodge of paper and pushing it into the incision he had made in the aneursymal sac. He preferred this over vitriol buttons or ligatures as it preserved the artery; if it failed, he resorted to the ligature[7]

Considering that modern surgery was still very much in its infancy, it seems distinctly odd that the incentive driving the search at this time for a reliable technique of vascular anastomosis was organ transplantation – a case of wanting to run before they could walk. But so it was, and foremost, by a long way, amongst the experimental surgeons was Alexis Carrel. He knew that transplantation would be impossible without a sure method of anastomosis, yet in 1902[8], when he reported his technique, only twenty-one 'successful' arterial sutures in man had been recorded. The underlying idea may have been acceptable but the method of execution most certainly was not. Small intestinal needles and thin gut were used, and the vessels stitched as though they were intestine – with conspicuous failure. Attempts to improve matters made little headway until 1905 when Carrel and Charles Guthrie, who were working together at the University of Chicago, perfected their technique. In this, the vessels were joined with a triple-threaded suture which, when drawn tightly, converted the lumen into an equilateral triangle so making suturing easier and ensuring a sound anastomosis without haemorrhage or thrombosis[9]. The stitches, taken through all coats of the vessel wall, were of fine silk thread or human hair, and were inserted using small tapered needles of polished steel.

On February 26, 1907, Carrel removed a segment of carotid artery from the body of a dog thirty-five minutes after its death, preserved it in Locke's solution in cold storage for eight days, and then transplanted it into the left carotid artery of another dog which remained in good health more than a year afterwards[10]. On numerous other occasions, and with a high rate of success, he transplanted sections of arteries and veins in experimental animals[11]; for this and for his work on organ transplantation and tissue culture he received the Nobel Prize for

Medicine or Physiology in 1912. Thus the foundations of modern blood-vessel surgery were laid, but the world was not yet ready; it did, indeed, have to learn to walk and the work of Alexis Carrel was destined to lie dormant for another forty years.

Just before the curtain fell there were four bright spots that helped keep hope alive. On February 27, 1912, in the Glasgow Royal Infirmary, James Hogarth Pringle operated on a nineteen-year-old blacksmith for a traumatic aneurysm of a brachial artery; he excised the aneurysm and restored continuity with a venous graft taken from the patient's right internal saphenous vein. On May 12 the man resumed his occupation 'and felt quite able for it.' Four days later Pringle repeated the performance on a forty-nine-year-old man who had a syphilitic aneurysm of his left popliteal artery. The venous graft was still patent nine months later[12]. The other surgeon to excise aneurysms and successfully replace them with vein grafts in 1912 was Erich Lexer in the February[13] and June[14] of that year. These were not Lexer's first expedition into this territory as, on February 22, 1907, he had resected a traumatic aneurysm of an axillary artery in a man of sixty-nine who had delirium tremens; he used a free graft of one of the man's saphenous veins to bridge the gap. All went well until the man died of his alcoholism five days later[15].

Blood-vessel surgery resurfaced in the 1940s when Crafoord and Gross, quite independently and almost simultaneously, announced that they had treated a coarctation of the aorta by excising the affected part and then stitching the cut ends together. The disease is a congenital malformation in which a section of the aorta in the chest is markedly narrowed. Clarence Crafoord's wealth of experience in chest surgery stood him in good stead when on October 19, 1944, he excised a coarctation in a twelve-year-old boy and joined the two cut ends of the aorta together. Twelve days later he repeated the performance on a twenty-seven-year-old farmer[16].

Meanwhile, in America, Robert Gross of Boston was bringing to fulfilment the experiments he had started in March 1938. At first he had followed in the steps of previous investigators by experimenting with tubes of various materials such as glass, aluminium, gold-plate and silver all lined with paraffin and all with the same unhappy result, thrombosis. He did find, however, that Lucite, a plastic, gave more promising results – a pointer, perhaps, to the way thoughts were turning to the new materials that had begun to appear since the early 1930s. Gross had later been joined by Charles Hufnagel and on June 28, 1945, they had operated on a five-year-old boy; regrettably the clamps used to seal off the blood flow were released too quickly and the lad died of cardiac dilatation. But, profiting from this error, they achieved complete success with their next patient, a girl of twelve. Her operation took place on July 6, and ten minutes of the three-and-a-half hour operation were spent in the slow removal of the clamps[17].

Modifications were later necessary to meet the demands imposed by coarctations in different parts of the aorta and especially to overcome the problems of a long stricture or a relatively inelastic aorta when the two ends could not be brought together. In the days before arterial grafting became commonplace recourse was had to a method devised by Alfred Blalock at Johns Hopkins. Having produced an experimental coarctation in dogs with elastic bands, he then bypassed it by freeing the left subclavian artery (which comes off the aorta before the coarctation in most human cases), ligating and dividing it at a suitable level, and anastomosing it end-to-side to the aorta below the stricture. The aorta itself was finally divided between ligatures at the level of narrowing[18]. For a few years other surgeons, such as Gordon Murray in Toronto, used this subclavian bypass operation as a routine in patients in whom the ends of the aorta could not be brought together[19]. However, it went out of fashion when arterial surgery was sufficiently advanced for grafts to be used instead.

In the early days it was hard to convince the medical profession that the aorta, the main artery of the body, could be anastomosed with just one row of fine stitches and still withstand the pressure of the blood flow. It took some time for it to sink in that the blood pressure in the upper part of the body, which is raised in patients with coarctation, falls, if not to normal, certainly to less dangerous levels once the obstruction has been relieved. By the time this was realized, surgeons were ready to insert grafts when necessary. The first to bridge the gap with a preserved human arterial graft was Gross on May 24, 1948; his patient was a seven-year-old boy and the graft was 5cm long[20]. Three months previously he had used a two-week-old preserved segment of adult iliac artery to anastomose the left pulmonary artery to the proximal end of the left subclavian artery in a five-year-old boy with Fallot's tetrad[21].

Grafts taken from the patient himself are the best for replacing excised portions of arteries, but since there are no expendable arteries, veins of appropriate calibre are used. When this is not practicable, healthy arteries removed from cadavers are suitable, and much research went into the best ways of obtaining these, and how to sterilize and preserve them. However, when it was found that the grafts from another person did not live in the patient, but only acted as scaffolding for Nature to build around, attention was focused on the use of prosthetic materials. In his experimental work on dogs, Arthur Blakemore inserted tubes made of Vinyon 'N', a fine mesh cloth, to bridge defects in the abdominal aorta. He found that these became infiltrated with fibroblasts which served as the basis for the formation of a functional intima[22]. Since then many other plastics have been tried, including nylon, orlon, dacron, Teflon, terylene. Besides being used to replace defects, grafts are also used to bypass a diseased area of artery. In this manner the strain on the vessel wall is relieved and the body's local adaptation to the disease is not compromised.

Excision with end-to-end anastomosis, endarterectomy (reboring), grafting and bypassing are applicable to other arteries besides those already mentioned.

For example, in 1954 Keasley Welch of Colorado was the first to excise a lesion of the middle cerebral artery in the brain[23]. These operations were not always successful and this Julius Jacobson of Vermont attributed to the inability of the surgeon to see clearly what he was doing. Accordingly, in 1962, he described an operating microscope to help in endarterectomy of these small blood vessels[24]. The operating microscope has since become of inestimable benefit to many surgical disciplines.

25

Organ transplantation

Christaan Barnard's operations at the Groote Schuur Hospital, Cape Town, brought home to the world in no uncertain manner the fact that a new era in surgery had arrived. Previously the public had not been unduly troubled by transplantation research; admittedly kidney grafting was making an impression for both ethical and financial reasons, but when a heart was transplanted mankind's emotions ran riot and it became impossible to assess the situation dispassionately. Did not Aristotle say that the heart was the seat of the soul, of the emotions, the very source of life? Traditional beliefs die hard and the Aristotelian outlook is still very close to the surface even in an educated and sophisticated society - is not the heart the shrine of romantic love? But functionally it is nothing more nor less than a remarkably efficient pump. The blood that it pumps brings life-giving oxygen to all parts of the body - and blood is transplanted by the gallon every day with approval from all except some religious sects.

Although the impact of organ transplantation is new, transplantation itself has a history extending far back in time. Legend would have us believe that a certain Chinese gentleman knew all the answers. Pien Ch'iao, who carried his secret to the grave in the third century BC, was an honourable and cultured doctor on terms of intimacy with a pixie who helped him to see through the human body and diagnose disease. On one occasion, for no reason other than the pixie's prompting, he gave two soldiers a knockout brew of narcotic wine and while they were sleeping he opened them up and swapped some of their internal organs, including their hearts. Three days later the soldiers awoke, none the worse for their experience. A little fairy, Chinese or otherwise with similar capabilities, would be of great assistance in the modern operating theatre.

Another miraculous operation was performed by two Arabian healers and wandering preachers of Christianity. In the third century of our era the twin brothers Cosmas and Damian amputated the cancerous leg of a white man and grafted in its place the leg of a Moor who had just died. We do not know the outcome of this heroic piece of surgery, but after their martyr's deaths by beheading the twins became the patron saints of surgery.

The first reliable documentation of a severed human limb being successfully reattached to its owner's body was in 1962 – technically a 'replantation', not a transplanation, but none the less dramatic for that. On May 23, a boy of twelve lost his right arm just below the shoulder in an accident. Thirty minutes later he was admitted to the Massachusetts General Hospital, Boston, where the arm was placed in an ice and salt mixture and its arteries perfused with a solution that would keep it nourished and free from clotting and infection. When the boy was ready for surgery, Ronald Malt and Charles McKhann first fixed the humerus with a nail through the marrow to give them the necessary stability for joining up all the muscles and blood vessels. The nerves they grafted three-and-a-half months later. Twenty months after this, the boy had sensation in his fingers, could write his name, and could lift 10-pound weights. In 1963 the two surgeons repeated the performance on a man of forty-four but, as they pointed out, the patients chosen for replantation must be those who would benefit more from having their own arms than artificial ones, and suitable for the arduous task of rehabilitation[1]. Not long afterwards a number of reports came from China of workers having hands and feet successfully replanted.

Research on transplantation began at the beginning of the 20th century with, as we saw in the last chapter, the work of Alexis Carrel and of Charles Guthrie, the Pittsburgh physiologist (so often neglected), first of all on blood vessel anastomosis, the sine qua non of transplantation surgery, and then on the transplantation of tissues, organs (kidney, ovary, thyroid and parathyroid) and limbs. Apart from showing the technical feasibility of such undertakings, their work demonstrated beyond doubt the surprising fact that nervous connections were unnecessary for the satisfactory functioning of transplanted organs.

Before moving on to discuss the problems of transplantation and what has been achieved, it would be as well to define the various procedures covered by the broad term 'transplantation'. Organs and tissues can be removed from an animal and put back into the same animal – replantation or autotransplantation, a technique often used at the beginning of research to discover the technical difficulties and assess the basic problems of function that may arise. Organs and tissues can be taken from one animal and transplanted into another of the same species – homotransplantation. Or they may be transplanted into an animal of a different species – heterotransplantation.

Finally, organs may be transplanted into their anatomically correct place in the recipient body or into another perhaps more convenient area. In one way or another all these procedures have been applied in human surgery.

Some of the transplantations and related work have been for academic research; indeed if one gives one's imagination full rein the implications could be quite horrifying. For example, in 1912 Guthrie told how he had kept the head of a puppy, grafted onto the side of the neck of an adult dog, alive for a few hours[2]. Between them, Guthrie and Carrel transplanted kidneys, adrenals, thyroids, parathyroids, ovaries, legs, arms, loops of intestines, the lower half of the body, the head and neck, and the heart[3]. The prime purpose of these experiments was to study the function of the transplanted tissues and organs, not to pave the way for transplantation surgery. Nevertheless, the possibility was not far from the front of their minds for, as Carrel wrote: 'Another difficulty would be that of finding organs suitable for transplantation into man. A process of immunization would no doubt be necessary before organs of animals would be suitable for transplantation into man. Organs from a person killed by accident would no doubt be suitable.'[4] Thirty-five years on, Vladimir Demikhov, a Russian, launched himself on another tidal wave of transplantation studies; among his experiments was a repeat of Guthrie's grafting of a puppy's head onto the neck of an adult dog. This time the puppy's head lived for twenty-nine days[5].

But to return to the practical problems of organ and tissue transplantation: Grafting of tissue from one part of a patient to another part of his own body is a common undertaking when skin and bone are used, and it is also practicable, to a more limited extent, in blood-vessel surgery; yet, however valuable these particular procedures are, there is obviously a limit to the amount of tissue that can be grafted and to which tissues can be used. An alternative is to take the graft from other human beings (or even animals), but here the big difficulty is met. For some reason not properly understood, the tissues of a human being are peculiar to its owner's body and when grafted onto another body they invoke what is known as an antibody reaction, with the result that the recipient body rejects the graft after a variable number of days. If the complex biochemical reaction could be elucidated and measures taken to overcome it, surgery could expand its scope immeasurably. One or two clues have been given by experimental work on animals and from grafting operations on patients whose body chemistry is disordered.

In the attempt to prevent rejection, tissues and organs are typed or matched before grafting, in much the same way as blood is grouped. A complete correspondence of all the many antigens is an impossibility (as far as we know) but when the tissue to be grafted or transplanted is in plentiful supply (all too rarely) it is often possible to match the major antigens. Exceptions to this are grafts between identical twins who, from the transplantation point of view, can be regarded as one person. Grafting of tissues from one person to another without generally encountering rejection problems is, however, possible when the graft is only required to act as scaffolding for the body to build around and is not called upon to continue functioning. Examples of this are bone and artery grafts, and the very special case of the cornea in the eye (see Chapter 16).

The endocrine organs have attracted the attention of transplant surgeons for a number of years, and although most of the work has been on experimental animals, a few operations have been performed clinically. One of the first concerned the adrenal glands which lie just above the kidneys. In 1946 Lennox Ross Broster, a surgeon, and Harold Gardiner-Hill, a physician, of London, removed an adrenal gland from a woman who was suffering from the effects of its overactivity, and grafted it onto the blood vessels inside another woman who was suffering from Addison's disease and whose own adrenal glands were inactive. Later tests on the patient showed either that the graft was functioning or that her own adrenals had recovered[6].

There has been only slight interest in transplanting the thyroid gland because of the ready availability of thyroid hormone as a drug but in 1890, before this appeared, Odilon Marc Lannelongue treated a cretin by thyroid transplantation[7].

Transplantation of the ovaries got off to a good start when, in 1906, Robert Morris of New York reported the birth of a living child to a woman whose ovaries had been removed and replaced with those of another four years previously[8]. Experimental work flourished in the first decade of the 20th century and then subsided until the 1960s. In 1964, for instance, James Hardy of the University of Mississippi reported the removal and replantation of the uterus and ovaries of a dog[9]. To emphasize the success of the procedure, the dog subsequently gave birth to a litter of healthy puppies. But despite this encouraging experimental work the idea was overtaken by events in the laboratory. It was simpler to remove eggs from a donor, fertilize them with the spouse's sperm and implant two or three in the woman's womb.

The bulk of the pancreas is concerned with the production of digestive juices but about 1 percent consists of the islets of Langerhans which secrete insulin. In the 1960s attempts were made to see whether grafting pancreatic tissue would help patients with diabetes mellitus[10] and in 1966 Richard Lillehei and William Kelly of Minnesota reported that they had developed two different techniques: in one they used the whole pancreas with its duct and the length of duodenum into which it secretes its digestive juices. In the other, only part of the pancreas was transplanted, the duct was closed and it was hoped that the secretion of digestive juices would be abolished, after transplantation, by radiotherapy which would not affect the secretion of insulin into the blood stream. Their first clinical operation made use of the second method, but although technically successful the radiation failed to stop the production of digestive juices, and the production of insulin soon failed. The twenty-eight-year-old diabetic patient also had chronic kidney failure and at the same operation she received a kidney transplant, but this too failed to function satisfactorily. Two months after the operation the two transplanted organs were removed and she was kept alive on an artificial kidney.

Lillehei and Kelly's next patient was a woman of thirty-two, a diabetic since the age of ten and in the last stages of kidney failure. On New Year's Eve, 1966, another woman died from a brain haemorrhage and one of her kidneys, her pancreas and a section of duodenum were used as grafts. The kidney was inserted into the recipient's right lower abdomen (iliac fossa) where it began to secrete urine as soon as its blood vessels had been anastomosed; the pancreas and duodenum were transplanted into the left iliac fossa and their blood vessels anastomosed. The top end of the duodenum was stitched closed and the lower end brought out at an opening on the skin surface. In earlier experiments the lower end had been anastomosed to the animal's small bowel for drainage of the digestive juices, but in this clinical case Lillehei and Kelly decided against it; the anastomosis would be done at a later operation. Four months after the double transplant the patient had weathered two rejection crises with the aid of drugs and no longer required insulin[11]. When the two surgeons were assessing the second operation, Lillehei remarked, 'I think we've overlooked the fact that we may also be proving that you can successfully transplant ten inches of bowel' – referring to the length of duodenum.

The origins of kidney transplantation can, like so much else in this field, be traced back to the opening years of the 20th century when, apart from the studies of Carrel and Guthrie, a fair amount of experimental work was being done. Possibly the first heterotransplant (from dog to goat) was reported in 1902 by Emerich Ullman in Austria; he put the dog's kidney in the goat's neck and used tubes for the anastomosis between the blood vessels[12]. Then came a scattering of human operations, all employing heterotransplants. In 1905, M. Princeteau of Bordeaux inserted two pieces of rabbit kidney into an incision in a child's kidney; the volume of urine temporarily increased but the child died sixteen days afterwards[13]. The following year Mathieu Jaboulay in Lyon grafted, first, a pig's kidney onto the arm blood vessels of a forty-eight-year-old woman; it secreted urine satisfactorily for two days, then failed. His second patient, a woman of fifty, received a goat's kidney on her arm which again functioned for two days before failing[14]. Difficulties with the arterial sutures explained the differences between his experimental results and those of Carrel. The first person to transplant a kidney into its correct anatomical place was N. Floresco, working with dogs in Jonnesco's clinic in Bucharest; the longest survival he achieved with one kidney was twelve days, and with two, 165 hours[15]. Ernst Unger, of the University of Berlin, in 1910 transplanted the kidney of a non-human primate into a patient who survived for thirty-two hours[16]. Harold Neuhof of New York in 1923 reported his use of lamb's kidneys as the graft for a patient whose own kidneys had failed as a result of mercury poisoning; his patient lived for nine days[17]. But despite Neuhof's expressed optimism for the future, the general feeling was one of despair until the 1950s.

Willem Kolff's invention, during World War II, of the artificial kidney machine (we will come back to this later) marked the turning point, as it enabled seriously ill patients to be brought to a reasonably fit state to withstand surgery. A modified version had been installed at the Peter Bent Brigham Hospital, Boston, in 1949, and three years later David Hume and John Merrill reported on their experience with six patients in advanced, irreversible, chronic kidney failure. The donor kidneys in three cases came from cadavers, and in the other three from surgical operations in which removal was necessary. In all cases the kidney was placed in the recipient's thigh, where it was anastomosed to the main blood vessels, and the ureter was brought out onto the skin surface. This procedure necessitated a skin graft to increase the diameter of the thigh. Three of the transplants never produced urine at all, but the other three did so until eventually destroyed by infection[18]. By 1955 Hume and Merrill had operated on three more patients, in only one of whom was there temporary success[19].

Next on the scene was the team at the Necker Hospital, Paris, under the physician Jean Hamburger. Marius R., a sixteen-year-old carpenter, seriously injured his right kidney, and it had to be removed. Then to everyone's horror he was found to have no left kidney. On Christmas night, 1952, his mother (who belonged to the same blood group) donated her right kidney which was grafted into Marius's right iliac fossa, where it functioned well for three weeks. Marius died from pulmonary oedema (waterlogged lungs) and failure of the graft[20].

Gordon Murray of Toronto, had, before World War II, been working on the autotransplantation of dogs' kidneys to their necks, and subsequently on the grafting of human kidneys to patients' arms as a temporary measure when normal renal function was expected to recover (a sort of non-artificial kidney machine). These grafts were not very satisfactory, although they did function to a certain degree. Then, in 1954, Murray reported that he had grafted a human kidney onto the external iliac vessels (in the pelvis) of a woman whose own kidneys had been steadily deteriorating for one and a half years. Within eight weeks she was out of bed, her health greatly improved and, at the time of the report, she had been back at work as a stenographer for fifteen months. She was his only success out of four similar operations[21].

But the operation that really put kidney grafting on the map took place on December 23, 1954, when John Merrill used the patient's identical twin brother as the donor, thus showing his faith in the technical aspects of the operation provided the problems of infection and rejection, which had plagued his previous attempts, could be overcome. The patient was a young man, twenty-four years old, dying from a severe disease of both kidneys. After extensive tests had shown that his twin brother was in fact his identical twin and had two healthy kidneys, the transplantation took place. The brothers were operated on in adjoining theatres and at 9:53a.m. the donor kidney arrived ready for grafting. It was anastomosed to blood vessels (the hypogastric artery and common iliac vein) in the pelvis, and the ureter was led into the bladder. The whole procedure took three-and-a-half hours. Thereafter, the patient steadily improved with his new kidney functioning perfectly, and at two subsequent dates his own useless kidneys were removed with further beneficial effects[22]. He later married his nurse and became a father[23].

By the end of the 1950s Peter Medawar's demonstration in 1944 that rejection of skin grafts was due to an immunological reaction[24] – he shared the 1960 Nobel Prize for Medicine or Physiology for his work – was beginning to bear fruit, particularly when the same mechanism was shown to be operative in the rejection of organs. Understanding the nature of a problem helps towards its solution, and the earliest attempts to suppress the immune reaction were made by subjecting the patient to whole-body irradiation before operation. In 1959 this method was used in the first kidney transplants between non-identical twins carried out by Merrill in Boston and by Hamburger in Paris. Merrill's patient received two doses of irradiation eight days apart, and after operation was nursed for a month in a room sterilized by detergent, with positive-inflow ventilation and an ultraviolet ray barrier. The diseased kidneys were later removed and the patient made a satisfactory recovery[25].

At this time drugs specially designed as immunosuppressive agents were making their appearance, which allowed surgeons to use a wider range of donor material – no longer did the donor have to be an identical twin or a close relative. Cadaver kidneys provided a valuable source of supply, and a great deal of work was done on methods of storage. In 1963 and 1964 there was a short-lived burst of enthusiasm for employing non-human primates as donors. For instance, Keith Reemtsma of Tulane University School of Medicine in June 1963 transplanted both kidneys from a chimpanzee into the right iliac region of a forty-three-year-old man. The kidneys functioned well and the patient overcame two episodes of rejection with the aid of drugs, but he died after two months from a lung infection; the transplanted kidneys showed no signs of rejection[26]. In 1966 Reemtsma reported that patients had survived up to nine months after receiving chimpanzee kidneys[27].

Before leaving the kidneys, a word must be said about the artificial kidney, as this has played a not inconsiderable part in preparing patients for surgery and in supporting them if the transplant fails. A kidney machine was used in laboratory experiments as long ago as 1913, but not until 1944 did the world learn of the first clinical application of such a machine when Willem Kolff published an amazing story. During the Nazi occupation of Holland, he had built, in the Municipal Hospital at Kampen, an artificial kidney and had used it successfully despite the fact that the dialysing membrane was composed of nothing more nor less than cellophane[28, 29].

The early kidney machines were unreliable and hazardous, but once their value was appreciated, technical developments proceeded apace and in the next decade many types of safe and efficient machines became available. The most important advances were the introduction of non-wettable plastic tubing, special cellophane membranes, and improved pumps and methods of sterilization. At first the artificial kidney was used only to treat patients with acute renal failure or poisoning by dialysable drugs. In these cases the idea was to keep the patient alive until the kidneys recovered from the acute episode. Then, in the early 1960s, Belding Scribner began treating patients with chronic renal failure by long-term, repeated, intermittent dialysis. This was made possible by the introduction of the Teflon-Silastic Scribner shunt which would remain patent for a long time when kept in veins or arteries. Previously, cannulae had clotted and had had to be reinserted every few weeks at a different site until eventually no suitable sites remained.

Other problems, such as infection and technical difficulties, were soon largely overcome, and chronic renal dialysis became a reality. It was then that considerations other than purely medical ones became only too apparent. The technique was costly, almost prohibitively so, and patients had to be selected. The chosen ones were admitted to hospital twice a week for some sixteen hours while dialysis took place. But for the remainder of the week, they were able to lead near-normal lives and earn their livings. In some hospitals, committees were set up to decide which patients should receive treatment, since it was felt the problem was one for society rather than medicine. Nevertheless, much thought was given to circumventing this unenviable situation, and in 1964 home dialysis using a simplified and largely automated machine was introduced. However, some surgeons, such as John Merrill, were seriously concerned about costs and regarded home dialysis as merely a short-term method of managing the patient in chronic renal failure outside hospital until a kidney suitable for grafting became available.

Animal experiments on homotransplantation of the lung were recorded by Vladimir Demikhov in 1947, although the Western world was not to learn of them until 1962 when the translation of his book, *Experimental transplantation of vital organs*[5], was published. For example, on one occasion he transplanted the right lower lobe of a dog's lung into the thoracic cavity of another; the recipient animal survived seven days. But in the meantime the West, too, had been testing the waters, and from 1950 onwards a steady stream of reports was published on the replantation and homotransplantation of dog lungs or lobes of lungs. Andre Juvenelle of Buffalo, New York, replanted the right lung of a dog in May 1950; the animal maintained good health and normal respiratory function until it was sacrificed thirty-five months later[30]. Homotransplantation, however, produced a multitude of problems, with the length of survival being measurable only in days.

Nevertheless, on June 11, 1963, James Hardy of the University of Mississippi Medical Center transplanted the lung of a man who had died from a heart attack into another patient. Hardy had previously done more than four hundred experiments on dogs and had decided that his first human transplant should be of the left lung, as it was technically easier than the right. For over a year he waited for a suitable case, and his eventual choice was a man of fifty-eight who fulfilled all the requirements and preferred the chance of a cure, however remote, to palliative radiotherapy. This patient, a heavy smoker, had a cancer obstructing the main bronchus with resulting chronic infection that had virtually destroyed the whole lung. His right lung was emphysematous and inefficient; his life expectancy was obviously limited. Unfortunately, he also had serious chronic renal disease which almost decided Hardy against the transplant.

The operation lasted three hours, and afterwards the patient was given drugs and cobalt radiotherapy to prevent rejection. The lung functioned well right from the start, but alas, the kidney disease sapped his strength and he died on the eighteenth day. Post-mortem examination revealed no evidence that the lung was being rejected (donor and recipient shared eight of the thirteen blood groups tested)[31].

Transplantation of the liver is beset with technical difficulties. The organ is bulky and there are many bothersome little anastomoses to be performed. Probably the first technically successful experimental homotransplantation was achieved in 1956 by Edward Goodrich of Albany Medical College. He drew attention to the particular sensitivity of the liver to lack of oxygen and to the presence (especially in dogs' livers) of bacteria that proliferate rapidly under anaerobic conditions. However, he managed to keep transplanted organs functioning in dogs for up to five days before they were rejected. The dogs' own livers were not removed[32]. In 1967 Thomas Starzl of the University of Colorado School of Medicine, Denver, reported on his own work to date and drew attention to the similar experiments carried out in Boston by Francis Moore and by workers in France[33]. Starzl transplanted the organ into its proper place after removal of the recipient's own liver. Initially the use of radiotherapy and immunosuppressive drugs did not materially affect the length of survival, even so, in 1967, he had several animals still living after three years.

In the spring and summer of 1963, Starzl made five attempts at human homotransplantation without a single success. The first case was a three-year-old boy whose bile ducts had failed to develop. Largely owing to the delay (seven hours) between death of the donor and completion of the anastomoses, the child only lived four hours before dying from operative haemorrhage. The remaining patients and two others operated on in Boston and Paris were all adults, mostly over fifty, with cancer of the liver, either primary or metastatic; the longest survival was twenty-two days. At the post-mortems there were relatively few signs of rejection, death being due in most instances to haemorrhage or infection.

Once a diseased liver has been removed the new liver has to function right from the start, particularly as there is invariably a co-existing complex metabolic disorder. To sidestep the hazard of possible failure, livers were grafted into other parts of the abdomen leaving the patient's liver undisturbed. Starzl recorded in his 1967 paper that he had transplanted an auxiliary liver into the lower abdomen in two patients dying from cirrhosis. The new livers functioned in both patients before death occurred from sepsis after twenty-three and thirty-five days.

Although there was no machine to support a patient in liver failure, unlike the kidney for which the artificial kidney was available, a method employing a pig's liver was developed, primarily to help a patient overcome temporary failure when there was a reasonable chance that his own liver would recover. Ben Eiseman of the University of Kentucky found pig's liver cheap, easy to maintain, and ideal for the purpose, as it is normally free from bacteria. After much experimentation, he first used the technique clinically on a man of forty-two in April 1964. The liver was removed from the pig, flushed through, connected up to arteries and veins in the patient's thigh (later, blood vessels in the arm were used) and placed in a special perfusion chamber. A pump was included in the extracorporeal circuit to pump the blood back into the patient's vein after it had passed through the liver. At first the patients chosen were judged to be moribund and the longest survival was twelve days. In 1966 Eiseman reported his total experience with forty-five patients; only eight recovered completely, but five of these, who were alcoholics, went back on the bottle as soon as they left hospital and died within a month or two[34].

Transplantation of the heart has a longer history than that of the liver, extending back as it does to the experiments of Carrel and Guthrie; but these were purely academic, as were those of Frank Mann of Georgetown University in 1933. The heart was usually placed in a pouch fashioned beneath the skin of the neck with the carotid artery of the host joined to the coronary arteries, and the coronary veins anastomosed to the external jugular vein. These workers had no intention of letting this extra heart support the animal's circulation. The experiments were simply designed to see what happened when the heart of one animal was transplanted to another: as Mann concluded, it behaved just the same as other organs[35].

By the 1950s, though, serious thought was being given to placing a donor heart in its correct anatomical site where it could replace the functions of the host's heart. For instance, Charles Bailey (then of Philadelphia) and his colleagues reported in 1952 how they had substituted a dog's heart and lungs in three experiments. They first devised a technique whereby the substitution could be done in less than fifteen minutes. Both donor and recipient dogs were cooled to 24°C for the operation, and in the most successful case the dog survived six hours with a normal electrocardiogram (for 24°C) and a return of reflexes and spontaneous breathing[36]. (Because of the anastomoses entailed, it was technically less difficult to transplant the heart and lungs as a unit rather than the heart on its own.)

Although a number of centres throughout the world were working on heart grafting, maximum survival times were all around the six-hour mark until Norman Shumway of Stanford University, California, in 1960 devised a vastly improved surgical technique. The essential aspects of this were to leave parts of the recipient animal's atria and atrial septum behind so as to reduce the number of vascular anastomoses required, and to improve the method of cannulation of the vessels so that the catheters did not obtrude into the surgical area and yet kept the heart nourished more efficiently. The donor hearts were cooled to 12–15°C and no attempt was made to alter the immune status of the animals. After the operations he used a machine to keep the recipient's circulation going until its new heart was fully able to do the necessary work. Survival times were greatly improved and some dogs lived for as long as twenty-one days. During this time the animals were normally active, but when the end came it was rapid due, Shumway presumed, to rejection of the homograft[37].

The studies that were to lead to the first human patient receiving another heart began in 1956. More than two hundred animal heart transplants were performed in his laboratory by James Hardy, in addition to which he removed and replaced the heart in many human cadavers. He even had what he called a 'dry run' with a heart operation going on at the same time as a suitable donor was dying. Had the patient required a new heart he could have had one. Thus Hardy was technically and organizationally equipped to carry out a heart transplant; the moral and ethical considerations had been discussed at length, and more than a year before it happened the decision had been taken to transplant a heart when all conditions were suitable[38].

On January 23, 1964, a man of sixty-eight was admitted to the University Hospital of the University of Mississippi Medical Center with hypertensive cardiovascular disease and severe coronary arteriosclerosis. His blood pressure had fallen to undetectable levels. The outlook was bad. However, he was put on a heart-lung machine as there was a young man in the recovery ward at death's door from irrecoverable brain damage. But the young man lingered on. When the patient's own heart action ceased, the situation became critical. So Hardy decided to use a chimpanzee's heart instead; in the circumstances he believed this would be well within ethical and moral boundaries. Unfortunately the chimp only weighed ninety-six pounds, considerably less than the patient, and although the heart beat well after transplantation it was too small to cope with the task required of it in spite of the fact that Hardy implanted pacemakers to boost its rate. It could not maintain the blood pressure and the patient died after a few hours. News of the operation leaked out to the press, which at first believed a human donor had been used; when the truth was told the excitement died down.

Later that year Shumway and Lower wrote: 'Perhaps the cardiac surgeon should pause while society becomes accustomed to resurrection of the mythological chimera.'[39] But he did not.

Even so the world should have been prepared for what was by then the inevitable. But it was not, either. The events at Groote Schuur Hospital, Cape Town, on December 3, 1967, shook a goodly proportion of doctors and laymen alike. On that day Christiaan Barnard and his team transplanted the heart of a girl of twenty-four, who had died from head injuries, into fifty-four-year-old Louis Washkansky. Washkansky was a diabetic who had had heart attacks in 1959, 1960 and 1965 – examination of his heart after removal showed that about 90 percent of the muscle had been destroyed and replaced by scar tissue. He was now in intractable heart failure and readily agreed to the hope offered by transplantation. This took place in the early hours of the morning, using the technique devised by Norman Shumway. Immunosuppressive drugs were given from the day of operation and the heart itself was, at intervals, locally irradiated from a cobalt source[40]. In a blaze of publicity that Barnard was powerless to prevent, Washkansky lived for eighteen days, with the heart performing well and correcting all the biochemical upsets brought about by the failure of his own heart, before dying from extensive bilateral pneumonia. At the post-mortem the transplanted heart was at first thought to show signs of rejection, but these were later proved to be due to the radiation[41]. (Contrary to rumours circulating at the time, Barnard had a sound experimental and clinical background for what he did[42].)

Meanwhile, on December 6, Adrian Kantrowitz in Brooklyn had transplanted the heart of an infant born with a grossly deficient brain into a two-and-a-half-week-old boy who had a lethal heart defect. This heart beat for only six-and-a-half hours[43].

The next operation, on January 2, 1968, was again carried out by Barnard's highly coordinated team; the recipient was Philip Blaiberg, a fifty-eight-year-old dentist, and the donor a Cape Coloured man of twenty-four who had died suddenly from a brain haemorrhage. Blaiberg successfully overcame a number of rejection crises and gave every indication of thoroughly enjoying his extra life, despite – or perhaps because of – being virtually a human pillbox. Blaiberg's progress confounded Barnard's critics and surprised and even puzzled his most ardent supporters. In June, 1969, Philip Blaiberg's health suddenly deteriorated and he died two months later, on August 17, having survived for five hundred and ninety-three days and having been transformed from a breathless cardiac cripple into a man able to look after himself, drive a car and bathe in the sea[44].

The world now at long last had woken up to the reality of heart transplantation and was going to have its say, belatedly maybe, on the moral, social, ethical, religious and economic issues involved. Comment by doctors and laymen alike was by no means entirely favourable and at times the criticism looked remarkably like hysteria born of fear – fear deeply rooted in the beliefs of mankind; fear that the heart would be used for transplantation before the body was dead. But despite this atmosphere, one hundred and forty-three operations were performed in countries all over the world in the opening twenty months after the first human heart homotransplantation. Twenty-nine of the one hundred and forty-one recipients (two patients had the operation twice) were still alive, and one of them had survived for longer than six months. More than half the transplantations (eighty-four) took place in the United States of America. Happily, many of the teams who jumped on the transplantation bandwagon inadequately prepared, realized what they were up against and withdrew from the fray: the one hundred and forty-three heart transplants were performed by fifty-six teams, but only about ten of them were still carrying on after those twenty months.

Amongst those well-qualified to continue was Norman Shumway who, on January 6, 1968, put into effect his years of experimental preparation when he transplanted the heart of a forty-three-year-old woman into Michael Kasperak who was dying from chronic viral myocarditis. Misfortune dogged the way from the start. The diseased heart was so enlarged that the space left after its removal was nearly three times the size of the donor heart. This gave rise to technical problems, and five hours after the operation the fifty-four-year-old patient had to be taken back to theatre where his chest was reopened and fluid removed from the pericardial cavity. Then, about two days later, his kidneys and liver began to fail – as a result of his long-standing heart condition their function was seriously impaired – and he began bleeding from his gastrointestinal tract, a manifestation of the liver failure. The kidney failure was treated by peritoneal dialysis and the bleeding by massive blood transfusion. Eight days later he had his gall-bladder removed under local anaesthetic, but the end was not far off and he died a few days later[45].

Another surgeon who was well prepared was Denton Cooley. He had graduated from Johns Hopkins University School of Medicine where, in due course, he became surgical resident to Alfred Blalock. Yet, with all his previous vast experience of cardiac surgery he admitted: 'Dr Barnard showed that a heart transplant patient could survive. Otherwise I would have hesitated.'[46] At the beginning of May, 1968, his team had been on twenty-four-hour alert for three months. Then by a remarkable coincidence he obtained three donors and three suitable recipients within a four-day period. The first patient, a man of forty-seven, on May 3 received the heart of a fifteen-year-old girl who had shot herself in the head. The second, another man of forty-seven, was operated on on May 5;

his heart came from a fifteen-year-old boy. And the third, a man of sixty-two, received his new heart on May 7[47]. In an addendum to the report of these cases, Cooley mentioned that one patient had received the heart of a sheep: he died. By the beginning of October, 1968, Cooley had performed ten human heart transplants with seven survivors at that time. Some of the patients had returned to work.

Cooley was renowned for his swiftness in operating, with not one unnecessary movement. 'Remember,' he said, 'that in surgery the longer you take, the sicker the patient gets.'[46] But he was not stressing speed for speed's sake. By sheer skill and organization he reduced the length of operation from about four-and-a-half hours to one hour and forty-five minutes, skin to skin. In certain respects his transplantation technique differed from that of others such as Barnard and Shumway. For instance, he neither cooled nor perfused the donor heart; this at first was a controversial point, but it was eventually endorsed by other cardiac surgeons.

On the same day (May 3, 1968) that Cooley carried out his first heart transplant, the first British operation was performed by Donald Ross at the National Heart Hospital in London. The recipient was a forty-five-year-old man who for three years had had a chronic heart condition and was now in severe congestive failure. Ross had been looking for a suitable donor for some time and during the previous week had been searching hard. Then on May 2, a man of twenty-six sustained serious head injuries in a fall on a building site. He was operated on at King's College Hospital but could not be saved. The following afternoon, Ross knew he had a donor, and all preparations were made while the body was rushed across London in an ambulance with the circulation maintained by external cardiac massage[48]. The recipient, Frederick West, lived for forty-five days.

Looking back over the achievements of the past one hundred and fifty years, since the discovery of anaesthesia heralded a new era in human endeavour, we can trace a number of fairly distinct phases that yet merge imperceptibly. When Lister gave realization to the possibilities opened up by anaesthesia, a period of intense activity followed, during which the basic principles of surgical technique were developed and specialization made its necessary appearance. During this period also, many 'modern' operations were introduced and a surprising number of apparently recent innovations first saw the light of day, only to fail because the human body was called upon to withstand too much unaided. The next phase was that of consolidation. In the years between the wars, blood transfusion, knowledge of fluid balance, advances in anaesthesia and the beginnings of chemotherapy, gave surgery a new lease of life. Public-health measures, antibiotics, and advances in medical diagnosis and treatment all helped to alter the conditions for which surgery was required. Diseases that are largely the result of infections, such as empyema, mastoiditis, osteomyelitis and the late ravages of venereal disease, that constituted a large part of surgical practice in years gone by, now came to occupy a place of minor importance in the general picture of surgery. They could be prevented or cured before a surgeon's knife was needed, and there would seem to be no reason why eventually the same could not apply to many of the diseases on a modern operating list. But lest we become too confident, it would be as well to remember that we really know very little about the human body: once one problem is overcome Nature has a peculiar propensity for producing something else just to keep the balance even.

The phase that occupied the last part of the 20th century still continues but in a state of transition. It was based upon the previous ones and was characterized by fresh progress in surgical techniques and the development of new operations. Much was unspectacular and concerned with improving the accepted routines and practices of surgery. Standing out, however, was the development of the use of the microscope. An important defining feature of the forthcoming phase will be minimally invasive laparoscopic surgery - keyhole surgery - the foundations of which were laid by Kurt Semm, a gynaecologist, in the 1970s and 1980s at the University of Kiel. Initially, his work was received with ridicule and scepticism, but he persevered and the technique has become standard practice for a surprising array of operations. Fibreoptics provide the illumination and a telescope transmits the image to a television screen. Also already on the scene is telemanipulation which enables surgeons (maybe miles away) to perform operations without putting their hands inside the body cavity concerned - for instance, coronary artery bypass, in which instruments are placed inside the chest through small incisions (ports) and the surgeon then sits at a console which faithfully transmits his hand movements to the instruments. Many other instances of surgery taking advantage of present and future scientific discoveries undoubtedly lie just around the corner.

In *Heart of Darkness* Joseph Conrad wrote: 'The mind of man is capable of anything - because everything is in it, all the past as well as all the future.' The prospect is exciting, indeed.

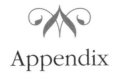

Appendix

Anatomy of the abdominal contents

The abdomen is home to a wonderful array of organs. Extending from the diaphragm in the north to the pelvic floor in the south, the gastrointestinal tract is the boiler house of the body. But the abdomen contains much else besides: on either side at the back are the kidneys (the left usually a little higher than the right) protected by the lower ribs in front and by powerful muscles behind. Sitting on top of them are the adrenal glands which produce important hormones. Lying behind the stomach on the left is the spleen – responsible for removing and destroying time-expired red blood cells and for the manufacture of the breed of white blood cells known as lymphocytes. And, more or less centrally down the back run the abdominal aorta carrying blood to the lower part of the body and (to its right) the inferior vena cava returning it to the heart when it has given up its oxygen and taken up waste carbon dioxide. Lastly, in the deep south of the pelvic cavity are found the bladder, receiving urine from the kidneys down the ureters, and the female organs of generation – the ovaries, fallopian tubes, the uterus and the vagina. The male organs, except for the prostate, the seminal vesicles and most of the connecting duct known as the vas deferens, made their escape to the relative coolness but apparent vulnerability of the scrotum before birth or soon after.

Forming a continuous lining to the walls of the abdominal cavity is the membranous peritoneum. It plasters the kidneys, major blood vessels and some other structures to the back wall with just sufficient firmness to allow whatever movement is required – for example, the kidneys can move up and down by 4 or 5cm, whereas the pancreas is virtually immovable. The peritoneum then roofs over the contents of the pelvic cavity, tucking itself in between the various organs to create pouches and folds, and is continued up the inside of the front of the abdominal wall to line the under surface of the diaphragm. The cavity it forms is the peritoneal cavity which, because it is filled with the gastrointestinal tract, the liver and gall-bladder, is more potential than real. The other digestive organ, the pancreas, is fixed behind the peritoneum. The spleen, which is not concerned with digestion, does, however, lie within the peritoneal cavity.

The structures within the cavity are, with one or two exceptions, completely covered in peritoneum which has been reflected from the back wall and returned to the same place when it has done its job. For instance, the small intestine is at least 4m long yet the peritoneum that fans out to surround it originates from, and returns to, an obliquely situated root of a mere 15cm or so. This great fan is known as its mesentery and brings it its blood vessels, lymph vessels and nerve supply. The appendix and the transverse and pelvic colons have their own, much smaller mesenteries.

In surrounding the structures within its cavity, the peritoneum forms a number of so-called 'ligaments' (not to be confused with those of the musculo-skeletal variety), sacs and folds. The ligaments serve to carry blood and lymphatic vessels and nerves to the various structures. The arrangement is highly complex and the only formation we need bother about is the greater omentum. This fold of peritoneum hangs down from the greater curvature of the stomach like a great apron before returning to envelop the transverse colon. It is burdened with greater or lesser amounts of fat. Frequently, however, the surgeon finds the apron folded in between coils of intestine or tucked into some other part of the cavity.

By secreting a sufficiency of serous fluid the peritoneum performs the extremely valuable function of allowing the organs to slide around and over one another. For instance, much of an empty stomach sits snugly under the rib cage, but after a good meal it may stretch down to the borders of the pelvic cavity. In similar fashion the downward curve of the transverse colon is exaggerated when loaded with faeces. The mobile structures within the cavity also slide about under the influence of gravity and the peritoneal fluid allows the waves of peristaltic activity to sweep unhindered down the small intestine during digestion.

The peritoneal cavity in the male is completely shut off from the outside world, but in the female the fallopian (uterine) tubes open into it close to the ovaries, ready to catch the ova when these are shed at the time of ovulation. Consequently there is a passage from the cavity along the tubes to the uterus and into the vagina and so to the exterior. Infection in the female genital tract may thus spread inwards and lead to adhesions (and, in consequence, perhaps to infertility) or evidence of peritonitis.

The reason for labouring the anatomy of the peritoneum is that it is of great importance to the surgeon since it can be a valuable ally in the healing process – when given a reasonable chance, it can put up a strong fight against infection. Apart from infection being introduced from outside, inflammation of the peritoneum (peritonitis) is nearly always secondary to inflammation of one of the organs it is in contact with. In these cases it produces an abundant exudation which helps with the healing process and may lead to the formation of adhesions to seal off the offending area. When infection is present the result is likely to be a suppurative peritonitis in which the pus may be sealed off or track from the original site to any of the various compartments of the peritoneal cavity.

And now a quick run down the gastrointestinal tract so that when we come to discuss surgical operations, the names of the structures may have a degree of familiarity. After piercing the diaphragm, the oesophagus has only a very short journey before it joins the stomach which, at its upper end, is firmly fixed to the posterior abdominal wall. This sac-like organ curves from left to right to end in the narrow pyloric canal and pyloric sphincter – a circle of muscle preventing food both rushing into the duodenum and regurgitating back into the stomach. The duodenum is roughly C-shaped, the first and short fourth parts of which are relatively mobile to allow for movement of the stomach and the jejunum, respectively. The second and third parts are firmly fixed to the back wall of the abdomen behind their covering of peritoneum. In the curve of the C lies the head of the pancreas, its tail reaching the spleen (besides producing digestive juices, the pancreas secretes the hormone insulin from what are known as its islet cells). The main duct of the pancreas joins with, but does not enter, the common bile duct to open into the second part of the duodenum at the duodenal papilla or ampulla of Vater (named after Abraham Vater who described it in 1720), guarded at the point of entry by another circle of muscle – the sphincter of Oddi (named after the Italian Ruggero Oddi who described it in 1887). An accessory pancreatic duct opens into the duodenum a short distance higher up.

The common bile duct is formed by the junction of the common hepatic duct (carrying bile directly from the liver) with the cystic duct (carrying bile from the gall-bladder). During meals the sphincter of Oddi relaxes to allow bile to flow into the duodenum; but between whiles it contracts so that the bile formed in the liver flows along the common hepatic duct to be stored in the gall-bladder.

The next part of the small intestine after the duodenum is the jejunum which merges imperceptibly into the ileum. After its run of four or more metres the small intestine ends at the ileo-caecal valve to enter the first part of the large intestine – the caecum, from the bottom of which hangs the appendix. This perverse little structure can cause the surgeon quite a few headaches: he may find it dangling where he hoped it would; however, it may have hidden itself away behind coils of intestine; it may have risen up behind the caecum; or it may have dropped into the pelvic cavity and in the female patient may be lying close to the right ovary creating problems of differential diagnosis. It may be stuck to its surroundings and it may have formed an abscess which may burst into the peritoneal cavity.

The large intestine continues, after the caecum, as the ascending colon (which has no mesentery and so is firmly secured); this takes a right-angled bend to the left to become the transverse colon (which has a mesentery). When it reaches its left extremity it, too, takes a right-angled turn, this time downwards to become the descending colon (again with no mesentery) which, at the pelvic rim becomes the pelvic colon (with a mesentery). This becomes the rectum which gradually loses its peritoneal covering until its third and last part comes to lie below and behind the peritoneal cavity. Faeces congregate in the pelvic colon until the time comes for them to enter the empty rectum and create the urge to defaecate. The end of the large intestine is the anal canal and anus with its sphincter muscle to prevent unwelcome accidents.

The terminology of some of the operations on the gastrointestinal tract is at first sight more than a little formidable; but taken slowly and with an understanding of how the names are formed - despite the combination of Latin and Greek roots - it becomes clear what has been done.

The names that cause the most bother are those ending in –stomy. This is derived from the Greek *stoma*, a mouth, and is applied to an opening made between two hollow organs or between one hollow organ and the skin. Thus gastrostomy is an opening between the stomach and the skin surface; a colostomy is an opening between the colon and the skin surface (this may be qualified according to the segment of colon involved; for example, transverse colostomy; descending colostomy and so on; or it may be qualified according to the position where it is fashioned as with inguinal colostomy); and an ileostomy is an opening between the ileum and the skin surface. When two hollow organs are involved each is named; for example, gastroduodenostomy (between stomach and duodenum); gastrojejunostomy (between stomach and jejunum); gastroenterostomy (between stomach and small intestine).

Also troublesome are words ending in –tomy. This is derived from the Greek *tomos*, cutting, and is confusing because of its resemblance to –stomy. (To make matters worse, in their early days colostomies were called colotomies.) However, -tomy is familiar in the well-known appendicectomy. An example of the use of the two suffixes is provided by a surgeon who performs a tracheotomy to give the patient a tracheostomy - he cuts into the trachea to give the patient a hole to breathe through.

Sources

CHAPTER 1: BY THE BANKS OF THE STYX

1   Hemlow J. ed. (1986). *Fanny Burney. Selected letters and journals.* Oxford; Clarendon. [See pp. 134–40.]

CHAPTER 2: A FALSE DAWN

1   Thedoric. *Cyrurgia.* Book 4, Ch. 8, f. 146. In: Chauliac G. de. (1498) *Cyrurgia Guidonis de Chauliaco, Et Cyrurgia Bruni Theodorici.* Venice; Bonetus Locatelli for Octavius Scotus. (For a translation, see: Campbell E, Colton J. (1960). *The surgery of Theodoric; ca AD 1257*, II, 213. New York; Appleton-Century Crofts.)

2   Priestley J. (1772). Observations on different kinds of air. *Philosophical Transactions of the Royal Society of London*, 62, 147–264.

3   Davy H. (1800). *Researches, chemical and philosophical; chiefly concerning nitrous oxide, or dephlogisticated nitrous air and its respiration.* London; Johnson. (See p. 556)

4   Hickman H. (1824). *A letter on suspended animation.* Ironbridge; Smith.

5   Antiquack. (1825–6). Letter to the editor: Surgical humbug. *Lancet,* 9, 646–7.

6   Long CW. (1849). An account of the first use of sulphuric ether by inhalation as an anaesthetic in surgical operations. *Southern Medical Journal*, 5, 705–13.

7   Pope E. Cited in: Lyman HM. (1881). *Artificial anaesthesia and anaesthetics.* New York; W Wood. [By this date William Clarke was physician in Chicago.]

8   Morton WTG. (1847). *Circular. Morton's Letheon.* 5th ed. Boston; Dutton and Wentworth. [First edition, 1846.]

9   Jackson CT, Morton WTG. (1846). United States Patent No. 4848 (November 12).

10 Oliver Wendell Holmes's letter of November 21, 1846, to Morton is cited in: Warren E. (1847). *Some account of the Lethēon: or, who is the discoverer?* 3rd ed. Boston; Dutton and Wentworth. [See pp. 84–85.]

11 Bigelow HJ. (1846). Insensibility during surgical operations produced by inhalation. *Boston Medical and Surgical Journal*, 35, 309–17.

12 Dana RH. (Editor). A history of the ether discovery. *Littell's Living Age*, 16, 529–71; 575. [Contains a memoir by Morton to the French Academy of Sciences, Paris, dated Boston, July 31, 1847, and a report of the Trustees of the Massachusetts General Hospital.]

13 Wells H. (1847). *A history of the discovery of the application of nitrous oxide gas, ether, and other vapors, to surgical operations.* Hartford; JG Wells.

14 Squire, W. (1888). On the introduction of ether inhalation as an anaesthetic in London. *Lancet*, 1, 1220–1.

15 Boott F. (1847). Surgical operations performed during insensibility, produced by the inhalation of sulphuric ether. *Lancet*, 1, 5–8.

16 Scott W. (1872). Letter to the Editor: The exhibition of ether as an anaesthetic. *Lancet,*

2, 585.

17 Snow J. (1858). *On chloroform and other anaesthetics: their action and administration*. Edited, with a memoir of the author, by Benjamin W Richardson, MD. London; Churchill.

18 Simpson JY. (1847). On a new anaesthetic agent, more efficient than sulphuric ether. *Lancet*, 2, 549-50.

19 Snow J. (1847). *On the inhalation of the vapour of ether in surgical operations: containing a description of the various stages of etherization*. London; Churchill.

20 Morton WTG. (1850). *On the physiological effects of sulphuric ether, and its superiority to chloroform*. Boston; Clapp.

21 Marc-Dupuy. (1847). Note sur les effets de l'injection de l'éther dans le rectum. *Comptes Rendus Hebdomadaires des Séances de l'Académie des Sciences*, 24, 605-7.

22 Pirogoff. (1847). Nouveau procédé pour produire, au moyen de la vapeur d'éther, l'insensibilité chez les individus soumis des opérations chirurgicales. *Comptes Rendus Hebdomadaires des Séances de l'Académie des Sciences*, 24, 789.

23 Pirogoff. (1847). Effets des vapeurs d'éther administrées par le rectum. *Comptes Rendus Hebdomadaires des Séances de l'Académie des Sciences*, 24, 1110.

24 Oré. (1872). Des injections intra-veineuses de chloral. *Bulletin et Mémoires de la Société de Chirurgie de Paris*, 1, 400-12.

25 Oré. (1874). De l'anesthésie produite chez l'homme par les injections de chloral dans les veines. *Comptes Rendus Hebdomadaires des Séances de l'Académie des Sciences*, 78, 515-7; 651-4.

26 Bernard C. (1869). Des effets physiologiques de la morphine et de leur combinaison avec ceux du chloroforme. *Bulletin de Générale Thérapie*, 77, 241-56.

CHAPTER 3: WHITEWASH TO CARBOLIC

1 Simpson WG. ed. (1871). *Anaesthesia, hospitalism hermaphroditism and a proposal to stamp out small-pox and other contagious diseases*. Vol. 2 of *The works of Sir James Young Simpson, Bart*. Edinburgh; Black. [See p. 291.]

2 Smith D. (1998). *The Greenhill Napoleonic Wars data book*. London; Greenhill: Pennsylvania; Stackpole. [See pp. 547-8.]

3 Aristotle. See *Historia animalium*, lib.V, 1, 19, 31; lib.VI, 15, 16. Translated by D'Arcy W Thompson (1910). Oxford; Clarendon.

4 Labarraque AG. (1826). *The use of the chlorate of soda, and the chlorate of lime*. Translated by James Scott. London; Highly. [Original French edition, 1825.]

5 Pouteau C. (1760). *Mélanges de chirurgie*. Lyon; Regnault. [See pp. 180 et seq.]

6 Clarke J. (1790). Observations on the puerperal fever, more especially as it has of late occurred in the Lying-in Hospital of Dublin. *(Edinburgh) Medical Commentaries*, (15) n.s. 5, 299-324.

7 Denman T. (1794-5). *An introduction to the practice of midwifery*. 2 vols. London; Johnson. [See vol. 2, pp. 477 et seq.]

8 Gordon A. (1795). *A treatise on the epidemic puerperal fever of Aberdeen*. London; Robinson. [See pp. 50 et seq.]

9 Collins R. (1835). *A practical treatise on midwifery, containing the result of sixteen thousand six hundred and fifty-four births, occurring in the Dublin Lying-in Hospital, during a period of seven years, commencing November 1826*. London; Longman, Rees, Orme, Browne, Green and Longman. [See pp. 388-9.]

10 Holmes OW. (1842-3). The contagiousness of puerperal fever. *New England Quarterly Journal of Medicine*, **1**, 503-30.

11 Kneeland S. (1846). On the contagiousness of puerperal fever. *American Journal of the Medical Sciences*, n.s. **11**, 45-63.

12 Kneeland S. (1846). On the connection between puerperal fever and epidemic erysipelas, in its origin and mode of propagation. *American Journal of the Medical Sciences*, n.s. **11**, 324-47.

13 Semmelweis IP. (1847). Höchst wichtige Erfahrungen über die Ätiologie der in Gebäranstalten epidemischen Puerperalfieber. *Zeitschrift der K. K. Gesellschaft der Aerzte in Wien*, **4**, Pt. 2, 242-4. (1849). **5**, Pt. 1, 64-5.

14 Semmelweis IP. (1861). *Die Aetiologie, der Begriff und die Prophylaxis des Kindbettfiebers*. Pest, Wien und Leipzig; Hartleben.

15 Pasteur L. (1862). Mémoir sur les corpuscles organisés qui existent dans l'atmosphère, examende la doctrine des générations spontanées. *Annales de Chimie et de Physique*, **64**, 5-110. [Contains the principal results of the presentation to the Academy of Sciences in 1860.]

16 Spalanzani. (1769). *Nouvelles recherches sur les découvertes microscopiques et la génération des corps organisés*. Vol. 1. Translated from the Italian by the Prince de Marsan with notes by Needham. London and Paris; Lacombe.

17 Schröder H, Dusch T von. (1854). Ueber Filtration der Luft in Beziehung auf Fäulniss und Gährung. *Annalen der Chemie und Pharmacie*, **89**, 232-43.

18 Küchenmeister F. (1860). Ueber Desinfectionsmittel im Allgemeinen, das Spirol und seine therapeutische Verwendung im Besondern. *Deutsche Klinik*, **12**, 123-4.

19 Lemaire J. (1860). *Du coaltar saponiné désinfectant énergique, arrêtant les fermentations. De ses applications a l'hygiène, a la thérapeutique, a l'histoire naturelle*. Paris; Baillière.

20 Lister J. (1867). On a new method of treating compound fracture, abscess, etc. with observations on the conditions of suppuration. *Lancet*, **1**, 326-9, 357-9, 387-9, 507-9; **2**, 95-6.

21 Lister J. (1867). On the antiseptic principle in the practice of surgery. *British Medical Journal*, **2**, 246-8. [Also in the *Lancet* (1867), **2**, 353-6.]

22 Lucas-Championnière J. (1876). *Chirurgie antiseptique. Principes, modes d'application et les résultats du pansement de Lister*. Paris; Baillière.

23 Lister J. (1869). Observations on ligature of arteries on the antiseptic system. *Lancet*, **1**, 451-5.

24 Lister J. (1881). President's address: On the catgut ligature. *Transactions of the Clinical Society of London*, **14**, xliii-lxiii.

25 Lister J. (1909). *The collected papers of Joseph, Baron Lister*. 2 vols. Oxford; Clarendon. [See vol. 2, pp. 279-80.]

26 Ref. 25 above, vol. 2, p.336.

27 Bruns V von. (1880). Fort mit dem Spray! *Berliner Klinischer Wochenschrift*, **17**, 609-11.

CHAPTER 4: STOMACH, GALL-BLADDER AND PANCREAS

1 Macewen W. (1880). Clinical observations on the introduction of tracheal tubes by the mouth instead of performing tracheotomy or laryngotomy. *British Medical Journal*, **2**, 122-4; 163-5.

2   McDowell E. (1817). Three cases of extirpation of diseased ovaria. *Eclectic Repertory and Analytical Review, Medical and Philosophy*, **7**, 242–4.

3   Wells TS. (1879). Remarks on forcipressure and the use of pressure-forceps in surgery. *British Medical Journal*, **1**, 926–8; **2**, 3–4.

4   Koeberlé E. (1893). *L'hémostatic définitive rapide par les pinces hémostatiques et la suppression de la ligature out été inventées à Strasbourg en 1867 par* ..... Strasbourg; Schultz.

5   Billroth T. (1863). *Die allgemeine chirurgische Pathologie und Therapie*. Berlin; Reimer.

6   Billroth T. (1881). *Clinical surgery. Extracts from the reports of surgical practice between the years 1860–1876*. Translated by CT Dent. London; New Sydenham Society. [See pp. 1–5.]

7   Billroth T. (1872). Ueber die Resection des Oesophagus. *Archiv für Klinische Chirurgie*, **13**, 65–69.

8   Watson PH. (1866). Reported by: Foulis, Czerny. (1881). *Diseases of the throat*. London; Kolckmann. [See pp. 57–72.]

9   Lembert M. (1826). Mémoire sur l'entéroraphie, avec la description d'un procédé nouveau pour pratiquer cette opération chirurgicale. *Repertoire Général d'Anatomie et Physiologie*, **2**, 100–7.

10 Péan JE. (1879). De l'ablation des tumeurs de l'estomac par la gastrectomie. *Gazette des Hôpitaux Civils et Militaires*, **52**, 473–5.

11 Rydygier. (1881). Exstirpation des carcinomatösen Pylorus. Tod nach zwölf Stunden. *Deutsche Zeitschrift für Chirurgie*, **14**, 252–60.

12 Billroth T. (1881). Offenes Schreiben an Herrn Dr. L. Wittelshöfer. *Wiener Medizinische Wochenschrift*, **31**, 162–5. [Billroth I.]

13 Gussenbauer C. Winiwarter A von. (1876). Die partielle Magenresection. Eine experimentelle, operative Studie, nebst einer Zusammenstellung der im pathologische-anatomischen Institute zu Wien in dem Zeitraume von 1817 bis 1875 beobachteten Magencarcinome. *Archiv für Klinische Chirurgie*, **19**, 347–80.

14 Hacker von. (1885). Zur Casuistik und Statistik der Magenresectionen und Gastroenterostomien. *Archiv für Klinische Chirurgie*, **32**, 616–25. [Billroth II. This was originally reported by von Hacker, an assistant in Billroth's clinic, to the 14th Congress of the German Surgical Society, held in Berlin, on April 10, 1885.]

15 Kocher T. (1893). Zur Technik und zu den Erfolgen der Magenresection. *Korrespondenzblatt für Schweizer Ärzte*, **23**, 682–94. [Modification of Billroth I.]

16 Stumpf R. (1908). Beitrag zur Magenchirurgie. *Beitrage zur Klinische Chirurgie*, **59**, 551–641. [Report of Max Friedrich Hofmeister's modification of Billroth II.]

17 Finsterer H. (1918). Ausgedehnte Magenresektion bei Ulcus duodeni statt der einfachen Duodenalresektion bzw. Pylorusausschaltung. *Zentralblatt für Chirurgie*, **45**, 434–5. [This type of modification became known as the Hofmeister-Finsterer gastroenterostomy.]

18 Mayo WJ. (1900). Malignant diseases of the stomach and pylorus. *Transactions of the American Surgical Association*, **18**, 97–123. [Modification of Kocher's modification; ref. 15 above.]

19 Pólya E. (1911). Zur Stumpfversorgung nach Magenresektion. *Zentralblatt für Chirurgie*, **38**, 892–4.

20 Schlatter C. (1897). Uber Ernährung und Verdauung nach vollständiger Entfernung des

Magens-Oesophagoenterostomie-beim Menschen. *Beitrage zur Klinische Chirurgie,* **19,** 157-76.

21 Rydygier. (1882). Die erste Magenresektion beim Magengeschwür. *Berliner Klinische Wochenschrift,* **19,** 39-41.

22 Doyen EL. (1895). *Traitment chirurgicale des affections de l'estomac et du duodénum.* Paris; Rueff. [See pp. 219 et seq.]

23 Dragstedt L. (1935). Some physiologic principles involved in the surgical treatment of gastric and duodenal ulcer. *Annals of Surgery,* **102,** 563-80.

24 Dragstedt LR, Owens FM Jr. (1943). Supra-diaphragmatic section of the vagus nerves in treatment of duodenal ulcer. *Proceedings of the Society for Experimental Biology and Medicine, New York,* **53,** 152-4.

25 Wangensteen OH, Root HD, Jenson CB, Imamoglu K, Salmon PA. (1958). Depression of gastric secretion and digestion by gastric hypothermia: Its clinical use in massive hematemesis. *Surgery,* **44,** 265-74.

26 Wangensteen OH, Peter ET, Nicoloff DM, Walder AI, Sosin H, Bernstein EF. (1964). Achieving 'physiological gastrectomy' by gastric freezing. A preliminary report of an experimental and clinical study. *Journal of the American Medical Association,* **180,** 439-44.

27 Winiwarter A von. (1878). *Beiträge zur Statistik der Carcinome.* Stuttgart; Enke.

28 Moynihan BGA. (1926). *Abdominal operations,* 4th ed., vol. 1, p. 244. Philadelphia and London; Saunders.

29 Wölfler A. (1881). Gastro-Enterostomie. *Zentralblatt für Chirurgie,* **8,** 705-8.

30 Courvoisier LG. (1883). Gastro-Enterostomie nach Wölfler bei inoperablem Pyloruscarcinom. *Zentralblatt für Chirurgie,* **10,** 794-7.

31 Senn N. (1888). An experimental contribution to intestinal surgery with special reference to the treatment of intestinal obstruction. *Archives of Surgery,* 7, 171-86.

32 Murphy JB. (1892). Cholecysto-intestinal, gastro-intestinal, entero-intestinal anastomosis, and approximation without sutures. (Original research.) *Medical Record, New York,* **42,** 665-76.

33 Mayo Robson AW. (1893). A method of performing intestinal anastomosis by means of decalcified bone bobbins. *British Medical Journal,* **1,** 688-9.

34 Mayo WJ. (1906). The technique of gastrojejunostomy. *Annals of Surgery,* **43,** 537-42.

35 Portis MM. (1906). Why gastroenterostomy is not a harmless operation. *Annals of Surgery,* **44,** 901-6.

36 Mikulicz J. (1897). Die chirurgische Behandlung des chronischen Magengeschwürs. *Zentralblatt für Chirurgie,* **24,** 69-98.

37 Heusner L. Cited by: Kriege H. (1892). Ein Fall von einem frei in die Bauchhöhle perforirten Magengeschwür. Laparotomie. Naht der Perforationsstelle. Heilung. *Berliner Klinische Wochenschrift,* **29,** 1244-7; 1280-4.

38 Mikulicz J. (1881). Ueber Gastroskopie und Oesophagoskopie. *Wiener Medizinische Presse,* **22,** 1405-8; 1437-43; 1473-7; 1505-7; 1537-41; 1573-7; 1629-31. [This last has the revised title: Zur Technik der Gastroskopie und Oesophagoskopie.]

39 Mikulicz J. (1897). Das Operieren in sterilisierten Zwirnhandschuhen und mit Mundbinde. *Zentralblatt für Chirurgie,* **24,** 713-17.

40 Herlin. (1767). Experiences sur l'ouverture de la vésicule du fiel, et sur son extirpation dans le chien et le chat. *Journal de Médecine, de Chirurgie, et Pharmacologie, Paris,* **27,** 463-70.

41 Bobbs JS. Case of lithotomy of the gall-bladder. *Transactions of the Indiana State Medical Society*, **18**, 68-73.

42 Sims JM. (1878). Remarks on cholecystotomy in dropsy of the gall-bladder. *British Medical Journal*, **1**, 811-15.

43 Tait RL. (1884). Note on cholecystotomy. *British Medical Journal*, **1**, 853.

44 Langenbuch CJA. (1882). Ein Fall von Exstirpation der Gallenblase wegen chronischer Cholelithiasis. Heilung. *Berliner Klinische Wochenschrift*, **19**, 725-7.

45 Tait L. (1885). Note on cholecystotomy. *British Medical Journal*, **1**, 275.

46 Kocher T. (1890). Cholelithothripsie bei Choledochusverschluss mit völliger Genesung. *Korrespondenzblatt für Schweizer Ärzte*, **20**, 97-106.

47 Abbe R. (1893). The surgery of gall-stone obstruction. *Medical Record, New York*, **43**, 548-52.

48 McBurney C. (1895). Removal of biliary calculi from the common duct by the duodenal route. *Annals of Surgery*, **28**, 481-6.

49 Kocher T. (1895). Ein Fall von Choledocho-Duodenostomia interna wegen Gallenstein. *Korrespondenzblatt für Schweizer Ärzte*, **25**, 193-7.

50 Kausch W. (1912). Das Carcinom der Papilla duodeni und seine radikale Entfernung. *Beitrage zur Klinische Chirurgie*, **78**, 439-86.

51 Whipple AO, Parsons WB, Mullins CR. (1935). Treatment of carcinoma of the ampulla of Vater. *Annals of Surgery*, **102**, 763-79.

52 Brunschwig A. (1937). Resection of head of pancreas and duodenum for carcinoma - pancreatoduodenectomy. *Surgery, Gynecology and Obstetrics*, **65**, 681-4.

CHAPTER 5: STONES IN THE BLADDER

1 *Diary of Samuel Pepys*. Everymans Library, No. 53, Vol. 1, p. 35. London; Dent.

2 Nicaise E. (1895). *Chirurgie de Pierre Franco de Turriers en Provence*. Chap. 33, p. 104. Paris; Felix Alcan.

3 Cheselden W. (1723). *A treatise on the high operation for the stone*. London; Osborn.

4 Reid A. (1748). A remarkable case of a person cut for the stone in the new way, commonly called the lateral, by William Cheselden. *Philosophical Transactions of the Royal Society of London*, 1746, pp. 33-35.

5 Civiale J. (1826). *Sur la lithotritie, ou broiement de la pierre dans la vessie*. Paris; Crochard.

6 Civiale J. (1837-42). *Traité pratique sur les maladies des organes genitourinaires*. 3 vols. Paris; Librarie de Fortin.

7 Brodie BC. (1849). *Lectures on the diseases of the urinary organs*. 4th ed. London; Longmans.

8 Bigelow HJ. (1878). Lithotrity by a single operation. *American Journal of Medical Science*, **75**, 117-34.

9 Haken FA. (1862). Dilatatorium urethrae zur Urethroscopy. *Wiener Medizinische Wochenschrift*, **12**, 177-9.

10 Bruck J. (1867). *Das Urethroscop und das Stomatoscop zur Durchleuchtung der Blase und der Zähne und ihrer Nachbarteile durch galvanisches Glühlicht*. Breslau; Maruschke and Berendt.

11 Nitze M. (1879). Eine neue Beobachtungs- und Untersuchungsmethode für Harnröhre, Harnblase und Rectum. *Wiener Medizinische Wochenschrift*, **29**, 649-52, 713-16, 779-82, 806-10. [Cystoscope illustrated in second part, showing Leiter's name on it.]

12 Nitze M. (1907). *Lehrbuch der Kystoscopie ihre technik und klinische bedetung.* 2nd ed. Weisbaden; Bergman.

CHAPTER 6: ASEPSIS AND STERILIZATION

1   Editorial (1879). *Lancet*, **2**, 246-7.
2   Koch R. (1878). *Untersuchungen über die Aetiologie der Wundinfections-krankheiten.* Leipzig; Vogel.
3   Cheyne WW. ed. (1886). *Recent essays by various authors on bacteria in relation to disease.* London; New Sydenham Society. [*Recent papers on disinfection.* II – Disinfection by hot air. Koch and Wolfhügel, pp. 519-25. III – *Disinfection by steam.* Koch, Gaffky and Loeffler, pp. 526-33.]
4   Henle J. (1840). *Pathologische Untersuchungen.* Berlin; Hirschwald.
5   Collins R. (1835). *A practical treatise on midwifery.* London; Longman, Rees, Orme, Browne, Green and Longman.
6   Henry W. (1831). Experiments on the healing powers of increased temperatures, with a view to the suggestion of a substitute for quarantine. *Philosophical Magazine and Annals of Philosophy*, n.s. **10**, 363-9.
7   Henry W. (1832). Further experiments on the disinfecting powers of increased temperatures. *Philosophical Magazine and Annals of Philosophy*, n.s. **11**, 22-31.
8   Chamberland C. Cited in: Bulloch W. (1938). *The history of bacteriology*, p. 234. London; Oxford University Press.
9   Redard P. (1888). De la désinfection des instruments chirurgicaux et des objets de pansement. *Révue de Chirurgie*, **8**, 360-71; 494-509.
10 Annotation (1889). Von Esmarch on the disinfecting action of steam. *Lancet*, **1**, 751.
11 Tomkins H. (1889). In report of a meeting of the Society of Medical Officers of Health. *Lancet*, **1**, 738.
12 Lockwood CB. (1896). *Aseptic surgery.* London; Pentland.
13 Schimmelbusch C. (1892). *Anleitung zur Aseptischen Wundbehandlung.* Berlin; Hirschwald. [*The aseptic treatment of wounds.* Translated by Rake T. (1894). London; Lewis.]
14 Halsted WS. (1894). The results of operations for the cure of cancer of the breast performed at the Johns Hopkins Hospital from June 1889 to January 1894. *Johns Hopkins Hospital Reports*, **4**, No. 6.
15 Mikulicz-Radecki J von. (1897). Das operieren in sterilisierten Zwirnhandschuhen und mit Mundbinde. *Zentralblatt für Chirurgie*, **24**, 713-7.
16 Carr WP. (1911). Saving the hundredth man. *Surgery, Gynecology and Obstetrics*, **13**, 434-9.
17 Rubbo SD, Gardner JF. (1965). *A review of sterilization and disinfection.* London; Lloyd-Luke.
18 Sykes G. (1972). *Disinfection and sterilization*, 2nd ed. London; Chapman and Hall.
19 Hart D. (1936). Sterilization of air in operating room by special bactericidal radiant energy; results of its use in extrapleural thoracoplasties. *Journal of Thoracic Surgery*, **6**, 45-81.
20 Charnley J, Eftekhar N. (1969). Post-operative infection in total arthroplasty of the hip with special reference to the bacterial content of the air. *British Journal of Surgery*, **56**, 641-9.
21 Schrader H, Bossert E. U.S. Patent No. 2,037,439, April 14, 1936, to Union Carbide and

Carbon Corp., U.S.A.

22 Gross PM, Dixon LF. Method of sterilizing. U.S. Patent 2,075,845, 1937.

23 Phillips CR, Kaye S. (1949). The sterilizing action of gaseous ethylene oxide. *American Journal of Hygiene*, **50**, 270-9.

24 Minck F. (1896). Zur Frage über einwirkung der Röntgen'schen Strahlen auf Bacterien und ihre eventuelle therapeutische Verwendbarkeit. *Münchener Medizinische Wochenschrift*, **43**, 101-2.

CHAPTER 7: APPENDICITIS: A 'NEW' DISEASE

1 Fitz RH. (1886). Perforating inflammation of the vermiform appendix; with special reference to its early diagnosis and treatment. *Transactions of the Association of American Physicians*, **1**, 107-44.

2 Fernel JF. (1567). *Universa medicina*. De partium quae sub diaphragmate sunt morbis, Liber VI. Cap IX, p. 303. Paris; Wechelus.

3 Amyand C. (1736). An inguinal rupture, with a pin in the appendix coeci, incrusted with stone; and some observations on wounds in the guts. *Philosophical Transactions of the Royal Society of London*, **39**, 329-42.

4 Mestivier. (1759). Observation sur une tumeur située proche de la région ombilicale, du côté droit, occasionée par une grosse épingle trouvée dans l'appendice vermiculaire du caecum. *Journal de Médecine, de Chirurgie et de Pharmacologie, Paris*, **10**, 441-2.

5 Mêlier F. (1827). Mémoire et observations sur quelques maladies de l'appendice coecale. *Journal Géneral de Médecine, de Chirurgie et de Pharmacie*, **100**, 317-45.

6 Parker W. (1867). An operation for abscess of the appendix vermiformis caeci. *Medical Record, New York*, **2**, 25-7.

7 Hancock H. (1848). Disease of the appendix caeci cured by operation. *London Medical Gazette*, **42**, 547-50.

8 Tait RL. (1890). The surgical treatment of typhlitis. *Birmingham Medical Review*, **27**, 26-34; 76-89.

9 Mikulicz J. (1850-1905). Ueber Laparotomie bei Magen- und Darmperforation. *Sammlung Klinische Vorträge,* No. **262**, Chir. No.**83**, 2307-34. [See pp. 2313-14.]

10 Krönlein RU. (1886). Ueber die operative Behandlung der acuten diffusen jauchig-eiterigen Peritonitis. *Archiv für Klinische Chirurgie*, **33**, 507-24.

11 Woodbury F. (1887). Cases of exploratory laparotomy followed by appropriate remedial operation. *Transactions of the College of Physicians, Philadelphia*, **9**, 183-93. [Records Morton's operation. Morton's remarks in discussion following paper.]

12 Sands HB. (1888). An account of a case in which recovery took place after laparotomy had been performed for septic peritonitis due to a perforation of the vermiform appendix. With remarks upon this and allied diseases. *New York Medical Journal*, **47**, 197-205.

13 McBurney C. (1889). Experience with early operative interference in cases of disease of the vermiform appendix. *New York Medical Journal*, **50**, 676-84.

14 Tait RL. (1889). Case of recurrent perityphlitis successfully treated by abdominal section. *British Medical Journal*, **2**, 763-4.

15 Treves F. (1888). Relapsing typhlitis treated by operation. *Medico-Chirurgical Transactions*, **71**, 165-72.

16 Murphy JB. (1889). The early treatment of perityphlitis. *Western Medical Reporter, Chicago*, **11**, 282.

17 McBurney C. (1894). The incision made in the abdominal wall in cases of appendicitis, with a description of a new method of operating. *Annals of Surgery*, **20**, 38-43.

18 Battle WH. (1895). Modified incision for removal of the vermiform appendix. *British Medical Journal*, **2**, 1360.

19 Jalaguier A. (1897). Traitement de l'appendicite. Procédé opératoire destiné à assurer la reconstitution solide de la paroi abdominale après l'excision à froid de l'appendicite. *Presse Médicale*, **5**, 53.

20 Kammerer F. (1897). A modified incision at the outer border of the rectus muscle for appendicitis. *Medical Record, New York*, **52**, 837-9.

21 Lennander KG. (1898). Über den Bauchschnitt durch eine Rectusscheide mit Verschiebung des medialen oder lateralen Randes des Musculus rectus. *Zentralblatt für Chirurgie*, **25**, 90-4.

22 McArthur LL. Choice of incisions of abdominal wall; especially for appendicitis. *Chicago Medical Recorder*, **7**, 289-92.

23 McArthur SW. (1937). The muscle-splitting or grid-iron incision for appendectomy. *Surgery, Gynecology and Obstetrics*, **65**, 714-16. [Includes a photograph of McBurney's letter to Lewis Linn McArthur acknowledging the latter's priority.]

24 Ochsner AJ. (1901). The cause of diffuse peritonitis complicating appendicitis and its prevention. *Journal of the American Medical Association*, **36**, 1747-54.

25 Sherren J. (1905). The causation and treatment of appendicitis. *Practitioner*, **74**, 833-44.

CHAPTER 8: ABDOMINAL WOUNDS AND EARLY COLOSTOMIES

1 Hippocrates. *The genuine works of Hippocrates* (1849). Translated from the Greek by F Adams. London; Sydenham Society. [See p. 755. Section VI, Aphorism 18.]

2 Celsus. *De medicina* with an English translation by WG Spencer (1935). London; Heinemann: Cambridge, Mass.; Harvard University Press. [See vol. 3, p. 385. Book VII, Section 16.]

3 Cheselden W. (1756). *The anatomy of the human body*, 7th ed. London; Hitch and Dodsley. [See Plate 40, facing p. 324.]

4 Le Dran H-F. (1740). *Observations in surgery*. Translated by JS, 2nd ed. London; Hodges. (See Observation 60.) [Original French edition, 1731.]

5 Le Dran. (1781). *The operations in surgery*. Translated by Mr Gateker, 5th ed. London; Dodsley and Law. [See pp. 59, 60.] [Original French edition, 1742.]

6 Heister L. (1743). *A general system of surgery in three parts*. Translated into English from the Latin. London; Innys, Davis, Clark, Manby, and Whiston. [See Book I, Chap. VI, p. 63.] [Original German edition, 1718.]

7 Desault PJ. (1813). Mémoire sur les anus contre nature. *Oeuvres chirurgicales*, 3rd ed. Paris; Méquignon. [See vol. 2, pp. 352-79.] [These *Works* were compiled after Desault's death by his pupil Xavier Bichat.]

8 Larrey DJ. (1812). *Mémoires de chirurgie militaire, et campagnes*. Paris; Smith and Buisson. [See vol. 2, pp. 160-1.]

9 Larrey DJ. (1823). *Surgical essays*. Translated from the French by J Revere. Baltimore; Maxwell. [See pp. 227 et seq.]

10 Lembert A. (1826). Mémoire sur l'entérorraphie, avec la description d'un procédé

nouveau pour pratiquer cette opération chirurgicale. *Repertoire Generale d'Anatomie et Physiologie*, **2**, 100-7.

11 Ogilvie WH. (1944). Abdominal wounds in the Western Desert. *Surgery, Gynecology and Obstetrics*, **78**, 225-38.

12 Littre. (1719). Diverses observations anatomiques. II. *Histoire de l'Académie Royale des Sciences, Paris,* for the year 1710, 36-7. [Edition published in1732.]

13 Caelius Aurelianus. (1772). *De morbis acutis et chronicis.* Amsterdam; Wetsteniana. [See Liber III, Caput XVII, p. 244.]

14 Dubois A. Reported by Allan (1797). *Recueil Périodique de la Société de Médecine de Paris*, **3**, 125. [Reprinted in Amussat (1839), pp. 95-99. Ref. 25, below.]

15 Martin. (1798). [See Amussat (1839), p. 84. Ref. 25, below.]

16 Pillore. Report published by Amussat (1839), pp. 85-88. [Ref. 25, below.]

17 Duret C. (1798). Observation sur un enfant né sans anus, et auquel il a été fait un ouverture pour y suppléer. *Recueil Périodique de la Société de Médecine de Paris*, **4**, 45-50.

18 Desault PJ. Reported by Leveille (1794). Opération d'anus artificiel, par la procédé de Littre, sur un enfant imperforé qui n'a vecu que quatre jours. *Journal de Chirurgicia de Desault*, **4**, 248. [Reprinted in Amussat (1839). pp. 91-4. Ref. 25, below.]]

19 Dumas CL. (1797). Observations et réflexions sur une imperforation de l'anus. *Receuil Périodique de la Société de Médecine de Paris*, **3**, 46. [Reprinted in Amussat (1839), pp. 95-9. Ref. 25, below.]

20 Fine. (1797). Mémoire et observation sur l'entérotomie. *Annales de la Société de Médecine de Montpellier*, **6**. [Reprinted in Amussat (1839), pp. 109-24. Ref. 25, below.]

21 Callisen H. (1800). *Systema Chirurgiae Hodiernae* (pars posterior). New edition. Hafniae; Proft and Storch. (See pp. 688-9.) [German edition in three volumes 1786-1792, *Grundsätze der heutigen Chirurgie.* Vienna; Hörling.]

22 Allan. (1797). Rapport sur les observations et réflexions de Dumas, relatives aux imperforations de l'anus. *Receuil Périodique de la Société de Médecine de Paris*, **3**, 123. [Reprinted in Amussat (1839), pp. 100-2. See p. 102. Ref. 25, below.]

23 Sabatier. (1810). De l'imperforation de l'anus. *De la médecine operatoire*, 2nd ed. Paris; Huillier. [See vol. 3, Section 5, p. 330.]

24 Dupuytren. (1839). *Leçons orales de clinique chirurgicale.* Recalled and published by Drs Bierre de Boismont and Marx. Paris; Baillière. [See vol. 3, p. 664.]

25 Amussat J-Z. (1839). *Mémoire sur la possibilité d'établir un anus artificiel dans la région lombaire sans pénétrer dans la péritoine.* Paris; Baillière. [See p. 183.]

26 Miriel. See Amussat (1839), pp. 136-7, 149, 150-1.

27 Freer G. See Pring (1821). [Ref. 28, below.]

28 Pring D. (1821). History of a case of the successful formation of an artificial anus in an adult, with an account of an analogous operation in two cases, by G. Freer, Esq. of Birmingham. *London Medical and Physical Journal*, **45**, 1-15.

29 Martland R. (1825). Case in which the operation for artificial anus was successfully performed. *Edinburgh Medical and Surgical Journal*, **24**, 271-6.

CHAPTER 9: LATER COLOSTOMIES

1 Dupuytren. (1829). Anus anormal. In *Dictionnaire de médecine et de chirurgie pratiques*. Vol. 3, pp. 117-62. Paris; Gabon, Méquignon-Marvis, Baillière. [See pp. 124-5.]

2   Amussat J-Z. (1839). *Mémoire sur la possibilité d'établir un anus artificiel dans la région lombaire sans pénétrer le péritoine.* Paris; Baillière.

3   Amussat J-Z. (1841). *Deuxiéme mémoire sur la possibilité d'etablir un anus artificiel dans les régions lombaires sans ouvrir le péritoine.* Paris; Baillière.

4   Erichsen J. (1841). On the formation of an artificial anus in adults, for the relief of retention of the faeces. *London Medical Gazette,* **28** (n.s. **2**), 189–92; 223–7.

5   Pennell C. (1850). A case of stricture of the rectum, wherein an artificial anus was successfully established in the left lumbar region; with remarks. *Lancet,* **1**, 628.

6   Allingham W. (1871). *Fistula, haemorrhoids, painful ulcer, stricture, prolapsus, and other diseases of the rectum, their diagnosis and treatment.* London; Churchill.

7   Bryant T. (1876). The operation of colotomy. *The practice of surgery,* 2nd ed. pp. 680–4. London; Churchill.

8   Lund E. (1883). On air-inflation of the bowel as a rule of practice in the operation of left lumbar colotomy. *Lancet,* **1**, 588–9.

9   Colley D. (1885). Colotomy with delayed opening of the bowel. (Clinical Society of London – report of meeting.) *Lancet,* **1**, 522–3.

10 Ball CB. (1887). Colotomy. *The rectum and anus. Their diseases and treatment.* Chapter 25, pp. 351–71. London, Paris, New York and Melbourne; Cassell.

11 Schinzinger. (1881). Zur Darmresektion. *Weiner Medizinische Wochenschrift,* **31**, 1041–4.

12 Madelung. (1884). Über eine Modifikation der Colotomie wegen Carcinoma recti. *Centralblatt für Chirurgie* (Congress addendum), **11**, 68–9.

13 Reeves HA. (1892). Letter to the Editor: Sigmoidoscopy simplified. *British Medical Journal,* **1**, 359–60.

14 Reeves HA. (1892). Sigmoidoscopy simplified. *British Medical Journal,* **1**, 66–7.

15 Maydl K. (1988). Zur Technik der Kolotomy. *Centralblatt für Chirurgie,* **15**, 433–9.

16 Kelsey CB. (1889). An improvement in the technique of inguinal colotomy. *Medical Record, New York,* **36**, 398.

17 Allingham HW, Jun. (1887). Inguinal colotomy: its advantages over the lumbar operation, with special reference to a method for preventing faeces passing below the artificial anus. *British Medical Journal,* **2**, 874–8.

18 Paul FT. (1891). A method of performing inguinal colotomy, with cases. *British Medical Journal,* **2**, 118–19.

19 Allingham HW. (1887). Letter to the Editor: Inguinal colotomy. *British Medical Journal,* **2**, 337–8.

20 Hughes ESR. (1957). *Surgery of anus anal canal and rectum.* Edinburgh and London; Livingstone.

CHAPTER 10: CANCER OF THE RECTUM AND COLON

1   Faget (1743). Remarques sur les abces qui arrivent au fondement. *Mémoires de l'Académie Royale de Chirurgie, Paris,* **1**, pt. II, 257–67.

2   Lisfranc J. (1833). Mémoire sur l'excision de la partie inférieure du rectum devenue carcinomateuse. *Mémoires de l'Académie Royale de Médecine, Paris,* **3**, 291–302.

3   Verneuil AA. (1873). Résection du coccyx pour faciliter la formation d'un anus périnéal dans les imperforations du rectum. *Bulletin de la Société de Chirurgie de Paris,* Ser.3, **2**, 288–308.

4   Amussat J-Z. (1843). *Troisième mémoire sur la possibilité d'établir un anus artificiel*

dans la région lombaire gauche, sans ouvrir le péritoine, chez les enfants imperforés. Paris; Baillière.

5   Kocher T. (1874). Die exstirpatio recti nach vorheriger Excision des Steissbeins. *Centralblatt für Chirurgie,* **1**, 145-7.

6   Kraske P. (1887). Die sacrale Methode der Exstirpation von Mastdarmkrebsen und die Resectio recti. *Berliner Klinische Wochenschrift.* **24**, 899-904.

7   Cripps WH. (1880). *Cancer of the rectum. Its pathology, diagnosis, and treatment.* London; Churchill. [See p. 161, and also pp. 132-42 for a discussion of colostomy.)

8   Paul FT. (1895). Remarks on excision of the rectum, with a report of fourteen cases, and a new rectal truss. *British Medical Journal,* **1**, 519-22.

9   Baum. (1879). Resection eines carcinomatösen Dickdarmstückes. *Centralblatt für Chirurgie,* **6**, 169-76.

10 Pollosson M. (1884). Nouvelle méthode opératoire pour la cure radicale du cancer du rectum. *Lyon Médicale,* **46**, 67-75.

11 Madelung. (1884). Über eine Modifikation der Colotomie wegen Carcinoma recti. *Centralblatt für Chirurgie* (Congess addendum), **11**, 68-9.

12 Schede. (1887). Zur Operation des Mastdarmkrebses. *Deutsche Medizinische Wochenschrift,* **13**, 1048-9.

13 Heineke W. (1886). *Compendium der Chirurgischen Operations und Verbandlehre,* vol. 2, pp. 728-33. Erlangen; Besold. [The date is sometimes given as 1884, but that refers to vol. 1 only.]

14 Bloch O. (1892). Om extra-abdominal Behandlung af cancer intestinalis (Rectum derfra undtaget). *Centralblatt für Chirurgie,* **19**, 628-9.

15 Paul FT. (1895). Colectomy. *Liverpool Medico-Chirurgical Journal,* **15**, 374-88.

16 Paul FT. (1900). Two cases of colectomy. *Liverpool Medico-Chirurgical Journal,* **20**, 55-60.

17 Mikulicz J von. (1903). Chirurgische Erfahrungen über das Darmcarcinom. *Archiv für Klinische Chirurgie,* **69**, 23-47.

18 Maunsell HW. (1892). A new method of excising the two upper portions of the rectum and the lower segment of the sigmoid flexure of the colon. *Lancet,* **2**, 473-6.

19 Lockhart Mummery P. (1907). An address on the operation for removal of the entire rectum and neighbouring lymphatic area for carcinoma. *British Medical Journal,* **1**, 1289-93.

20 Bloodgood JC. (1906). The surgery of carcinoma of the upper portion of the rectum and the sigmoid colon with special reference to the combined sacral and abdominal operation for the resection of these tumors. *Surgery, Gynecology and Obstetrics,* **3**, 284-95.

21 Czerny. (1897). Therapie der krebsigen Stricturen des Oesophagus, des Pylorus und des Rectum. *Berliner Klinische Wochenschrift,* **34**, 779-83.

22 Miles WE. (1908). A method of performing abdomino-perineal excision for carcinoma of the rectum and of the terminal portion of the colon. *Lancet,* **2**, 1812-13.

23 Kirschner. (1934). Das synchrone Kombinierte Verfahren bei der Radikalbehandlung des Mastdarmkrebses. *Archiv für Klinische Chirurgie,* **180**, 296-308.

CHAPTER 11: MORE ABDOMINAL DISEASES

1   Morgagni. (1769). *The seats and causes of disease.* Translated from the Latin by B. Alexander. London; Millar, Cadell, Johnson and Payne. [See Book 3, Letter 31, Article 14

    – vol. 2, p. 75.]

2   Wilks S. (1859). *Lectures on pathological anatomy*. London; Longman, Brown, Green, Longmans, and Roberts. [See section on: Diseases of the alimentary canal and peritoneum; p. 253 – and especially pp. 290 et seq.]

3   Robson M. (1893). Case of colitis with ulceration treated by inguinal colotomy and local treatment of the ulcerated surfaces, with subsequent closure of the artificial anus. *Transactions of the Clinical Society of London*, **26**, 213-15.

4   Keith S. (1895). Letter to the Editor: The treatment of membranous colitis. *Lancet*, **1**, 639.

5   Weir RF. (1902). A new use for the useless appendix, in the surgical treatment of obstinate colitis. *Medical Record, New York*, **62**, 201-2.

6   Allison CC. (1909). Cecostomy – the operation of choice for temporary drainage of the colon. *Journal of the American Medical Association*, **53**, 1562.

7   Lilienthal H. (1903). Extirpation of the entire colon, the upper portion of the sigmoid flexure, and four inches of ileum for hyperplastic colitis. *Annals of* Surgery, 37, 616-17.

8   Brown JY. (1913). The value of complete physiological rest of the large bowel in the treatment of certain ulcerative and obstructive lesions of this organ. *Surgery, Gynecology and Obstetrics*, **16**, 610-13.

9   Discussion (1940). On the surgical treatment of idiopathic ulcerative colitis and its sequelae. *Proceedings of the Royal Society of Medicine*, **33**, 637-48. [Discussants: LEC Norbury; WH Ogilvie; WB Gabriel; Sir Arthur Hurst; R Corbett; JP Lockhart-Mummery; M Smythe; and SW Patterson.]

10   Corbett R. (1945). A review of the surgical treatment of chronic ulcerative colitis. *Proceedings of the Royal Society of Medicine*, **38**, 277-90.

11   Ravitch MM. (1948). Anal ileostomy with sphincter preservation in patients requiring total colectomy for benign conditions. *Surgery*, **24**, 170-87.

12   Nissen. (1933). Demonstrations of operative surgery, no. 39. *Zentralblatt für Chirurgie*, **60**, 888.

13   Miller GG, Gardner CMcG, Ripstein CB. (1949). Primary resection of the colon in ulcerative colitis. *Canadian Medical Association Journal*, **60**, 584-5.

14   Strauss AA, Strauss SF. (1944). Surgical treatment of ulcerative colitis. *Surgical Clinics of North America*, **24**, 211-24.

15   Gardner C, Miller GG. (1951). Total colectomy for ulcerative colitis. *Archives of Surgery*, **63**, 370-2.

16   Dragstedt LR, Dack GM, Kirsner JB. (1941). Chronic ulcerative colitis. *Annals of Surgery*, **114**, 653-62

17   Monroe CW, Olwin JH. (1949). Use of an abdominal flap graft in construction of a permanent ileostomy. *Archives of Surgery*, **59**, 565-77.

18   Brooke BN. (1952). The management of an ileostomy including its complications. *Lancet*, **2**, 102-4.

19   Crohn BB, Ginzburg L, Oppenheimer GD. (1932). Regional ileitis. A pathologic and clinical entity. *Journal of the American Medical Association*, **99**, 1323-9.

20   Goligher JC, de Dombal FT, Burton I. (1971). Surgical treatment and its results. In: *Regional enteritis (Crohn's disease)*. A Skandia International Symposium edited by A. Engel and T. Larsson. Stockholm; Nordiska Bokhandelns. [See p. 168.]

21   Crohn BB, Yarnis H. (1958). *Regional ileitis*, 2nd ed. New York and London; Grune and

Stratton.

22 Homans J, Hass GM. (1933). Regional ileitis: a clinical, not a pathological entity. *New England Journal of Medicine*, **209**, 1315-24.

23 Clute HM. (1933). Regional ileitis: a report of two cases. *Surgical Clinics of North America*, **13**, 561-7.

24 Koster H, Kasman LP, Sheinfeld W. (1936). Regional ileitis. *Archives of Surgery*, **32**, 789-809.

25 Clark RL, Dixon CF. (1939). Regional enteritis. *Surgery*, **5**, 277-304.

26 Marshall SF. (1943). Regional ileitis: surgical management and results of operation. *Surgical Clinics of North America*, **23**, 873-880.

27 Truelove SC, Ellis H, Webster CU. (1965). Place of double-barrelled ileostomy in ulcerative colitis and Crohn's disease of the colon: a preliminary report. *British Medical Journal*, **1**, 150-3.

28 Simon J. (1855). Congenital imperfection of the urinary organs treated by operation. *Transactions of the Pathological Society, London*, **6**, 256-8.

29 Smith T. (1879). An account of an unsuccessful attempt to treat extroversion of the bladder by a new operation. *St. Bartholomew's Hospital Reports*, **15**, 29-35.

30 Verhoogen J, Graeuwe A de. (1909). La cystectomie totale. *Folia Urologica*, **3**, 629-78.

31 Coffey RC. (1911). Physiological implantation of the severed ureter or common bile duct into the intestine. *Journal of the American Medical Association*, **56**, 397-403.

32 Bardenheuer B. (1887). *Die Extraperitoneale Explorativschnitt*. Stuttgart; Enke. [See p. 273.]

33 Coffey RC. (1927). Completed aseptic technique for the implantation of the ureter into the large bowel. *Surgery, Gynecology and Obstetrics*, **45**, 816-19.

34 Haffner HE. Cited by: Bricker EM. (1950). (Ref. 35, below.)

35 Bricker EM. (1950). Bladder substitution after pelvic evisceration. *Surgical Clinics of North America*, **30**, 1511-21.

36 Kennedy CS, Miller EB, McLean DC, Perlis MS, Dion RM, Horvitz VS. (1960). Lumbar amputation or hemicorporectomy for advanced malignancy of the lower half of the body. *Surgery*, **48**, 357-65.

37 Aust JB, Absolon KB. (1962). A successful lumbosacral amputation, hemicorporectomy. *Surgery*, **52**, 756-9.

38 Miller TR. (1966). Translumbar amputation for advanced cancer: indications and physiologic alterations in four cases. *Annals of Surgery*, **164**, 514-21.

CHAPTER 12: HERNIAS

1 Niemann A. (1860). *Ueber eine neue organische Base in den Cocablättern*. Göttingen; Huth.

2 Anrep B von. (1880). Ueber die physiologische Wirkung des Cocaïn. *Archiv für Gesammte Physiologie* (Pflüger's), **21**, 38-77.

3 Koller C. (1884). Vorläufige Mittheilung über locale Anästhesirung am Auge. *Klinische Monatsblatter für Augenheilkunde*, **22**, Beilageheft 60-3.

4 Halsted WS. (1885). Practical comments on the use and abuse of cocaine; suggested by its invariably successful employment in more than a thousand minor surgical operations. *New York Medical Journal*, **42**, 294-5.

5 Halsted WS. (1887). Circular suture of the intestine: an experimental study. *American Journal of Medical Science*, **94**, 436-61.

6   Marcy HO. (1878).The radical cure of hernia by the antiseptic use of carbolized catgut ligature. *Transactions of the American Medical Association*, **29**, 295-305.

7   Marcy HO. (1881). The cure of hernia by the antiseptic use of animal ligature. *Transactions of the International Medical Congress*, 7 session, **2**, 446-8.

8   Marcy HO. (1920). Letter to the Editor:Anecdotes of Baron Larrey. *Boston Medical and Surgical Journal*, **182**, 310.

9   Macewen W. (1886). On the radical cure of oblique inguinal hernia by internal abdominal peritoneal pad, and the restoration of the valved form of the inguinal canal. *Annals of Surgery*, **4**, 89-119.

10 Bassini E. (1889). *Nuovo metodo per la cura radicale dell'ernia crurale*. Padova; Prosperini.

11 Bassini E. (1890). Ueber die Behandlung des Leistenbruches. *Archiv für Klinische Chirurgie*, **40**, 429-76.

12 Halsted WS. (1889). The radical cure of hernia. (Report of a case.). *Johns Hopkins Hospital Bulletin*, **1**, 12-13; 111-12.

13 Halsted WS. (1893). The radical cure of inguinal hernia in the male. *Johns Hopkins Hospital Bulletin*, **4**, 17-24.

14 Lotheissen G. (1898). Zur Radikaloperation der Schenkelhernien. *Zentralblatt für Chirurgie*, **25**, 548-50.

15 Babcock WW. (1927).The ideal in herniorrhaphy.A new method efficient for direct and indirect inguinal hernia. *Surgery, Gynecology and Obstetrics*, **45**, 534-40.

16 McArthur LL. (1901). Autoplastic suture in hernia, and other diastases – preliminary report. *Journal of the American Medical Association*, **37**, 1162-5.

17 Kirschner M. (1910). Die praktischen Ergebnisse der freien Fascien-Transplantation. *Archiv für Klinische Chirurgie*, **92**, 889-912.

18 Gallie WE, Le Mesurier AB. (1921). The use of living sutures in operative surgery. *Canadian Medical Association Journal*, **2**, 504-13.

19 Gallie WE, Le Mesurier AB. (1924). The transplantation of the fibrous tissues in the repair of anatomical defects. *British Journal of Surgery*, **12**, 289-320.

20 Masson JC. (1933). A new instrument for securing fascia lata for repair of hernia. *Proceedings of the Staff Meetings of the Mayo Clinic*, **8**, 528-30.

21 Koontz AR. (1927). Dead (preserved) fascia grafts for hernia repair: clinical results. *Journal of the American Medical Association*, **89**, 1230-5.

22 Annandale T. (1875-6). Case in which a reducible oblique and direct inguinal and femoral hernia existed on the same side, and were successfully treated by operation. *Edinburgh Medical Journal*, **21**, 1087-91.

23 Ruggi G. (1893). *Del metodo inguinale nelle cura radicale dell'ernia crurale*. Bologna; Zanichelli.

CHAPTER 13: CANCER OF THE BREAST

1   Halsted WS. (1894). The results of operations for the cure of cancer of the breast performed at the Johns Hopkins Hospital from June 1889 to January 1894. *Johns Hopkins Hospital Reports*, **4**, 297-350.

2   Meyer W. (1894).An improved method of the radical operation for carcinoma of the breast. *Medical Record, New York*, **46**, 746-9.

3   Moore CH. (1867). On the influence of inadequate operations on the theory of cancer. *Medico-Chirurgical Transactions*, **50**, 254-80.

4   Heath C. (1871). A course of lectures on diseases of the breast. *Lancet*, **1**, 847-50.

5   Volkmann R von. (1875). *Beitrage zur Chirurgie*. Leipzig; Breitkoff und Härtel. [His follow-up statistics of cancer of the breast on p. 329.]

6   Halsted WS. (1890). The treatment of wounds with especial reference to the value of the blood clot in the management of dead spaces. IV Operations for carcinoma of the breast. *Johns Hopkins Hospital Reports*, **2**, 255-314.

7   Halsted WS. (1898). A clinical and histological study of certain adenocarcinomata of the breast: and a brief consideration of the supraclavicular operation and of the results of operations for cancer of the breast from 1889 to 1898 at the Johns Hopkins Hospital. *Annals of Surgery*, **28**, 557-76.

8   Ruge C, Veit J. (1878). Zur Pathologie der Vaginalportion. *Zeitschrift für Geburtshulfe und Gynakologie*, **2**, 415.

9   Cullen TS. (1895). A rapid method of making permanent specimens from frozen sections by the use of formalin. *Bulletin of the Johns Hopkins Hospital*, **6**, 67-73.

10 Handley WS. (1927). Parasternal invasion of the thorax in breast cancer and its suppression by the use of radium tubes as an operative precaution. *Surgery, Gynecology and Obstetrics*, **45**, 721-8.

11 Handley RS, Thackray AC. (1947). Invasion of the internal mammary lymph glands in carcinoma of the breast. *British Journal of Cancer*, **1**, 15-20.

12 Wangensteen OH. (1950). In discussion (pp. 839-41) following: Taylor GT, Wallace RH. (1950). Carcinoma of the breast: Fifty years experience at the Massachusetts General Hospital. *Annals of Surgery*, **132**, 833-7.

13 Urban JA, Baker HW. (1952). Radical mastectomy in continuity with en bloc resection of internal mammary lymph node chain: New procedure for primary operable cancer of the breast. *Cancer*, **5**, 992-1008.

14 McWhirter R. (1949). Treatment of cancer of the breast by simple mastectomy and roentgenotherapy. *Archives of Surgery*, **59**, 830-42.

15 Schinzinger A. (1889). Über carcinoma mammae. *Centralblatt für Chirurgie*, **16**, 55 (Suppl. 29).

16 Beatson GT. (1896). On the treatment of inoperable cancer of the mamma; suggestions for a new method of treatment, with illustrative cases. *Lancet*, **2**, 104-7; 162-5.

17 Huggins C, Stevens RE, Hodges CV. (1941). Studies on prostatic cancer. II. The effects of castration on advanced carcinoma of the prostate gland. *Archives of Surgery*, **43**, 209-23.

18 Huggins C, Scott WW. (1945). Bilateral adrenalectomy in prostatic cancer. *Annals of Surgery*, **122**, 1031-41.

19 Huggins C, Bergenstal DM. (1951). Surgery of the adrenals. *Journal of the American Medical Association*, **147**, 101-6.

20 Shimkin MB, Boldrey EB, Kelly KH, Bierman HR, Ortega P, Naffziger HC. (1952). Effects of surgical hypophysectomy in a man with malignant melanoma. *Journal of Clinical Endocrinology*, **12**, 439-53.

21 Luft R, Olivecrona H, Sjögren B. (1952). Hypofysektomi på människa. *Nordisk Medicin*, **47**, 351-4.

22 Luft R, Olivecrona H. (1953). Experiences with hypophysectomy in man. *Journal of Neurosurgery*, **10**, 301.

CHAPTER 14: EPILEPSY, TRIGEMINAL NEURALGIA AND PAIN

1 Broca P. (1861). Remarques sur le siège de la faculté du language articulé, suivie d'une observation d'aphémie (perte de la parole). *Bulletin de la Société Anatomique de Paris*, **36**, 330-57.

2 Fritsch G, Hertzig E. (1870). Ueber die elecktrische Erregbarkeit des Grosshirns. *Archiv für Anatomie und Physiologie*, **37**, 300-32.

3 Ferrier D. (1873). Experimental researches in cerebral physiology and pathology. *West Riding Lunatic Asylum Medical Reports*, **3**, 30-96.

4 Ferrier D. (1874). On the localization of the functions of the brain. *Proceedings of the Royal Society of London*, **22**, 229-32.

5 Ferrier D. (1874-5). Experiments on the brain of monkeys. *Proceedings of the Royal Society of London*, **23**, 409-31.

6 Bartholow R. (1874). Experimental investigation into the functions of the human brain. *American Journal of Medical Sciences*, **67**, 305-13.

7 Macewen W. (1879). Tumour of the dura mater; convulsions; removal of tumour by trephining; recovery. *Glasgow Medical Journal*, **12**, 210-13.

8 Macewen W. (1885). Cases illustrative of cerebral surgery. *Lancet*, **1**, 881-3; 934-6.

9 Macewen W. (1893). *Pyogenic infective diseases of the brain and spinal cord*. Glasgow; Maclehose.

10 Durante F. (1885). Estirpazione di un tumore endocranioco. *Bolletino della Accademia Medica Roma*, **11**, 247-52. [See also *Lancet* (1887). Contribution to endocranial surgery. **2**, 654-5.]

11 Bennett AH, Godlee RJ. (1884). Reported in: A mirror of hospital practice. (1884). Excision of a tumour from the brain. *Lancet*, **2**, 1090-1. [See also: *Lancet*, Nov. 29, 1884; Jan. 3, 1885; *The Times*, Dec. 11, 1884. – Letter from F.R.S. (Sir James Crichton-Browne) and subsequent correspondence which was linked to vivisection.]

12 Horsley V. (1886). Brain surgery. *British Medical Journal*, **2**, 670-5.

13 Horsley V. (1887). Remarks on ten consecutive cases of operations upon the brain and cranial cavity to illustrate the details and safety of the method employed. *British Medical Journal*, **1**, 863-5.

14 Birdsall WR, Weir RF. (1887). Brain surgery. Removal of a large sarcoma causing hemianopsia, from the occipital lobe. *Medical News, New York*, **50**, 421-8.

15 Weir RF, Seguin EC. (1888). Contribution to the diagnosis and surgical treatment of tumours of the cerebrum. *American Journal of Medical Sciences*, n.s. **96**, 25-38; 109-38; 219-32.

16 Keen WW. (1888). Three successful cases of cerebral surgery including (1) the removal of a large intracranial fibroma, (2) exsection of damaged brain tissue and (3) exsection of the cerebral center for the left hand. With remarks on the general technique of such operations. *Transactions of the American Surgical Association*, **6**, 293-347.

17 Wagner W. (1889). Die temporäre Resektion der Schädeldaches an Stelle der Trepanation. *Zentralblatt für Chirurgie*, **16**, 833-8.

18 Gigli L. (1898). Zur Technik der temporären Schädelresektion mit meiner Drahtsäge. *Zentralblatt für Chirurgie*, **25**, 425

19 McBurney C. Cited in: Starr MA. (1893). *Brain surgery*. London; Baillière, Tindall and Cox.

20 Krynauw RA. (1950). Infantile hemiplegia treated by removing one cerebral hemisphere. *Journal of Neurology, Neurosurgery and Psychiatry*, **13**, 243-67.

21 Dandy W. (1928). Removal of right cerebral hemisphere for certain tumors with hemiplegia. Preliminary report. *Journal of the American Medical Association*, **90**, 823-5.

22 van Wagenen WP, Herren RY. (1940). Surgical division of commissural pathways in the corpus callosum. Relation to spread of an epileptic attack. *Archives of Neurology and Psychiatry*, **44**, 740-59.

23 Lizars J. (1821). Neuralgia of the inferior maxillary nerve 'nervus mandibulo-labialis' cured by operation. *Edinburgh Medical Journal*, **17**, 529-37.

24 Carnochan JM. (1858). Exsection of the trunk of the second branch of the fifth pair of nerves, beyond the ganglion of Meckel, for severe neuralgia of the face; with three cases. *American Journal of Medical Sciences*, n.s. **35**, 134-43.

25 Pancoast J. (1871-2). New operation for the relief of persistent facial neuralgia. *Philadelphia Medical Times*, **2**, 285-7.

26 Rose W. (1890). Removal of the Gasserian ganglion for severe neuralgia. *Lancet*, **2**, 914-5.

27 Horsley V, Taylor J, Coleman WS. (1891). The various surgical procedures devised for the relief or cure of trigeminal neuralgia (tic douloureux). *British Medical Journal*, **2**, 1139-43; 1191-93; 1249-53.

28 Hartley F. (1892). Intracranial neuroectomy of the second and third divisions of the fifth nerve. A new method. *New York Medical Journal*, **55**, 317-19.

29 Krause F. (1892). Resection des Trigeminus, innerhalb der Schaedelhoehle. *Archiv für Klinische Chirurgie*, **44**, 821-32.

30 Cushing HW. (1900). A method of total extirpation of the gasserian ganglion for trigeminal neuralgia. By a route through the temporal fossa and beneath the middle meningeal artery. *Journal of the American Medical Association*, **34**, 1035-41.

31 Spiller WG, Frazier CH. (1901). The division of the sensory root of the trigeminus for the relief of tic douloureux; an experimental, pathological and clinical study, with a preliminary report of one successful case. *University of Pennsylvania Medical Bulletin*, **14**, 341-52.

32 Cushing HW. (1905). The surgical aspects of major neuralgia of the trigeminal nerve. A report of twenty cases of operation on the gasserian ganglion, with anatomic and physiologic notes on the consequences of its removal. *Journal of the American Medical Association*, **44**, 773-8; 860-5; 920-9; 1002-8; 1088-93.

33 Cushing HW. (1907). Remarks on some further modifications in the gasserian ganglion operation for trigeminal neuralgia (sensory-root evulsion). *Transactions of the Southern Surgical Association*, **19**, 480-5.

34 Frazier CH. (1925). Subtotal resection of sensory root for relief of major neuralgia. *Archives of Neurology and Psychiatry, Chicago*, **13**, 378-84.

35 Frazier CH. (1934). Bilateral trigeminal neuralgia. *Annals of Surgery*, **100**, 770-8.

36 Cushing HW. (1916). Cited in: Horrax G. (1952). *Neurosurgery: An historical sketch*. Springfield, Ill.; Thomas.

37 Peet MM. (1918). Tic douloureux and its treatment with a review of the cases operated upon at the University Hospital in 1917. *Journal of the Michigan Medical Society*, **17**, 91-9.

38 Taarnhøj P. (1952). Decompression of the trigeminal root and the posterior part of the ganglion as treatment in trigeminal neuralgia. Preliminary communication. *Journal of Neurosurgery*, **9**, 288-90.

39 Sheldon CH, Pudenz RH, Freshwater DB, Crue BL. (1955). Compression rather than decompression for trigeminal neuralgia. *Journal of Neurosurgery*, **12**, 123-6.

40 Abbe R. (1889). A contribution to the surgery of the spinal cord. *Transactions of the Medical Society of the State of New York*, Communication XVIII, 204-11.

41 Spiller WG. (1905). The location within the spinal cord of the fibers for pain and temperature sensations. *Journal of Nervous and Mental Diseases*, **32**, 318-20.

42 Spiller WG, Martin E. (1912). The treatment of persistent pain of organic origin in the lower part of the body by division of the anterolateral column of the spinal cord. *Journal of the American Medical Association*, **58**, 1489-90.

43 Frazier CH. (1920). Section of the anterolateral columns of the spinal cord for the relief of pain. *Archives of Neurology and Psychiatry, Chicago*, **13**, 378-84.

CHAPTER 15: TUMOURS OF THE BRAIN, HYDROCEPHALUS AND PSYCHOSURGERY

1 Gowers WR, Horsley V. (1888). A case of tumour of the spinal cord. Removal; recovery. *Medico-Chirurgical Transactions*, **53**, 377-430.

2 Macewen W. (1884). Trephining of the spine for paraplegia. *Glasgow Medical Journal*, n.s. **22**, 55-8.

3 Macewen W. (1885). Two cases in which excision of the laminae and portions of the spinal vertebrae had been performed in order to relieve pressure on the spinal cord causing paraplegia. *Glasgow Medical Journal*, n.s. **25**, 210-12.

4 Macewen W. (1888). Surgery of the brain and spinal cord. *Lancet*, **2**, 254-61. [Also: *British Medical Journal*, **2**, 302-9.]

5 Cushing HW. (1902). On the avoidance of shock in major amputations by cocainization of large nerve-trunks preliminary to their division. With observations on blood-pressure changes in surgical cases. *Annals of Surgery*, **36**, 321-45.

6 Cushing HW. (1905). The establishment of cerebral hernia as a decompressive measure for inaccessible brain tumors; with the description of intermuscular methods of making the bone defect in temporal and occipital regions. *Surgery, Gynecology and Obstetrics*, **1**, 297-314.

7 Cushing HW. (1910). Recent observations on tumours of the brain and their surgical treatment. *Lancet*, **1**, 90-4.

8 Cushing HW. (1911). The control of bleeding in operations for brain tumors. With the description of silver 'clips' for the occlusion of vessels inaccessible to the ligature. *Annals of Surgery*, **54**, 1-19.

9 Cushing HW. (1915). Concerning the results of operations for brain tumor. *Journal of the American Medical Association*, **64**, 189-95.

10 Redford LL, Cushing HW. (1909). Is the pituitary gland essential to the maintenance of life? *Johns Hopkins Hospital Bulletin*, **20**, 105-7.

11 Cushing HW. (1909). Partial hypophysectomy for acromegaly with remarks on the function of the hypophysis. *Annals of Surgery*, **50**, 1002-17.

12 Cushing HW. (1912). *The pituitary body and its disorders*. Philadelphia and London; Lippincott.

13 Cushing HW. (1927). Acromegaly from a surgical standpoint. *British Medical Journal* , **2**, 1-9; 48-55.

14 Frazier CH. (1913). An approach to the hypophysis through the anterior cranial fossa. *Transactions of the Philadelphia Academy of Surgery*, **15**, 215-21.

15 Cushing HW. (1917). *Tumors of the nervus acusticus and the syndrome of the*

   cerebellopontile angle. Philadelphia and London; Saunders.

16 Gwathmey JT. (1913). Oil-ether anaesthesia. *Lancet*, **2**, 1756–8.

17 Lundy JS. (1935). Intravenous anesthesia: preliminary report of the use of two new thiobarbiturates. *Proceedings of the Staff Meetings of the Mayo Clinic*, **10**, 536–43. [Introduction of thiopental sodium – Pentothal.]

18 Rowbotham ES, Magill IW. (1921). Anaesthetics in the plastic surgery of the face and jaws. *Proceedings of the Royal Society of Medicine*, **14**, 17–27.

19 Dandy WE. (1918). Ventriculography following the injection of air into the cerebral ventricles. *Annals of Surgery*, **68**, 5–11.

20 Moniz E. (1927). L'encéphalographie artérielle, son importance dans la localisation des tumeurs cérébrales. *Revue Neurologique*, **2**, 72–90.

21 Cushing HW, Bovie WT. (1928). Electro-surgery as an aid to the removal of intracranial tumors. *Surgery, Gynecology and Obstetrics*, **47**, 751–84.

22 Quincke H. (1891). Die Lumbalpunction des Hydrocephalus. *Berliner Klinische Wochenschrift*, **28**, 929–33; 965–8.

23 Ferguson AH. (1898). Intraperitoneal diversion of the cerebrospinal fluid in cases of hydrocephalus. *New York Medical Journal*, **67**, 902.

24 Kausch W. (1908). Die Behandlung des Hydrocephalus der kleinen Kinder. *Archiv für Klinische Chirurgie*, **87**, 709–96.

25 Cushing HW. (1905). The special field of neurological surgery. *Cleveland Medical Journal*, **4**, 1–25.

26 Gärtner (1895). Cited by Kausch W. (Ref. 24, above.)

27 Payr E. (1908). Drainage der Hirnventrikel mittelst frei transplantirter Blutgefässe; Bemerkungen über Hydrocephalus. *Archiv für Klinische Chirurgie*, **87**, 801–85.

28 Payr E. (1911). Ueber Ventrikeldrainage bei Hydrocephalus. *Verhandlungender Gesellschaft für Chirurgie*, **40**, 515–35.

29 McClure RD. (1909). Hydrocephalus treated by drainage into a vein in the neck. *Johns Hopkins Hospital Bulletin*, **20**, 110–13.

30 Cone WV. (1948). Cited in: Jackson IJ, Snodgrass SR. (1955). Peritoneal shunts in the treatment of hydrocephalus and increased intracranial pressure. A four year survey of 62 patients. *Journal of Neurosurgery*, **12**, 216–22.

31 Matson DD. (1949). A new operation for the treatment of communicating hydrocephalus. *Journal of Neurosurgery*, **6**, 238–47.

32 Heile B. (1925). Ueber neue operative Wege zur Druckentlastung bei angeborenem Hydrocephalus (Ureter-Duraanastomose). *Zentralblatt für Chirurgie*, **52**, 2229–36.

33 Matson DD. (1951). Ventriculo-ureterostomy. *Journal of Neurosurgery*, **8**, 398–404.

34 Harsh GR. (1954). Peritoneal shunt for hydrocephalus utilizing the fimbria of the fallopian tube for entrance to the peritoneal cavity. *Journal of Neurosurgery*, **11**, 284–94.

35 Nosik WA. (1950). Ventriculomastoidostomy. Technique and observations. *Journal of Neurosurgery*, **7**, 236–9.

36 Ransohoff J. (1954). Ventriculo-pleural anastomosis in treatment of midline obstructional neoplasms. *Journal of Neurosurgery*, **11**, 295–8.

37 Pudenz RH, Russell FE, Hurd AH, Shelden CH. (1957). Ventriculo-auriculostomy. A technique for shunting cerebrospinal fluid into the right auricle. Preliminary report. *Journal of Neurosurgery*, **14**, 171–9.

38 Burckhardt G. (1891). Ueber Rindenexcisionen, als Beitrag zur operativen Therapie der

Psychosen. *Allgemeine Zeitschrift für Psychiatrie*, 47, 463-548.

39 Moniz E. (1936). *Tentatives operatoires dans le traitement de certaines psychoses.* Paris; Masson.

40 Freeman W, Watts JW. (1936). Prefrontal lobotomy in agitated depression. Report of a case. *Medical Annals of the District of Columbia*, 5, 326-8.

41 Fiamberti AM. (1937). Proposta di una tecnica operatoria modificata e semplificata per gli interventi alla Moniz sui lobi prefrontali in malati di menti. *Rassagna di Studi Psichiatrici*, 26, 797-805.

42 Lyerly JG. (1939). Transsection of the deep association fibers of the prefrontal lobes in certain mental disorders. *Southern Surgeon*, 8, 426-34.

43 Poppen JL. (1948). Technic of prefrontal lobotomy. *Journal of Neurosurgery*, 5, 514-20.

CHAPTER 16: SPECIALIZATION

1 Kocher T. (1880). Ueber Radicalheilung des Krebses. *Deutsche Zeitschrift für Chirurgie*, 13, 134-66.

2 Kocher T. (1878). Exstirpation einer Struma retrooesophagea. *Korrespondenzblatt für Schweizer Ärtze*, 8, 702-5.

3 Kocher T. (1883). Ueber Kropfexstirpation und ihre Folgen. *Archiv für Klinische Chirurgie*, 29, 254-337.

4 Kocher T. (1898). Eine neue Serie von 600 Kropfoperationen. *Korrespondenzblatt für Schweizer Ärtze*, 28, 545.

5 Rehn L. (1884). Ueber die Extirpation des Kropfs bei Morbus basedowii. *Berliner Klinisch Wochenschrift*, 21, 163-6.

6 Murray GR. (1884). Note on the treatment of myxoedema by hypodermic injections of an extract of the thyroid gland of a sheep. *British Medical Journal*, 2, 796-7.

7 Eiselsberg A von. (1890). Ueber erfolgreiche Einheilung der Katzenschilddrüse in die Bauchdecke und Auftreten von Tetanie nach deren Exstirpation. *Wiener Klinische Wochenschrift*, 5, 81-5.

8 Mayo CH. (1907). Goiter. With preliminary report of three hundred operations on the thyroid. *Journal of the American Medical Association*, 48, 273-7.

9 Halsted WS. (1920). The operative story of goitre. *Johns Hopkins Hospital Reports*, 19, 17-257.

10 Dunhill TP. (1907). Exophthalmic goitre - partial thyroidectomy under local anaesthesia. *Intercolonial Medical Journal of Australia*, 12, 569-72.

11 Dunhill TP. (1908). Surgical treatment of exophthalmic goitre. *Intercolonial Medical Journal of Australia*, 13, 293-9.

12 Dunhill TP. (1909). Remarks on partial thyroidectomy, with special reference to exophthalmic goître, and observations on 113 operations under local anaesthesia. *British Medical Journal*, 1, 1222-5.

13 Helmholtz H von. (1851). *Beschreibung eines Augen-Spiegels zur Untersuchung der Netzhaut im lebenden Auge.* Berlin; Förstner.

14 Graefe A von. (1857). Ueber die Iridectomie bei Glaucom und über den glaucomatösen Process. *Archiv für Ophthalmologie*, 3: 2 Abth., 456-560.

15 Wells TS. Cited by: Allbutt TC. (1871). *The use of the ophthalmoscope in diseases of the nervous system and of the kidneys, and also in certain general disorders.* London and New York; Macmillan.

16 Koller C. (1884). Vorläufige Mittheilung über locale Anästhesirung am Auge. *Klinische Monatsblatter für Augenheilkunde*, **22**, Beilageheft 60-3.

17 Helmholtz H von. (1852). Ueber die Theorie der zusammengesetzten Farben. *Archiv für Anatomie, Physiologie und Wissenshaftliche Medizin*, 87, 461-82.

18 Young T. (1801). On the theory of light and colours. *Philosophical Transactions of the Royal Society of London*, **92**, 12-48. [See also *Nicholson's Philosophical Journal* (1801).]

19 Helmholtz H von. (1863). *Die Lehre von den Tonempfindungen als physiologische Grundlage für die Theorie der Musik.* Braunschweig; Wiewig.

20 Hippel A von. (1888). Eine neue methode der hornhauttransplantation. *Archiv für Ophthalmologie*, **34**, Abt 1, 108-30.

21 Power H. (1873). On transplantation of the cornea. *Report of the Fourth International Ophthalmological Congress, held in London, August, 1872*, pp. 172-6. London; Savill, Edwards.

22 Zirm E. (1906). Eine erfolgreiche totale Keratoplastik. *Archiv für Ophthalmologie*, **64**, 580-93.

23 Zirm E. (1907). Ueber Hornhautpfrapfung. *Wiener Klinische Wochenschrift*, **20**, 61-5.

24 Barraquer JI. (1967). Keratomileusis. *International Surgery*, **1**, 103-17.

25 Barraquer JI. (1968). Keratophakia for the correction of high hyperopia. *Journal of Cryosurgery*, **1**, 39-46.

26 Strampelli B. (1963). Osteo-odonto-cheratoprostesi. *Annali di Ottalmologica e Clinica Oculista*, **89**, 1039-44.

27 Hofmann F. (1841). See: Leading Article (1911). Zur Erinnerung an Friedrich Hofmann. *Zeitschrift für Laryngologie und Rhinologie*, **4**, 237.

28 Politzer A. (1865). *Atlas der Beleuchtungsbilder des Trommelfells im gesunden und kranken Zustande für praktische Aertze und Studierende.* Vienna; Braumuller.

29 Schwartze H, Eysell A. (1873). Ueber die künstliche Eröffnung des Warzenfortsatzes. *Archiv für Ohrenheilkunde*, **1**, 157-87.

30 Zaufal E. (1884). Sinusthrombose in Folge von Otitis media. [Trepanation des Proc. mastoid mit Hammer und Miesel.] *Prager Medizinische Wochenschrift*, **9**, 474-5.

31 Bergmann E von. (1888). Krankenvorstellung: Geheilter Hirnabscess. *Berliner Klinische Wochenschrift*, **25**, 1054-6.

32 Küster E. (1889). Ueber die Grundsätze der Behandlung von Eiterungen in starrwandigen Hölen, mit besonderer Berücksichtigung des Empyems der Pleura. *Deutsche Medizinische Wochenschrift*, **15**, 254-7.

33 Holmgren G. (1923). Some experiences in the surgery of otosclerosis. *Acta Otolaryngologica (Stockholm)*, **5**, 460-6.

34 Sourdille MLJM. (1937). New technique in the surgical treatment of severe and progressive deafness from otosclerosis. *Bulletin of the New York Academy of Medicine*, **13**, 673-91.

35 Lempert J. (1938). Improvements of hearing in cases of otosclerosis: a new, one-stage surgical technic. *Archives of Otolaryngology, Chicago*, **28**, 42-97.

36 Survey (1943). Carried out by Dr Marvin Fisher Jones of New York at the request of the American Academy of Ophthalmology and Otolaryngology.

37 Zöllner F. (1951). Die Bisherigen ergebnisse der Schallsondenuntersuchungen. *Archiv für Ohren-, Nasen und Kehlkopfheilkunde*, **159**, 358-64.

38 Wüllstein H. (1952). Funktionelle Operationen im Mittelohr mit hilfe des freien

Spaltlappen-Transplantates. *Archiv Ohren-, Nasen und Kehlkopfheilkunde*, **161**, 422-35.

39 Rosen S. (1952). Palpation of the stapes for fixation: Preliminary procedure to determine fenestration suitability in otosclerosis. *Archives of Otolaryngology, Chicago*, **56**, 610-15.

40 Rosen S. (1953). Mobilization of the stapes to restore hearing in otosclerosis. *New York Medical Journal*, **53**, 2650-3.

41 Kessel J. (1876). Über das Ausschneiden des Trommelfelles und Mobilisieren des Steigbügels. *Archiv für Ohren-, Nasen und Kehlkopfheilkunde*, **11**, 199.

42 Garcia M. (1856). Observations on the human voice. *Proceedings of the Royal Society of London*, **7**, 399-410.

43 Türck L. (1860). *Praktische Anleitung zur Laryngoskopie.* Vienna; Braumuller.

44 Czermak JN. (1858). Ueber den Kehlkopfspiegel. *Wiener Medizinische Wochenschrift*, **8**, 196-8.

45 Kirstein A. (1895). Autoskopie des Larynx und der Trachea (Laryngoscopia directa, Euthyskopie, Besichtigung ohne Spiegel). *Archiv für Laryngologie und Rhinologie*, **3**, 156-6.

46 Killian G. (1898). Ueber directe Bronchoskopie. *Münchener Medizinische Wochenschrift*, **45**, 844-7.

47 Jackson C. (1907). *Tracheo-bronchoscopy, esophagoscopy, and gastroscopy.* St Louis; The Laryngoscope Company.

CHAPTER 17: GYNAECOLOGY

1   Wells TS. (1873). *Diseases of the ovaries.* New York; Appleton.

2   Sims JM. (1852). On the treatment of vesico-vaginal fistula. *American Journal of Medical Sciences*, n.s. **23**, 59-82.

3   Sims JM. (1858). *Silver sutures in surgery.* New York; Wood.

4   Collis MH. (1857). Cases of vesico-vaginal fistula. *Dublin Quarterly Journal of Medical Sciences*, **23**, 119-32.

5   Collis MH. (1861). Further remarks upon a new and successful mode of treatment for vesico-vaginal fistula. *Dublin Quarterly Journal of Medical Sciences*, **31**, 302-16.

6   Mackenrodt AK. (1896). Ueber den künstlichen Ersatz der Scheide. *Zentralblatt für Gynaekologie*, **20**, 546-50.

7   Allbutt TC. (1884). *On visceral neuroses, being the Gulstonian Lecture on neuralgia of the stomach and allied disorders.* London; Macmillan.

8   Simpson JY. (1872). *Clinical lectures on the diseases of women, posthumously collected and edited by Alexander R. Simpson.* 3 vols. Edinburgh; Black. [See vol. 3. pp. 169-70.]

9   Alexander W. (1882). A new method of treating inveterate and troublesome displacements of the uterus. *Medical Times and Gazette*, **1**, 327-8.

10 Sutton JB. (1890). Cited by: Bett WR. (1956). *Sir John Bland-Sutton. 1855-1936.* Edinburgh and London; Livingstone.

11 Emmet TA. (1868-9). Surgery of the cervix in connection with the treatment of certain uterine diseases. *American Journal of Obstetrics*, **1**, 339-62.

12 Emmet TA. (1874-5). Laceration of the cervix uteri as a frequent and unrecognised cause of disease. *American Journal of Obstetrics*, **7**, 442-56.

13 Simpson JY. (1872). See ref. 8 above, vol. 3, p. 696.

14 Freund WA. (1878). Eine neue Methode der Extirpation des ganzen Uterus. *Sammlung Klinische Vorträge*, No. **133** (Gynaek. No. **41**), 911-24.

15 Ries E. (1895). Eine neue Operationsmethode des Uteruscarcinoms. *Zeitschrift für Geburtshilfe und Gynäkologie*, **32**, 266-74.

16 Wertheim E. (1900). Zur Frage der Radicaloperation beim Uteruskrebs. *Archiv für Gynäkologie*, **61**, 627-68.

17 Wertheim E. (1902). Ein neuer Beitrag zur Frage der Radikaloperation beim Uteruskrebs. *Archiv für Gynäekologie*, **65**, 1-39.

18 Wertheim E. (1905). A discussion on the diagnosis and treatment of cancer of the uterus. B*ritish Medical Journal*, **2**, 689-95.

19 Wertheim E. (1911). *Die erweiterte abdominale Operation bei Carcinoma colli uteri (auf Grund von 500 Fällen)*. Berlin; Urban und Schwartzenberg.

20 Ritgen FA. (1825). Geschichte eines mit ungünstigem Erfolge verrichteten Bauchscheidenschnitts und Folgerung daraus. *Heidelberger Klinische Annalen*, **1**, 263-77.

21 Porro E. (1876). *Dell'amputazione uter-ovarica come complemento di taglio cesareo*. Milan; Rechiedei.

22 Sänger M. (1882). *Der Kaiserschnitt bei Uterusfibromen, nebst verrgleichender Methodik der Sectio caesarea und der Porro-Operation. Kritiken Studien und Vorschläge zur Verbesserung des Kaiserschnitts*. Leipzig; Breitkopf and Hartel.

23 Thomas TG. (1870). Gastro-elytrotomy; a substitute for the caesarean section. *American Journal of Obstetrics and Diseases of Women*, **3**, 125-39.

24 Holland E. (1921). Methods of performing caesarean section. *Journal of Obstetrics and Gynaecology of the British Empire*, **28**, 349-57.

25 Kerr JMM. (1921). Indications for caesarean section. *Journal of Obstetrics and Gynaecology of the British Empire*, **28**, 338-48.

CHAPTER 18: ORTHOPAEDICS AND X-RAYS

1 Andry N. (1741). *L'orthopédie ou l'art de prevenir et de corriger dans les enfants, les difformités du corps*. 3 vols. Paris; La Veuve Alix.

2 Syme J. (1831). T*reatise on the excision of diseased joints*. Edinburgh; Black.

3 Stromeyer GFL. (1833). Die Durchschneidung der Achillessehne, als Heilmethode des Klumpfusses, durch zwei Fälle erläutert (1831-32). *Magazin für die Gesammte Heilkunde (Berlin)*, **39**, 195-218.

4 Little WJ. (1853). *On the nature and treatment of the deformities of the human frame*. London; Longman.

5 Langenbeck B. (1854). Die subcutane Osteotomie. *Deutsche Klinik*, **6**, 327.

6 Little LS. (1868). Cited by: Jones AR. (1956). A review of orthopaedic surgery in Britain. *Journal of Bone and Joint Surgery*, **37B**, 27-45.

7 Billroth T, Winiwarter v. A. (1884). *General surgical pathology and therapeutics*. Translated from the 4th edition and revised from the 10th by C. E. Hackney. London; Lewis.

8 Macewen W. (1878). Lecture on antiseptic osteotomy for genu valgum, genu varum, and other osseous deformities. *Lancet*, **2**, 911-14; (1879) **1**, 586-7.

9 Annandale T. (1885). An operation for displaced semilunar cartilage. *British Medical Journal*, **1**, 779.

10 Lorenz A. (1897). Zur congenitalen Luxation des Hüftgelenkes. *Berliner Klinische*

Wochenschrift, **34**, 112-14.

11 Hoffa A. (1890). Zur operativen Behandlung der angeborenen Hüftgelenksverrenkungen. *Verhandlungen der Deutschen Gesellschaft für Chirurgie*, **19**, 44-53.

12 Eaton W. (1795). Account of the Arabian mode of curing fractured limbs. *Medical Commentaries for the year 1794*. Philadelphia, **41**; 167.

13 Mathijsen, A. (1852). *Nieuwere wijze van aawending van het gipsverband bij beenbreuken; eere bidrage tot de militaire chirurgie*. Haarlem; van Loghem.

14 Mathysen A. (1854). *Du bandage plâtré et de son application dans le traitement des fractures*. Liége; Grandmont-Donders.

15 Hilton J. (1863). *Rest and pain*. London; Bell.

16 Thomas HO. (1875). *Diseases of the hip, knee and ankle joints, with their deformities, treated by a new and efficient method; (enforced, uninterrupted and prolonged rest)*. Liverpool; Dobb.

17 Albert E. (1882). Einige Fälle von kunstlicher Ankylosenbildung an paralytischen Gliedmassen. *Wiener Medizinische Presse*, **23**, 725-8.

18 Jones R. (1908). An operation for paralytic calcaneo-cavus. *American Journal of Orthopaedic Surgery*, **5**, 371-6.

19 Nicoladoni C. (1882). Nachtrag zum Pes calcaneus und zur Transplantation der Peronealsehnen. *Archiv für Klinische Chirurgie*, **27**, 660-6.

20 Parrish BF. (1892). A new operation for paralytic talipes valgus, and the enunciation of a new surgical principle. *New York Medical Journal*, **56**, 402-3.

21 Eve F. (1897). Cited by: Jones AR. (1956). Ref. 6, above.

22 Tubby AH, Jones R. (1903). *Modern methods in the surgery of paralyses*. London; Macmillan.

23 Guericke O von. (1672). *Experimenta nova (ut vocantur) Magdeburgica de vacuo spatio*. Amstelodami; Jan Jansson à Waesberge.

24 Röntgen WC. (1895). Ueber eine neue Art von Strahlen. *Sitzungsberichte der Physikalisch-Medizinischen Gesellschaft*, **29**, 132-41.

25 Burry J. (1896). A preliminary report on the Roentgen or x rays. *Journal of the American Medical Association*, **26**, 402-4.

26 Jones R, Lodge O. (1896). The discovery of a bullet lost in the wrist by means of the Roentgen rays. *Lancet*, **1**, 476-7.

27 Lane WA. (1894). A method of treating simple oblique fractures of the tibia and fibula more efficient than those in common use. *Transactions of the Clinical Society of London*, **27**, 167-75.

28 Lane WA. (1907). Clinical observations in the operative treatment of fractures. *British Medical Journal*, **1**, 1037-8.

29 Lister J. (1884). On the treatment of fracture of the patella. *Proceedings of the Medical Society of London*, **7**, 12-23.

30 Albee FH. (1911). Transplantation of a portion of the tibia into the spine in Pott's disease. *Journal of the American Medical Association*, **57**, 885.

31 Albee FH. (1915). *Bone-graft surgery*. Philadelphia; Saunders.

32 Smith-Petersen MN, Cave EF, Van Gorder GW. (1931). Intracapsular fractures of the neck of the femur. Treatment by internal fixation. *Archives of Surgery*, **23**, 715-59.

33 Langenbeck B von. (1878). In discussion of: Trendelenburg F. (1878). Vorstellung eines Fälles von veraltetem Querbruch der Patella. *Verhandlung der Deutsche Gesellschaft*

für Chirurgie, 7 Cong., 1, 92–3.

34 Steinmann F. (1907). Eine neue Extensionsmethode in der Frakturenbehandlung. *Zentralblatt für Chirurgie*, 34, 938–42.

35 Johansson S. (1932). On the operative treatment of medical fractures of the neck of the femur. *Acta Orthopaedica Scandinavica*, 3, 362–92.

36 Smith-Petersen MN. (1939). Arthroplasy of the hip. A new method. *Journal of Bone and Joint Surgery*, 21, 269–88.

37 Judet J, Judet RL. (1950). The use of an artificial femoral head for arthroplasty of the hip joint. *Journal of Bone and Joint Surgery*, 32B, 166–73.

CHAPTER 19: FIELDS OF BATTLE

1 Richardson RG, ed. (1977). *Nurse Sarah Anne: with Florence Nightingale at Scutari.* London; Murray. [Sarah Anne Terrot was one of eight Sellonite Sisters who proved the most valuable of the thirty-eight women as they had already had experience of epidemics of cholera in the slums of Plymouth.]

2 *Report of the Commissioners appointed to inquire into the regulations affecting the sanitary condition of the army, the organization of military hospitals, and the treatment of the sick and wounded; with evidence and appendix.* (1858). London; Eyre and Spottiswoode.

3 Pirogoff NI. (1864). *Grundzüge der Allgemeine Kriegschirurgie.* Leipzig; Vogel.

4 Dunant JH. (1862). *Un souvenir de Solferino.* Genève; Fick.

5 Chisholm JJ. (1862). *A manual of military surgery for the use of surgeons in the Confederate States army.* Richmond, Virginia; West and Johnson.

6 Wells TS. (1859). Three cases of tetanus in which 'Woorara' was used. *Proceedings of the Royal Medical and Chirurgical Society of London*, 3, 142–57.

7 Esmarch JFA von. (1869). *Der erste Verband auf dem Schlachtfelde.* Kiel; Schwers.

8 Vanghetti G. (1898). *Amputazione, disarticulazione e protesi.* Firenze.

9 Vanghetti G. (1906). *Plastica e protesi cinematische. Nuova teoria sulle amputazioni e sulla protesi.* Empoli; Travesari.

10 Ceci A. (1906). Tecnica generale della amputazioni mucosi. Amputazioni plastico-ortopediche con metodo proprio secundo la proposta de Vanghetti. Dimostrazioni pratiche. *Archivo ed Atti della Società Italiana di Chirurgica, Roma*, 19, 171.

11 Ceci A. (1906). Procédés originaux d'amputation plastico-cinétiques ou plastico-orthopédiques. *Presse Médicale*, 14, 745–7.

12 Putti V. (1917). Plastiche e protesi cinematische. *Chirurgica degli Organi di Movimento*, 1, 419–92.

13 Putti V. (1918). The utilization of the muscles of a stump to actuate artificial limbs: cinematic amputations. *British Medical Journal*, 1, 635–8.

14 Sauerbruch F. (1916). *Die Willkürlich bewegbare künstliche Hand. Eine Anleitung für Chirurgen und Techniker.* Berlin; Springer.

15 Sauerbruch EF, ten Horn C. (1923). *Die Willkürlich bewegbare künstliche Hand.* Berlin; Springer.

16 Marquardt E. (1961). Experiments on substitution and utilization of surface sensitivity in arm prostheses. *Archiv für Orthopädische und Unfallchirurgie*, 53, 64–71.

17 Wright AE, Leishman WB. (1900). Remarks on the results which have been obtained by the antityphoid inoculations. *British Medical Journal*, 1, 122–9. [See also: Preliminary note (1896). *Lancet*, 2, 807.]

18 Gedroitz VI. Cited by: Fraser J. in: Bailey H. (1941). *Surgery of modern warfare*, p. 198. Edinburgh; Livingstone.

19 Dakin HD. (1915). On the use of certain antiseptic substances in the treatment of infected wounds. *British Medical Journal*, **2**, 318-20.

20 Carrel A. (1916). Carrel-Dakin solution. *Journal of the American Medical Association*, **67**, 1777-8.

21 Carrel A, Dehelly G. (1917). *The treatment of infected wounds*. Translated by Herbert Child. New York; Hoeber.

22 Baer WS. (1931). The treatment of chronic osteomyelitis with the maggot (larva of the blow fly). *Journal of Bone and Joint Surgery*, **13**, 438-75.

23 Cummins SL. (1921). Tetanus in the British army during the European war (August 1914 to November 1918). *Cinquième Congrès du Société Internationale de Chirurgie, Paris, 19-23 Juillet 1920.* pp. 608-35. Bruxelles; Hayez.

24 Davis GG. (1916). Roentgen-ray diagnosis of gas and pus infections as complications of wounds with deeply buried bullets or shell fragments. *Surgery, Gynecology and Obstetrics*, **22**, 635-7.

25 Weinberg M, Séguin P. (1915). Le *B. oedematiens* et la gangrène gazeuse. *Comptes Rendus des Séances de la Société de Biologie et de ses Filiales*, **78**, 507.

26 Botallo L. (1660). De curandis vulneribus sclopetorum. In: *Opera omnia*, pp. 599-801. Lugdini Batavorum; Danielis and Abrahami. [Originally published in 1560 in Lyons.]

27 Desault PJ. (1803). *Cours théorique et pratique de clinique externe.* Des maladies par solution de continuité, **2**, 147 et seq. Paris; Delaplace.

28 Larrey DJ. (1812-17). *Mémoires de chirurgie militaire, et campagnes.* 4 vols. Paris; Smith.

29 Richardson R. (2000). *Larrey: Surgeon to Napoleon's Imperial Guard*. London; Quiller.

30 Friedrich PL. (1898). Die aseptishe Versorgung frischer Wunden, unter Mittheilung von Thier-Versuchen über die Auskeimungszeit von Infectionserregern in frischen Wunden. *Archiv für Klinische Chirurgie*, **57**, 288.

31 Hughes B, Banks HS. (1918). *War surgery. From firing-line to base.* London; Baillière, Tindall and Cox.

32 Orr HW. (1927). The treatment of osteomyelitis and other infected wounds by drainage and rest. *Surgery, Gynecology and Obstetrics*, **45**, 446-64.

33 Albert E. (1876). Cited by: Keith A. (1919). *Menders of the maimed*. London; Henry Frowde, Hodder and Stoughton.

34 Robson AWM. (1888). Cited by: Keith A. (1919). Ref. 33, above.

35 Ballance CA, Ballance HA, Stewart P. (1903). Remarks on the operative treatment of chronic facial palsy of peripheral origin. *British Medical Journal*, **1**, 1009-13.

36 Platt H, Bristow WR. (1924). Remote results of operations for injuries of peripheral nerves. *British Journal of Surgery*, **11**, 535-67.

37 Tagliacozzi G. (1597). *De curtorum chirurgia per insitionem.* Venetiis; apud G. Bindonum, jun.

38 Reverdin JL. (1869). Greffe épidermique. Expérience faite dans le service de M le docteur Gryon à l'hôpital Necker. *Bulletin-Société de Chirurgie de Paris*, 2 sèr., **10**, 511-15.

39 Ollier L. (1872). Greffes cutanées ou autoplastiques. *Bulletin de la Société Academique de Paris*, 2 sèr. **1**, 243-50.

40 Thiersch C. (1874). Ueber die feinerem anatomischen Veränderungen bei Aufheilung von Haut auf Granulationem. *Verhandlungen der Deutschen Gesellschaft für Chirurgie*, **3**, 69-75.

41 Krause F. (1893). Ueber die Transplantation grosser ungestielter Hautlappen. *Verhandlungen der Deutschen Gesellschaft für Chirurgie*, **22**, pt 2, 46-51.

42 Wolfe JR. (1875). A new method of performing plastic operations. *British Medical Journal*, **2**, 360-1.

43 Gillies H, Millard DR. (1957). *The principles and art of plastic surgery*. London; Butterworth.

CHAPTER 20: CONSOLIDATION

1 Libavius A. (1613). *Syntagma arcanorum et commentationum chymicorum*. 2 vols. Francofurti; Nicolaus Hoffman for Petrus Kopf.

2 Harvey W. (1628). *Exercitatio anatomica de motu cordis et sanguinis in animalibus*. Francofurti; Guilielmi Fitzeri.

3 Lower R. (1666). The method observed in transfusing the bloud out of one animal into another. *Philosophical Transactions of the Royal Society of London*, **1**, 353-8.

4 Lower R, King E. (1667). An account of the experiment of transfusion practised upon a man in London. *Philosophical Transactions of the Royal Society of London*, **2**, 557-64.

5 Denis JB. (1667). Extract of a letter written by Denis: Touching a late cure of an inveterate phrensy by the transfusion of blood. *Philosophical Transactions of the Royal Society of London*, **2**, 617-24.

6 Blundell J. (1828-9). Observations on transfusion of blood. *Lancet*, **2**, 321-4.

7 Landois L. (1875). *Die Transfusion des Blutes*. Leipzig; Vogel.

8 Landsteiner K. (1901). Ueber Agglutinationserscheinungen normalen menschlichen Blutes. *Wiener Klinische Wochenschrift*, **14**, 1132-4.

9 Bordet J, Gengou O. (1901). Recherches sur la coagulation du sang et les sérums anticoagulants. *Annales de l'Institut Pasteur*, **15**, 129-44.

10 Hustin A. (1914). Note sur une nouvelle méthode de transfusion. *Bulletin des Séances de la Société Royale des Sciences Médicales et Naturelles de Bruxelles*, **72**, 104-11.

11 Lewisohn R. (1915). A new and greatly simplified method of blood transfusion. A preliminary report. *Medical Record, New York*, **87**, 141-2.

12 Agote L. (1914-5). Nuevo procédimiento para la transfusion del sangre. *Anales del Instituto Modelo de Clinica Médico (B. Aires)*, **1**, 24-31.

13 Marriott HL, Kekwick A. (1935). Continuous drip blood transfusion. *Lancet*, **1**, 977-81.

14 Yudin SS. (1936). Transfusion of cadaver blood. *Journal of the American Medical Association*, **106**, 997-9.

15 Fantus B. (1937). The therapy of the Cook County Hospital. Blood preservation. *Journal of the American Medical Association*, **109**, 128-31.

16 Landsteiner K, Wiener AS. (1940). Agglutinable factor in human blood recognized by immune sera for rhesus blood. *Proceedings of the Society for Experimental Biology, New York*, **43**, 233.

17 Lane WA. Cited by: Layton TB. (1956). *Sir William Arbuthnot Lane; an enquiry into the mind and influence of a surgeon*. Edinburgh and London; Livingstone.

18 Murphy JB. (1909). Proctoclysis in the treatment of peritonitis. *Journal of the American Medical Association*, **52**, 1248-50.

19 Matas R. (1924). The continued intravenous 'drip' with remarks on the value of continued gastric drainage and irrigation by nasal intubation with gastroduodenal tube, (Jutte) in surgical practice. *Annals of Surgery*, **79**, 643-61.

20 Ryle JA. (1921). Studies in gastric secretion. *Guy's Hospital Reports*, **71**, 42-4.

21 Wangensteen OH. (1932). The early diagnosis of acute intestinal obstruction with comments on pathology and treatment. With a report of successful decompression of three cases of mechanical bowel obstruction by nasal catheter suction siphonage. *Western Journal of Surgery, Obstetrics and Gynecology*, **40**, 1-17.

22 Miller TG, Abbott WO. (1934). Intestinal intubation: a practical technique. *American Journal of Medical Sciences*, **187**, 595-9.

23 Domagk G. (1935). Ein Beitrag zur Chemotherapie der bakteriellen Infektionen. *Deutsche Medizinische Wochenschrift*, **61**, 250-3.

24 Colebrook L, Kenny M. (1936). Treatment of human puerperal infections, and of experimental infections in mice, with prontosil. *Lancet*, **1**, 1279-86.

25 Colebrook L, Buttle GAH, O'Meara RAQ. (1936). The mode of action of p-aminobenzenesulphonamide and prontosil in haemolytic streptococcal infections. *Lancet*, **2**, 1323-6.

CHAPTER 21: THE LAST FRONTIER

1 Béhier LJ. (1873). *Pleurésies à épanchements modérés. Thoracentèse avec trocarts capillaires et aspiration; appareils divers.* Paris; Pougin.

2 Bowditch HI. (1884). The aspiration in pleural effusion. *Boston Medical and Surgical Journal*, **140**, 572-3.

3 Schede M. (1890). Die Behandlung der Empyeme. *Verhhandlungen der Deutscher Kongress für Innere Medizin*, **9**, 41-100.

4 Estlander JA. (1879). Résection des côtes dans l'empyéme chronique. *Revue Mensuelle de Médecine et de Chirurgie*, **3**, 157-70; 885-8.

5 Lane WA. (1883). Cases of empyema in children treated by removal of a portion of rib. *Guy's Hospital Reports*, **41**, 45-6.

6 Bülau G. (1891). Für die Heber-Drainage bei Behandlung des Empyems. *Zeitschrift für Klinische Medizin*, **18**, 31-45.

7 Carson J. (1822). *Essays, physiological and practical.* Liverpool; Wright.

8 Stokes W. (1837). *A treatise on the diagnosis and treatment of diseases of the chest.* Dublin; Hodges and Smith.

9 Forlanini C. (1882). A contribuzione della terapie chirurgica della tisi ablazione del polmone? Pneumotrace artificiale? *Gazzetta degli Ospedali e delle Clinische, Agosto*, Sett.-Ott. Nov. **3**, 537, 585, 601, 609, 617, 625, 641, 657, 665, 689, 705.

10 Cerenville E de. (1885). De l'intervention opératoire dans les maladies du poumon. *Revue Médicale de la Suisse Romande, Genève*, **5**, 441-67.

11 Gourdet J. (1895). *Etude sur l'aplatissement comparé du thorax par les différents procédés de résection costale, et specialement sur un nouveau procédé de thoracoplastie.* Thèse de Paris, n.361.

12 Brauer L. (1908). Indications du traitement chirurgicale de la tuberculose pulmonaire. *Congres Association Français de Chirurgie*, **21**, 569-74.

13 Sauerbruch F. (1913). Die Beeinflussung von Lungenerkrankungen durch künstliche Lähmung des Zwerchfells (Phrenikotomie). *Münchener Medizinische Wochenschrift*, **60**, 625-6.

14 Stürtz CAE. (1912). Experimenteller Beitrag zur Zwerch fellbewegung nach einseitiger. Phrenicusdurchtrennung. *Deutsche Medizinische Wochenschrift*, **38**, 897-900.

15 Friedrich PL. (1915). Cited by: Blades B. (1955). Intrathoracic surgery (lungs, heart, and great vessels: surgical management of the diseases of the esophagus), 1905-1955. *Surgery, Gynecology and Obstetrics, International Abstracts of Surgery*, **100**, 413-24.

16 Tuffier T. (1897). *Chirurgie du poumon en particulier dans les cavernes tuberculeuses et la gangrène pulmonaire*. Paris; Masson. [See p. 31.]

17 Macewen W. (1906). On some points in the surgery of the lung. *British Medical Journal*, **2**, 1-7. [The left 'pneumonectomy' for tuberculosis took place on April 24, 1895. The patient was still alive in 1940.]

18 Mikulicz-Radecki J von. (1886). Ein Fall von resection des carcinomatösen Oesophagus mit plastischem Ersatz des exciderten Stückes. *Prager Medizinische Wochenschrift*, **11**, 93-4.

19 Sauerbruch. (1904). Zur Pathologie des offenen Pneumothorax und die Grundlagen meines Verfahrens seiner Ausschaltung. *Mitteilungen aus den Grenzebietender Medizin und Chirurgie*, **13**, 399-482.

20 Trendelenburg. (1871). Beitrage zu den Operationem an den Luftwegen. *Archiv für Klinische Chirurgie*, **12**, 112-33.

21 Macewen W. (1880). Clinical observations on the introduction of tracheal tubes by the mouth instead of performing tracheotomy or laryngotomy. *British Medical Journal*, **2**, 122-4; 163-5.

22 Matas R. (1900). Intralaryngeal insufflation. For the relief of acute surgical pneumothorax. Its history and methods with a description of the latest devices for this purpose. *Journal of the American Medical Association*, **34**, 1371-5; 1468-73.

23 O'Dwyer J. (1887). Fifty cases of croup in private practice treated by intubation of the larynx, with a description of the method and of the dangers incident thereto. *Medical Record, New York*, **32**, 557-61.

24 Fell GE. (1887). Forced respiration in opium poisoning - its possibilities, and the apparatus best adapted to produce it. *Buffalo Medical and Surgical Journal*, **27**, 145-57.

25 Tuffier, Hallion. (1896). Opérations intrathoraciques avec respiration artificielle par insufflation. *Comptes Rendus des Séances de la Société de Biologie et ses Filiales*, 10s, **3**, 951-3.

26 Kirstein A. (1895). Autoskopie des Larynx und der Trachea (Laryngoscopia directa, Euthyskopie, Besichtigung ohne Spiegel). *Archiv für Laryngologie und Rhinologie*, **3**, 156-64.

27 Kuhn F. (1902). Die pernasale Tubage. *Münchener Medizinische Wochenschrift*, **49**, 1456-7.

28 Bartélemy, Dufour. (1907). L'anesthésie dans la chirurgie de la face. *Presse Médicale*, **15**, 475-6.

29 Volhard F. (1908). Ueber künstliche Atmung durch Ventilation der Trachea und eine einfache Vorrichtung zur rhytmischen künstlichen Atmung. *Münchener Medizinische Wochenschrift*, **55**, 205-11.

30 Meltzer SJ, Auer J. (1909). Continuous respiration without respiratory movements. *Journal of Respiratory Medicine*, **11**, 622-5.

278

31 Elsberg CA. (1910). The value of continuous intratracheal insufflation of air (Meltzer) in thoracic surgery: with description of an apparatus. *Medical Record, New York*, **77**, 493-5.

32 Rowbotham ES, Magill IW. (1921). Anaesthetics in the plastic surgery of the face and jaws. *Proceedings of the Royal Society of Medicine*, **14**, 17-27.

33 Magill IW. (1936). Anaesthesia in thoracic surgery, with special reference to lobectomy. *Proceedings of the Royal Society of Medicine*, **29**, 643-53.

34 Waters RM. (1924). Clinical scope and utility of carbon dioxid [*sic*] filtration in inhalational anesthesia. *Anesthesia and Analgesia; Current Researches*, **3**, 20-22, 26.

35 Crafoord C. (1938). On the technique of pneumonectomy in man. A critical survey of the experimental and clinical development and a report of the author's material and technique. *Acta Chirurgica Scandinavica*, **81**, suppl. 54, p.142.

36 Nosworthy MD. (1941). Anaesthesia in chest surgery, with special reference to controlled respiration with cyclopropane. *Proceedings of the Royal Society of Medicine*, **34**, 479-505.

37 Griffith HR, Johnson GE. (1942). The use of curare in general anesthesia. *Anesthesiology*, **3**, 418-20.

38 Sicard JA, Forestier J. (1924). L'exploration radiologique des cavités broncho-pulmonaires par les injections intra-trachéales d'huile iodée. *Journal Médical Français*, **13**, 3-9.

39 Sicard JA, Forestier J. (1921). Méthode radiographique d'exploration de la cavité épidurale par le lipiodol. *Revue Neurologique*, **28**, 1264-6.

40 Graham EA. (1923). Pneumonectomy with the cautery: a safer substitute for the ordinary lobectomy in cases of chronic suppuration of the lung. *Journal of the American Medical Association*, **81**, 1010-12.

41 Whittemore W. (1927). The treatment of such cases of chronic suppurative bronchiectasis as are limited to one lobe of the lung. *Annals of Surgery*, **86**, 219-26.

42 Brunn HB. (1929). Surgical principles underlying one-stage lobectomy. *Archives of Surgery*, **18**, 490-515.

43 Nissen R. (1931). Exstirpation eines ganzen Lungenflugels. *Zentralblatt für Chirurgie*, **58**, 3003-6.

44 Shenstone NS, Janes RM. (1932). Experiences in pulmonary lobectomy. *Canadian Medical Association Journal*, **27**, 138-45.

45 Davies HM. (1913). Recent advances in the surgery of the lung and pleura. *British Journal of Surgery*, **1**, 228-58.

46 Edwards AT. (1932). The surgical treatment of intrathoracic new growths. *British Medical Journal*, **1**, 827-30.

47 Graham EA, Singer JJ. (1933). Successful removal of an entire lung for carcinoma of the bronchus. *Journal of the American Medical Association*, **101**, 1371-4.

48 Rienhoff WF Jr. (1933). Pneumonectomy. A preliminary report of the operative technique in two successful cases. *Bulletin of the Johns Hopkins Hospital*, **53**, 390-3.

49 Rienhoff WF. (1939). A two-stage operation for total pneumonectomy in the treatment of carcinoma of the lung, demonstrating a new technique for closure of the bronchus. *Journal of Thoracic Surgery*, **8**, 254-71.

50 Waters RM, Schmidt ER. (1934). Cyclopropane anesthesia. *Journal of the American Medical Association*, **103**, 975-83.

51 Lundy JS. (1935). Intravenous anesthesia: preliminary report of the use of two new

barbiturates. *Proceedings of the Staff Meetings of the Mayo Clinic*, **10**, 536-43.

52 Pelouze, Bernard C. (1850). Reserches sur le curare. *Comptes Rendus Hebdomadaires des Séances de l'Académie des Sciences*, **31**, 533-7.

53 Overholt RH, Langer L, Szypulski JT, Wilson NJ. (1946). Pulmonary resection in the treatment of tuberculosis: present-day technique and results. *Journal of Thoracic Surgery*, **15**, 384-413.

54 Churchill ED, Belsey R. (1939). Segmental pneumonectomy in bronchiectasis: the lingula segment of the left upper lobe. *Annals of Surgery*, **109**, 481-99.

55 Kirschner M. (1920). Ein neus Verfahren der Oesophagoplastik. *Archiv für Klinische Chirurgie*, **114**, 606-63.

56 Ohsawa T. (1930). Über die freie ventro-arco-diaphragmale Thorakolaparotomie bzw. Laparothorakotomie. *Zentralblatt für Chirurgie*, **57**, 2467-72.

57 Ohsawa T. (1933). The surgery of the oesophagus. *Archiv für Japanische Chirurgie*, **10**, 605-95.

58 Evans A. (1913). In: *Transactions of the XVII International Congress of Medicine*, **7**, part 2, 125.

59 Evans A. (1933). A rubber oesophagus. *British Journal of Surgery*, **20**, 388-92.

60 Torek F. (1913). The first successful case of resection of the thoracic portion of the oesophagus for carcinoma. *Surgery, Gynecology and Obstetrics*, **16**, 614-17.

61 Garlock JH. (1944). The re-establishment of esophagogastric continuity following resection of esophagus for carcinoma of middle third. *Surgery, Gynecology and Obstetrics*, **78**, 23-8.

CHAPTER 22: MORE IN A MILITARY VEIN

1 Böhler L. (1929). *Technik der Knochenbruchbehandlung*. Wien; Maudrich.

2 Trueta J. (1939). *Treatment of war wounds and fractures, with special reference to the closed method as used in the war with Spain*. London; Hamilton.

3 Macintosh RR, Mendelssohn K. (1941). The quantitative administration of ether vapour. *Lancet*, **2**, 61-2.

4 Epstein HG, Macintosh RR, Mendelssohn K. (1941). The Oxford vaporiser no. 1. *Lancet*, **2**, 62-4.

5 Cowan SL, Scott RD, Suffolk SF. (1941). The Oxford vaporiser no. 2. *Lancet*, **2**, 64-6.

6 Epstein HG, Pask EA. (1941). The performances of the Oxford vaporisers with ether. *Lancet*, **2**, 66-7.

7 Ehrlich P, Hata S. (1910). *Die experimentelle Chemotherapie der Spirillosen (Syphilis, Rückfallfieber, Hühnerspirillose, Frambösie)*. Berlin; Springer.

8 Domagk G. (1935). Ein Beitrag zur Chemotherapie der bakteriellen Infektionen. *Deutsche Medizinische Wochenschrift*, **61**, 250-3.

9 Tréfouël J, Tréfouël T, Nitti F, Bovet D. (1935). Activité du p-aminophénylsulfamide sur les infections streptococciques expérimentales de la souris et du lapin. *Comptes Rendus Hebdomadaires des Séances de la Société de Biologie et de ses Filiales*, **120**, 756-8.

10 Colebrook L, Buttle GAH, O'Meara RAQ. (1936). The mode of action of p-aminobenzenesulphonamide and prontosil in haemolytic streptococcal infections. *Lancet*, **2**, 1323-6.

11 Finland M, Strauss E, Peterson OL. (1941). Sulfadiazine. Therapeutic evaluation and toxic effects on four hundred and forty-six patients. *Journal of the American Medical*

Association, **116**, 2641-7.

12 Cope Z, ed. (1953). *History of the Second World War. Surgery*. London; HMSO.

13 Lister J. (1876). A contribution to the germ theory of putrefaction and other fermentation changes, and to the natural history of torulae and bacteria. *Transactions of the Royal Society of Edinburgh*, **27**, 313-44. [The paper was read in 1873.]

14 Roberts W. (1874). Studies on biogenesis. *Philosophical Transactions of the Royal Society of London*, **164**, 457-77.

15 Tyndall J. (1876). Optical deportment of the atmosphere in relation to the phenomena of putrefaction and infection. *Philosophical Transactions of the Royal Society of London*, **166**, 27-74.

16 Fleming A. (1929). On the antibacterial action of cultures of a penicillium, with special reference to their use in the isolation of *B. influenzae*. *British Journal of Experimental Pathology*, **10**, 226-36.

17 Abraham EP, Chain E, Fletcher CM, Florey HW, Gardner AD, Heatley NG, Jennings MA. (1941). Further observations on penicillin. *Lancet*, **2**, 177-88.

18 Ogilvie WH. (1944). Abdominal wounds in the Western Desert. *Surgery, Gynecology and Obstetrics*, **78**, 225-38.

19 Harken DE. (1947). The removal of foreign bodies from the pericardium and heart. A moving picture demonstration. *Journal of Thoracic Surgery*, **16**, 701-4.

20 Miscall L. In discussion following Harken DE. (1947). Ref. 19 above.

21 Padgett EC. (1939). Calibrated intermediate skin grafts. *Surgery, Gynecology and Obstetrics*, **69**, 779-93.

22 Gabarro P. (1943). A new method of grafting. *British Medical Journal*, **1**, 723-4.

23 Bodenham DC. (1943). The problem of fractures with associated burn injuries: principles of treatment. *Proceedings of the Royal Society of Medicine*, **36**, 657-62.

24 McIndoe AH. (1943). Skin grafting in the treatment of wounds. *Proceedings of the Royal Society of Medicine*, **36**, 647-56.

25 Wright D. (1956). Commonwealth surgery in the Korean war. *Lancet*, **2**, 505-10.

26 Hughes CW. (1958). Arterial repair during the Korean war. *Annals of Surgery*, **147**, 555-61.

CHAPTER 23: SURGERY OF THE HEART

1 Larrey DJ. (1810). Sur une blessure du péricarde, suivie d'hydro-péricardie. *Bulletin des Sciences Médicales*, **6**, 255-73.

2 Hilsmann FA. (1875). Ueber die paracentese des perikardiums. *Schriften der Universität zu Kiel*, **22**, No. 7. [His father's operation was the basis for FA Hilsmann's inaugural thesis.]

3 Langenbeck B von. (1888). *Vorlesungen über Akiurgie*, pp.449-50. Berlin; Hirschwald.

4 Dieulafoy G. (1873). *A treatise on the pneumatic aspiration of morbid fluids*, pp.219-44. London; Smith, Elder.

5 Cappelen A. (1896). Valvus cordis; sutur of hjertet. *Norsk Magazin for Laegevidenskaben*, **57**, 285-8.

6 Farina G. (1896-7). Sutura del ventricolo destro. *Bulletino di Accademia Medica di Roma*, **23**, 248.

7 Rehn. (1896). Fall von penetrirender Stichverletzung des rechten Ventrikel's Herznaht. Versammlung der Gesellschaft deutscher Naturforscher und Ärzte in Frankfurt a/M. vom 21. Bis 26. September 1896. *Zentralblatt für Chirurgie*, **23**, 1048-9.

8 Milton H. (1897). Mediastinal surgery. *Lancet*, 1, 873-5.

9 Samways DW. (1898). Mitral stenosis: A statistical inquiry. *British Medical Journal*, 1, 364-5.

10 Lane WA. (1902). Letter to the Editor: Surgical operation for mitral stenosis. *Lancet*, 1, 547.

11 Brunton L. (1902). Letter to the Editor: Surgical operation for mitral stenosis. *Lancet*, 1, 547.

12 Tuffier, Hallion. (1898). De la compression rythmée du coeur dans la syncope cardiaque par embolie. *Bulletin de la Société de Chirurgie de Paris*, 24, 937-9.

13 Igelsrud K. (1904). Abdominal hysterectomy; chloroform collapse; massage of the heart; recovery. Personal communication to WW Keen, published in: Keen WW. (1904). A case of total laryngectomy (unsuccessful) and a case of abdominal hysterectomy (successful), in both of which massage of the heart for chloroform collapse was employed, with notes of 25 other cases of cardiac massage. *Therapeutic Gazette*, 28, 217-30. [See p.220.]

14 Starling EA, Lane WA. (1902). Reflex inhibition of the heart during administration of ether in which manual compression of the heart was successful in restoring the circulation. *Lancet*, 2, 1397.

15 Beck CS, Pritchard WH, Feil HS. (1947). Ventricular fibrillation of long duration abolished by electric shock. *Journal of the American Medical Association*, 135, 985-6.

16 Kouwenhoven WB, Jude JR, Knickerbocker GG. (1960). Closed-chest cardiac massage. *Journal of the American Medical Association*, 173, 1064-7.

17 Brauer. (1902). Ueber chronischer adhäsive Mediastino-Perikarditis und deren Behandlung. *Münchener Medizinische Wochenschrift*, 49, 1072.

18 Morison A. (1908). On thoracostomy in heart disease. *Lancet*, 2, 7-12.

19 Delorme (1898). Sur un traitement chirurgical de la symphyse cardo-péricardique. *Bulletin et Mémoires de la Société de Chirurgie de Paris*, 24, 918-22.

20 Rehn L. (1913). Die Chirurgie des Herzens und des Herzbeutels. *Berliner Klinische Wochenschrift*, 50, 241-6.

21 Sauerbruch F, O'Shaughnessy L. (1937). *Thoracic surgery*. London; Arnold.

22 Trendelenburg F. (1908). Ueber die operative Behandlung der Embolie der Lungenarterie. *Archiv für Klinische Chirurgie*, 86, 686-700.

23 Kirschner M. (1924). Ein durch die Trendelenburgsche Operation geheilter Fall von Embolie der Art. pulmonalis. *Archiv für Klinische Chirurgie*, 133, 312-59.

24 Crafoord C. (1929). Two cases of obstructive pulmonary embolism successfully operated upon. *Acta Chirurgica Scandinavica*, 64, 172-86.

25 Steenburg RW, Warren R, Wilson RE, Rudolf LE. (1958). A new look at pulmonary embolectomy. *Surgery, Gynecology and Obstetrics*, 107, 214-20.

26 Cooley DA, Beall SC Jr, Alexander JK. (1961). Acute massive pulmonary embolism: successful surgical treatment using temporary cardiopulmonary bypass. *Journal of the American Medical Association*, 177, 283-6.

27 Munro JC. (1907). Ligation of the ductus arteriosus. *Annals of Surgery*, 46, 335-8.

28 Tuffier T. (1913). Etat actuel de la chirurgie intrathoracique. *Transactions of the XVII International Medical Congress, London*. Section 7, surgery, pp.247-327.

29 Doyen E. (1913). Reported in: Association Française de Chirurgie XXVIe Congrès (Paris 6-11 Octobre 1913). *Presse Médicale*, 21, 860.

30 Allen DS, Graham EA. (1922). Intracardiac surgery – a new method. Preliminary report. *Journal of the American Medical Association*, 79, 1028-30.

31 Cutler EC, Levine SA. (1923). Cardiotomy and valvulotomy for mitral stenosis. Experimental observations and clinical notes concerning an operated case with recovery. *Boston Medical and Surgical Journal*, 188, 1023-7.

32 Beck CS, Cutler EC. (1924). A cardiovalvulotome. *Journal of Experimental Medicine*, 40, 375-9.

33 Souttar HS. (1925). The surgical treatment of mitral stenosis. *British Medical Journal*, 2, 603-6.

34 Pribram BO. (1926). Die operative Behandlung der Mitralstenose. *Archiv für Klinische Chirurgie*, 142, 458-65.

35 Bleichröder F. (1912). Intraarterielle Therapie. *Berliner Klinische Wochenschrift*, 49, 1503-4.

36 Forssmann W. (1929). Die Sondierung des Rechten Herzens. *Klinische Wochenschrift*, 8, 2085-7; 2287.

37 Robb GP, Steinberg I. (1938). A practical method of visualization of the chambers of the heart, the pulmonary circulation, and the great blood vessels in man. *Journal of Clinical Investigation*, 17, 507.

38 Cournand A, Ranges HA. (1941). Catheterization of the right auricle in man. *Proceedings of the Society for Experimental Biology and Medicine*, 46, 462-6.

39 Sones FM, Shirey EK. (1962). Cine coronary arteriography. *Modern Concepts of Cardiovascular Disease*, 31, 735-8.

40 Jonnesco T. (1920). Angine de poitrine guérie par la résection du sympathique cervico-thoracique. *Bulletin de l'Académie de Médecine*, 84, 93-102.

41 François-Franck. (1899). Signification physiologique de la résection du sympathique dans la maladie de Basedow, l'epilepsie, l'idiotie et le glaucome. *Bulletin de l'Académie de Médecine*, 41, 565-94.

42 Mayo CH. In discussion following: Lilienthal H. (1925). Cervical sympathectomy in angina pectoris. A report of three cases. *Archives of Surgery*, 10, 531-43. [See p.541.]

43 Beck CS. (1935). The development of a new blood supply to the heart by operation. *Annals of Surgery*, 102, 801-13.

44 O'Shaughnessy L. (1937). Surgical treatment of cardiac ischaemia. *Lancet*, 1, 185-94.

45 Beck CS, Stanton E, Batiuchok W, Leiter E. (1948). Revascularization of heart by graft of systemic artery into coronary sinus. *Journal of the American Medical Association*, 137, 436-42.

46 Harken DE, Black H, Dickson JF, Wilson HE. (1955). De-epicardialization: A simple, effective treatment for angina pectoris. *Circulation*, 12, 955-62.

47 Vineberg AM. (1946). Development of an anastomosis between the coronary vessels and a transplanted internal mammary artery. *Canadian Medical Association Journal*, 55, 117-19.

48 Vineberg AM. (1954). Internal mammary artery implant in the treatment of angina pectoris: A three year follow up. *Canadian Medical Association Journal*, 70, 367-78.

49 Vineberg A, Pifarre R, Mercier C. (1962). An operation designed to promote the growth of new coronary arteries, using a detached omental graft: A preliminary report. *Canadian Medical Association Journal*, 86, 1116-18.

50 Absolon KB, Aust JB, Varco RL, Lillehei CW. (1956). Surgical treatment of occlusive coronary artery disease by endarterectomy or anastomotic replacement. *Surgery,*

Gynecology and Obstetrics, **103**, 180-5.

51 May AM. (1957). Coronary endarterectomy. Curettement of coronary arteries in dogs. *American Journal of Surgery*, **93**, 969-73.

52 Bailey CP, May AM. (1957). Survival after coronary endarterectomy in man. *Journal of the American Medical Association*, **164**, 641-6.

53 Senning Å. (1961). Strip grafting in coronary arteries. Report of a case. *Journal of Thoracic and Cardiovascular Surgery*, **41**, 542-9.

54 Sawyer PH, Kaplitt MJ, Sobel S, Di Maio D. (1967). Application of gas endarterectomy to atherosclerotic peripheral vessels and coronary arteries: Clinical and experimental results. *Circulation* (suppl. 1), **35, 36**, 163-8.

55 Favaloro R. (1970). *The surgical treatment of arteriosclerosis*, ch. 5, pp.39-66. Baltimore; Williams and Wilkins. [See p.47.]

56 Grüntzig A. (1978). Letter to the Editor: Transluminal dilatation of coronary-artery stenosis. *Lancet*, **1**, 263.

57 Gross RE, Hubbard JP. (1939). Surgical ligation of a patent ductus arteriosus: Report of first successful case. *Journal of the American Medical Association*, **112**, 729-31.

58 Blalock A, Taussig HB. (1945). The surgical treatment of malformations of the heart in which there is pulmonary stenosis or pulmonary atresia. *Journal of the American Medical Association*, **128**, 189-202.

59 Potts WJ, Smith S, Gibson S. (1946). Anastomosis of the aorta to a pulmonary artery. *Journal of the American Medical Association*, **132**, 627-31.

60 Brock RC. (1948). Pulmonary valvotomy for the relief of congenital pulmonary stenosis. Report of three cases. *British Medical Journal*, **1**, 1121-6.

61 Sellors TH. (1948). Surgery of pulmonary stenosis. A case in which the pulmonary valve was successfully divided. *Lancet*, **1**, 988-9.

62 Lillehei CW, Cohen M, Warden HE, Read RC, Aust JB, De Wall RA, Varco RL. (1955). Direct vision intracardiac surgical correction of the tetralogy of Fallot, pentalogy of Fallot, and pulmonary atresia defects. Report of first ten cases. *Annals of Surgery*, **142**, 418-45.

63 Smithy HG, Boone JA, Stallworth JM. (1950). Surgical treatment of constrictive valvular disease of the heart. *Surgery, Gynecology and Obstetrics*, **90**, 175-92.

64 Bailey CP. (1949). Surgical treatment of mitral stenosis. Mitral commissurotomy. *Diseases of the Chest*, **15**, 377-97.

65 Harken DE, Ellis LB, Ware PE, Norman LR. (1948). The surgical treatment of mitral stenosis. I. Valvuloplasty. *New England Journal of Medicine*, **239**, 801-9.

66 Baker C, Brock RC, Campbell M. (1950). Valvulotomy for mitral stenosis. Report of six successful cases. *British Medical Journal*, **1**, 1283-93.

67 Murray G. (1948). Closure of defects in cardiac septa. *Annals of Surgery*, **128**, 843-53.

68 Gross RE, Pomeranz AA, Watkins E, Goldsmith EI. (1952). Surgical closure of defects of the interauricular septum by use of an atrial well. *New England Journal of Medicine*, **247**, 455-60.

69 Bigelow WG, Lindsey WK, Greenwood WF. (1950). Hypothermia. Its possible role in cardiac surgery: an investigation of factors governing survival in dogs at low body temperatures. *Annals of Surgery*, **132**, 849-66.

70 McQuiston WO. (1950). Anesthesia in cardiac surgery. Observations on three hundred and sixty-two cases. *Archives of Surgery*, **61**, 892-9.

71 Lewis FJ, Taufic M. (1953). Closure of atrial septal defects with the aid of hypothermia;

experimental accomplishments and report of one successful case. *Surgery*, **33**, 52-9.

72 Swan H, Zeavin I, Blount SG, Virtue RW. (1953). Surgery by direct vision in the open heart during hypothermia. *Journal of the American Medical Association*, **153**, 1081-5.

73 Boerema I, Wildschut A, Schmidt WJH, Broekhuysen L. (1951). Experimental researches into hypothermia as an aid in surgery of the heart. *Archivum Chirurgicum Neerlandicum*, **3**, 25-34.

74 Delorme EJ. (1952). Experimental cooling of the blood stream. Preliminary communication. *Lancet*, **2**, 914.

75 Ross DN. (1954). Venous cooling. A new method of cooling the blood-stream. *Lancet*, **1**, 1108-9.

76 Drew CE, Anderson IM. (1959). Profound hypothermia in cardiac surgery. Report of three cases. *Lancet*, **1**, 748-50.

77 Gibbon JH. (1937). Artificial maintenance of the circulation during experimental occlusion of the pulmonary artery. *Archives of Surgery*, **34**, 1105-31.

78 Gibbon JH. (1954). Application of a mechanical heart and lung apparatus to cardiac surgery. *Minnesota Medicine*, **37**, 171-80.

79 Björk VO. (1948). An artificial heart or cardiopulmonary machine: performance in animals. *Lancet*, **2**, 491-3.

80 Gerbode F, Osborn JJ, Melrose DG, Perkins HA, Norman A, Baer DM. (1958). Extracorporeal circulation in intracardiac surgery: a comparison between two heart-lung machines. *Lancet*, **2**, 284-6.

81 Melrose DG. Personal communication. [Melrose did not publish an account of the first clinical elective cardiac arrest.]

82 Sergeant CK, Geoghegan T, Lam CR. (1956). Further studies in induced cardiac arrest using the agent acetylcholine. *Surgical Forum*, **7**, 254-7.

83 Lillehei CW, Warden HE, DeWall R, Stanley P, Varco RL. (1957). Cardiopulmonary by-pass in surgical treatment of congenital or acquired cardiac disease. *Archives of Surgery*, **75**, 928-45.

84 Andreasen AT, Watson F. (1952). Experimental cardiovascular surgery. *British Journal of Surgery*, **39**, 548-51.

85 Campbell GS, Crisp NW Jr, Brown EB Jr. (1955). Maintenance of respiratory function with isolated lung lobes during cardiac inflow occlusion. *Proceedings of the Society for Experimental Biology and Medicine*, **88**, 390-3.

86 De Wall RA, Warden HE, Read RC, Gott VL, Ziegler NR, Varco RL, Lillehei CW. (1956). A simple, expendable, artificial oxygenator for open heart surgery. *Surgical Clinics of North America*, **36**, 1025-34.

87 Kirklin JW, Donald DE, Harshbarger HG, Hetzel PS, Patrick RT, Swan HJC, Wood EH. (1956). Studies in extracorporeal circulation. I. Applicability of Gibbon-type pump-oxygenator to human intracardiac surgery. 40 cases. *Annals of Surgery*, **144**, 709-21.

88 Brock RC. (1950). The arterial route to the aortic and pulmonary valves. The mitral route to the mitral valve. *Guy's Hospital Reports*, **99**, 236-46.

89 Bailey CP, Bolton HE, Jamison WL, Larzelere HB. (1953). Commissurotomy for aortic stenosis. *Journal of the International College of Surgeons*, **20**, 393-408.

90 Hufnagel CA, Harvey WP, Rabil PJ, McDermott TF. (1954). Surgical treatment of aortic insufficiency. *Surgery*, **35**, 673-83.

91 Murray G. (1956). Homologous aortic-valve-segment transplants as surgical treatment

for aortic and mitral insufficiency. *Angiology*, **7**, 466–71.

92 Kantrowitz A, Akutsu T, Chaptal P-A, Krakauer J, Kantrowitz AR, Jones RT. (1966). Clinical experience with an implanted mechanical auxiliary ventricle. *Journal of the American Medical Association*, **197**, 525–9.

93 Liotta D, Hall CW, Henly WS, Cooley DA, Crawford ES, De Bakey ME. (1963). Prolonged assisted circulation during and after cardiac or aortic surgery. Prolonged partial left ventricular bypass by means of intracorporeal circulation. *American Journal of Cardiology*, **12**, 399–405

94 De Bakey ME. (1967–8). In: *The year book of general surgery*, p.46. Chicago; Year Book Medical Publishers.

95 Nosé Y, Topaz S, SenGupta A, Tretbar LL, Kolff WJ. (1965). Artificial hearts inside the pericardial sac in calves. *Transactions. American Society for Artificial Organs*, **11**, 255–62.

96 Atsumi K. (1967). Personal communication.

[For a fuller account of the history of cardiac surgery, see: Richardson R. (2001). *Heart and scalpel*. London; Quiller.]

CHAPTER 24: ARTERIAL SURGERY

1   Matas R. (1888). Traumatic aneurism of the left brachial artery. Failure of direct and indirect pressure; ligation of the artery immediately above tumor; return of pulsation on the tenth day; ligation immediately below tumor; failure to arrest pulsation; incision and partial excision of sac; recovery. *Medical News (Philadelphia)*, **53**, 462–6.

2   Matas R. (1908). The statistics of endoaneurismorrhaphy, or the radical cure of aneurism by intrasaccular suture. Summary of cases reported up to June 1, 1908. *Journal of the American Medical Association*, **51**, 1667–71.

3   Jaboulay M, Briau E. (1896). Recherches expérimentales sur la suture et la greffe artérielles. *Lyon Médicale*, **81**, 97–9.

4   Murphy JB. (1897). Resection of arteries and veins injured in continuity – end-to-end suture – experimental and clinical research. *Medical Record, New York*, **51**, 73–88.

5   Nitze T. (1897). Demonstration at the XII international medical congress in Moscow, 19–26 August 1897. *Zentralblatt für Chirurgie*, **24**, 1042.

6   Payr E. (1900). Beiträge zur Technik der Blutgefäss-und Nervennaht nebst Mittheilungen über die Verwendung eines resorbirbaren Metalles in der Chirurgie. *Archiv für Klinische Chirurgie*, **62**, 67–93.

7   Dionis (1710). *A course of chirurgical operations demonstrated in the Royal Garden at Paris*. Translated from the Paris edition. London; Tonson. [See p.389.]

8   Carrel A. (1902). La technique opératoire des anastomoses vasculaires et la transplantation des viscères. *Lyon Médicale*, **98**, 859–64.

9   Carrel A, Guthrie CC. (1906). Anastomoses des vaisseaux sanguins. *XV Congrès International de Médecine* (Lisbon, April 1906). Section de Chirurgie, 238–49.

10 Carrel A. (1908). Results of the transplantation of blood vessels, organs and limbs. *Journal of the American Medical Association*, **51**, 1662–7.

11 Guthrie CC. (1912). *Blood-vessel surgery and its applications*. London; Arnold. [Describes in detail his and Carrel's method of vascular anastomosis and the many uses in transplantation to which they put it.]

12 Pringle JH. (1913). Two cases of vein-grafting for the maintenance of a direct arterial circulation. *Lancet*, **1**, 1795–6.

13 Lexer E. (1912). Zur Gesichtsplastik. *Verhandlungen der Deutschen Gesellschaft für Chirurgie*, **41**, pt 1, 132-3.

14 Lexer E. (1913). Ideale Aneurysmaoperation und Gefässtransplantation. *Verhandlungen der Deutschen Gesellschaft für Chirurgie*, **42**, pt 1, 113-16.

15 Lexer E. (1907). Die ideale Operation des arteriellen und des arteriell-venösen Aneurysma. *Archiv für Klinische Chirurgie*, **83**, 459-77.

16 Crafoord C, Nylin G. (1945). Congenital coarctation of the aorta and its surgical treatment. *Journal of Thoracic Surgery*, **14**, 347-61.

17 Gross RE. (1945). Surgical correction for coarctation of the aorta. *Surgery*, **18**, 673-8.

18 Blalock A, Park EA. (1944). The surgical treatment of experimental coarctation (atresia) of the aorta. *Annals of Surgery*, **119**, 445-56.

19 Murray G. (1950). Vascular surgery. In: *British surgical practice*, ed. Carling ER, Ross JP. Vol. 8, pp. 489-528. London; Butterworth.

20 Gross RE. (1950). Coarctation of the aorta. Surgical treatment of one hundred cases. *Circulation*, **1**, 41-55.

21 Gross RE, Bill AH, Peirce EC. (1949). Methods for preservation and transplantation of arterial grafts. Observations on arterial grafts in dogs. Report of transplantation of preserved arterial grafts in 9 human cases. *Surgery, Gynecology and Obstetrics*, **88**, 689-701.

22 Voorhees AB, Jaretzki A, Blakemore AW. (1952). The use of tubes constructed of Vinyon "N" cloth in bridging arterial defects. *Annals of Surgery*, **135**, 332-6.

23 Welch K. (1956). Excision of occlusive lesions of the middle cerebral artery. *Journal of Neurosurgery*, **13**, 73-80.

24 Jacobson JH II, Wallman LJ, Schumacher GA, Flanagan M, Suarez EL, Donaghy RM. (1962). Microsurgery as an aid to middle cerebral artery endarterectomy. *Journal of Neurosurgery*, **19**, 108-15.

CHAPTER 25: ORGAN TRANSPLANTATION

1 Malt RA, McKhann CF. (1964). Replantation of severed arms. *Journal of the American Medical Association*, **189**, 716-22.

2 Guthrie CC. (1912). *Blood-vessel surgery and its applications*. London; Arnold.

3 Carrel A. (1907). The surgery of blood vessels, etc. *Bulletin of the Johns Hopkins Hospital*, **18**, 18-28.

4 Carrel A. (1906). Surgery of the blood-vessels and its application to changes of circulation and transplantation of organs. *Bulletin of the Johns Hopkins Hospital*, **17**, 236-7.

5 Demikhov VP. (1962). *Experimental transplantation of vital organs*. Translated by B. Haigh. New York; Consultants Bureau.

6 Broster LR, Gardiner-Hill H. (1946). A case of Addison's disease successfully treated by a graft. *British Medical Journal*, **2**, 570-2.

7 Lannelongue OM. (1890). Transplantation du corps thyroïde sur l'homme. *Bulletin Médicale*, **4**, 225.

8 Morris RT. (1906). A case of heteroplastic ovarian grafting, followed by pregnancy, and the delivery of a living child. *Medical Record, New York*, **69**, 697-8.

9 Hardy JD. (1964). The transplantation of organs. *Surgery*, **56**, 685-705.

10 Lillehei RC, Manax WG. (1966). Organ transplantation.....a review of past accomplishments, present problems and future hopes. *Anesthesia and Analgesia;*

Current Researches, **45**, 707-32.

11 Kelly WD, Lillehei RC, Merkel FK, Idezuki Y, Goetz FC. (1967). Allotransplantation of the pancreas and duodenum along with the kidney in diabetic nephropathy. *Surgery*, **61**, 827-37.

12 Ullman E. (1902). Experimentell nierentransplantation: Verläufige mitteilung. *Wiener Klinische Wochenschrift*, **15**, 281-2.

13 Princeteau M. (1905). Greff rénale. *Journal de Médecine de Bordeaux*, **26**, 549.

14 Jaboulay M. (1906). Greffe de reins au pli du coude par soudures artérielles et veineuses. *Lyon Médicale*, **107**, 575-7.

15 Floresco N. (1905). Recherches sur la transplantation du rein. *Journal de Physiologie et de Pathologie Générale*, **7**, 47-59.

16 Unger E. (1910). Nierentransplantationen. *Klinische Wochenschrift*, **47**, 573-8.

17 Neuhof H. (1923). *Transplantation of tissues*. New York; Appleton. [See p.260.]

18 Hume DM, Merrill JP, Miller BF. (1952). Homologous transplantation of human kidneys. *Journal of Clinical Investigation*, **31**, 640-1.

19 Hume DM, Merrill JP, Miller BF, Thorn GW. (1955). Experiences with renal homotransplantation in the human: report of nine cases. *Journal of Clinical Investigation*, **34**, 327-82.

20 Michon L, Hamburger J, Oeconomos N, Delinotte P, Richet G, Vaysse J, Antione B. (1953). Une tentative de transplantation rénale chez l'homme. Aspects médicaux et biologiques. *Presse Médicale*, **61**, 1419-23.

21 Murray G, Holden R. (1954). Transplantation of kidneys, experimentally and in human cases. *American Journal of Surgery*, **87**, 508-15.

22 Merrill JP, Murray JE, Harrison JH, Guild WR. (1956). Successful homotransplantation of the human kidney between identical twins. *Journal of the American Medical Association*, **160**, 277-82.

23 Murray JE, Merrill JP, Harrison JH. (1958). Kidney transplantation between seven pairs of identical twins. *Annals of Surgery*, **148**, 343-59.

24 Medawar PB. (1944). The behaviour and fate of skin autografts and skin homografts in rabbits. *Journal of Anatomy*, **78**, 176-99.

25 Merrill JP, Murray JE, Harrison JH, Friedman EA, Dealy JB, Dammin GJ. (1960). Successful homotransplantation of the kidney between nonidentical twins. *New England Journal of Medicine*, **262**, 1251-60. [See also: Annotation (1959). Successful kidney homograft. *Lancet*, **1**, 874.]

26 Reemtsma K, McCracken BH, Schlegel JU, Pearl MA, DeWitt CW, Creech O Jr. (1964). Reversal of early graft rejection after renal heterotransplantation in man. *Journal of the American Medical Association*, **187**, 691-6.

27 Reemtsma K. (1966). Renal heterotransplantation. *Advances in Surgery*, **2**, 285-93.

28 Kolff WJ, Berk HTJ, ter Welle M, van Noordwijk J. (1944). The artificial kidney: a dialyser with a great area. *Acta Medica Scandinavica*, **117**, 121-34.

29 Kolff WJ. (1946). *The artificial kidney*. Kampen; Kok.

30 Juvenelle AA, Citret C, Wiles CE, Stewart JD. (1951). Pneumonectomy with replantation of the lung in the dog for physiologic study. *Journal of Thoracic Surgery*, **21**, 111-15.

31 Hardy JD, Webb WR, Dalton ML Jr, Walker GR. (1963). Lung homotransplantation in man. Report of the initial case. *Journal of the American Medical Association*, **186**, 1065-74.

32 Goodrich EO, Welch HF, Nelson JA, Beecher TS, Welch CS. (1956). Homotransplantation

of the canine liver. *Surgery*, **39**, 244-51.

33 Starzl TE, Marchioro TL, Porter KA, Brettschneider L. (1967). Homotransplantation of the liver. *Transplantation*, **5**, 790-803.

34 Eisman B. (1966). Treatment of hepatic coma by extracorporeal liver perfusion. *Annals of the Royal College of Surgeons of England*, **38**, 329-48.

35 Mann FC, Priestley JT, Markowitz J, Yater WM. (1933). Transplantation of the intact mammalian heart. *Archives of Surgery*, **26**, 219-24.

36 Cookson BA, Neptune WB, Bailey CP. (1952). Hypothermia as a means of performing intracardiac surgery under direct vision. *Diseases of the Chest*, **22**, 245-60.

37 Lower RR, Shumway NE. (1960). Studies on orthotopic homotransplantation of the canine heart. *Surgical Forum*, **11**, 18-19.

38 Hardy JD, Chavez CM, Kurrus FD, Neely WA, Eraslan S, Turner MD, Fabian LW, Labecki TD. (1964). Heart transplantation in man. Developmental studies and report of a case. *Journal of the American Medical Association*, **188**, 1132-40.

39 Shumway NE, Lower RR. (1964). Special problems in transplantation of the heart. *Annals of the New York Academy of Sciences*, **120**, 773-7.

40 Barnard CN. (1967). A human cardiac transplant: an interim report of a successful operation performed at Groote Schuur Hospital, Cape Town. *South African Medical Journal*, **41**, 1271-4.

41 Thomson JG. (1968). Heart transplantation in man – necropsy findings. *British Medical Journal*, **2**, 511-17.

42 Shrire V, Barnard CN. (1966). An analysis of cardiac surgery at Groote Schuur Hospital, Cape Town, for the 14 years April 1951 – April 1965. *South African Medical Journal*, **40**, 279-84; 461-7.

43 Kantrowitz A, Haller JD, Joos H, Cerruti MM, Carstensen HE. (1968). Transplantation of the heart in an infant and an adult. *American Journal of Cardiology*, **22**, 782-90.

44 Barnard CN. (1968). Human cardiac transplantation. An evaluation of the first two operations performed at the Groote Schuur Hospital, Cape Town. *American Journal of Cardiology*, **22**, 584-96.

45 Stinson EB, Dong E Jr, Schroeder JS, Harrison DC, Shumway NE. (1968). Initial clinical experience with heart transplantation. *American Journal of Cardiology*, **22**, 791-803.

46 Cooley DA. (1968). Quotations from an exclusive Tribune interview. *Medical Tribune*, June 20, 1968, pp. 1, 18.

47 Cooley DA, Bloodwell RD, Hallman GL, Nora JJ. (1968). Transplantation of the human heart. Report of four cases. *Journal of the American Medical Association*, **205**, 479-86.

48 Ross D. (1968). Report of a heart transplant operation. *American Journal of Cardiology*, **22**, 838-9.

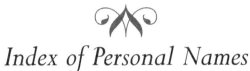

Index of Personal Names

Bowditch, Henry Ingersoll, 1808-92, 187-8
Boyle, Robert, 1627-91, 182
Bramann, Fritz, 1854-1913, 147
Brauer, Ludolph, 1865-1951, 188-9, 213
Bricker, Eugene (1950), 103
Bristow, Walter Rowley, 1882-1947, 178
Broca, Pierre Paul, 1824-80, 122
Brock, *Lord* Russell Claude, 1903-80, 218, 219, 222
Brodie, *Sir* Benjamin Collins, 1783-1862, 48
Brooke, Bryan Nicholas (1952), 100
Broussais, François Joseph Victor, 1772-1838, 83
Broster, Lennox Ross, 1889-1965, 233
Brown, John Young (1913), 97-8
Bruck, Julius, 1840-1902, 51
Brunn, Harold, 1874-1950, 193-4
Bruns, Viktor von, 1812-83, 31
Brunschwig, Alexander, 1901-69, 45, 104
Brunton, *Sir* Thomas Lauder, 1844-1916, 212
Bryant, Thomas, 1828-1914, 85
Bülau, Gotthard, 1835-1900, 188
Burckhardt, Gottlieb, 1836-1907, 136
Burney, Frances (Fanny), Madame Alexandre d'Arblay, 1752-1840, 1, 2, 117
Buttle, Gladwin Albert Hurst, 1899-1983, 203

Callisen, Hendrik, 1740-1824, 78-9
Calvin, John, 1509-64, 18
Cappelen, Axel, ?-1919, 211
Carnochan, John Murray, 1817-87, 126
Carr, W.P. (1911), 57
Carrel, Alexis, 1873-1944, 135, 171, 226-7, 231, 232, 234, 239
Carson, James, 1772-1843, 188
Cavour, *Count* Camillo Benso di, 1810-61, 167
Ceci, Antonio, 1852-1920, 169
Celsus, 53 BC-AD 7, 69
Cerenville, Edouard de, 1843-1915, 188
Chadwick, *Sir* Edwin, 1800-90, 167
Chain, Ernst Boris, 1906-79, 204
Chamberland, Charles (1884), 55
Championnière, Just Marie Marcellin Lucas, 1843-1913, 30
Chauliac, Guy de, 1300-68, 6, 115
Cheselden, William, 1668-1752, 48, 70
Chisholm, J.J. (1862), 168
Churchill, Edward Delos, 1895-?, 196

Civiale, Jean, 1792-1867, 48-9
Clark, R. Lee (1939), 101
Clarke, Joseph, 1758-1834, 22
Clarke, William E. (1842), 10
Clover, Joseph Thomas, 1825-82, 49, 50
Clute, Howard Merrill, 1890-1946, 101
Coffey, Robert Calvin, 1869-1933, 103
Cohn, Ferdinand Julius, 1828-98, 54
Colebrook, *Sir* Leonard, 1883-1967, 201
Collins, Robert, 1801-68, 22-3, 54, 59
Collis, Maurice Henry, 1824-69, 149
Colton, Gardner Quincy, 1814-?, 10
Cone, William Vernon, 1897-?, 135
Cooley, Denton A., b.1920, 213, 242-3
Corbett, Rupert Shelton (1945), 99
Cosmas, *Saint*, c. AD 303, 231
Cournand, André Frédéric, 1895-1988, 215
Courvoisier, Ludwig G., 1843-1918, 42
Crafoord, Clarence, 1899-?, 192, 213, 227
Crampton, *Sir* Philip (1846), 49
Cripps, William Harrison, 1850-1923, 91
Crohn, Burrill Bernard, 1884-?, 101-2
Crookes, *Sir* William, 1832-1919, 159
Cullen, Thomas Stephen, 1868-1953, 119
Cushing, Harvey Williams, 1869-1939, 118, 119, 127-8, 131-4, 135, 138, 140
Cutler, Elliott Carr, 1888-1947, 214
Czermak, Johann Nepomak, 1828-73, 146
Czerny, Vincenz, 1842-1916, 94

Dakin, Henry Drysdale, 1880-1952, 171-2
Damian, *Saint*, c. AD 303, 231
Dana, Richard Henry, 1815-82, 12
Dandy, Walter Edward, 1886-1946, 126, 134
Davies, Hugh Morriston, 1879-1965, 194
Davies-Colley, John Neville Colley, 1842-1900, 85-6
Davy, *Sir* Humphry, 1778-1829, 9, 10
De Bakey, Michael Ellis, b.1908, 223
Delorme, Edmond, 1847-1929, 213
Delorme, Edmund Joseph, b.1911, 220
Demikhov, Vladimir Petrovitch (1946), 232, 237
Denis, Jean Baptiste, ?-1704, 182
Denman, Thomas, 1733-1815, 22
Desault, Pierre Joseph, 1744-95, 72, 77, 173
Dieulafoy, Georges, 1839-1911, 211
Dionis, Pierre, 1645-1718, 226
Dioscorides, Pedacius, c. AD 60, 8
Dittel, Leopold Ritter von, 1815-98, 51

Dixon, Claude Frank, 1893-?, 101
Dixon, L.F. (1937), 59
Domagk, Gerhard, 1895-?, 201
Doyen, Eugène Louis, 1859-1916, 40, 214
Dragstedt, Lester Reynold, 1893-1975, 40, 100
Drew, Charles Edwin, 1916-87, 220
Dubois,Antoine, 1756-1837, 1, 2, 74
Duchainois (1767), 44
Dufour (1907), 191
Dumas, Charles Louis, 1765-1813, 77-8, 89
Dunant, Jean Henri, 1828-1910, 167
Duncan, James Matthews, 1826-90, 17, 151
Dunhill, *Sir*, Thomas Peel, 1876-1957, 140
Durante, Francesco, 1844-1934, 123
Duret, C. (1793), 76-7, 79
Dusch, Theodor von, 1824-90, 26
Dupuytren, Guillaume, 1777-1835, 75, 79, 82

Eberth, Carl Joseph, 1835-1926, 56
Edward VII, 1841-1910, 67
Edwards, Arthur Tudor, 1890-1946, 195
Ehrlich, Paul, 1854-1915, 201
Eiselsberg, Anton Freiheer von, 1860-1939, 139
Eiseman, Ben, b.1917, 239
Elderton, John (1817), 48
Elisha, *c.* 895 BC, 213
Elsberg, Charles Albert, 1871-1948, 191
Emmet, Thomas Addis, 1828-1919, 151
Erichsen, *Sir* John Eric, 1818-96, 46, 83, 84
Esmarch, Johann Friedrich August von, 1823-1908, 55, 168
Estlander, Jakob August, 1831-81, 188
Evans, Arthur (1909), 197
Eve, *Sir* Frederic Samuel, 1853-1916, 159

Faget, Jean F. (1739), 90
Fallot, Etienne Louis Arthur, 1850-1911, 218
Fantus, Bernard, 1874-1940, 184
Faraday, Michael, 1791-1867, 10
Farina, Guido (1896), 211
Favaloro, René, 1923-2000, 217
Fell, George Edward, 1850-1918, 190
Ferguson, Alexander Hugh, 1853-1912, 135
Fergusson, *Sir* William, 1808-87, 32
Fernel, Jean François, 1497-1558, 61-2
Ferrier, *Sir* David, 1843-1928, 122
Fiamberti, A. Mario (1937), 136-7

Fine, Pierre, 1760-1814, 75, 78
Fitz, Reginald Heber, 1843-1913, 61, 64-5
Fleming, *Sir* Alexander, 1881-1955, 204
Floresco, N. (1905), 234
Florey, *Lord* Howard Walter, 1898-1968, 204
Flugge, Carl (1897), 56
Forestier, Jacques, 1890-?, 192
Forlanini, Carlo, 1847-1918, 188
Forssmann, Werner Theodor Otto, 1904-79, 215
Franco, Pierre, 1500-61, 48
François-Franck, Charles Emile, 1849-1921, 215
Frazier, Charles Harrison, 1870-1936, 128, 129, 131, 133
Frederick III, Emperor of Germany, 1831-88, 147
Freeman, Walter Jackson, 1895-?, 136
Freer, George R.V., ?-1867, 79
Frère Jacques (Jacques de Beaulieu), 1651-1719, 48
Freund, Wilhelm Alexander, 1833-1918, 151
Friedrich, Paul L. (1898), 173, 189
Fritsch, Gustav Theodor, 1838-97, 122

Gabarro, P. (1943), 208
Gabriel, William Bahall, 1893-1975, 98
Galen, 130-c..200, 69, 225
Gallie, William Edward, 1882-1959, 133-14
Garcia, Manuel, 1805-1906, 145-6
Garcia, Manuel del Popolo Vicente, 1775-1832, 145
Gardiner-Hill, Harold, 1891-1982, 233
Gardner, Campbell (1951), 100
Garlock, John Harry, 1896-?, 197
Gärtner (1895), 135
Gatling, Richard Jordan, 1818-1903, 168
Gedroitz, *Princess* Vera Ignatievna (1905), 170-1
Gengou, Octave, 1875-?, 183
Gerhardt, Karl Adolph Christian Jacob, 1833-1902, 147
Gibbon, John Heysham Jr, 1903-73, 221
Gigli, Leonardo, 1863-1908, 124
Gillies, *Sir* Harold Delf, 1882-1960, 179, 191, 207
Godlee, *Sir* Rickman John, 1849-1925, 124
Goodrich, Edward O. (1956), 238
Gordon, Alexander, 1752-99, 22, 23
Gourdet, J. (1895), 188

Kelsey, Charles B. (1889), 87

Kennedy, Charles S., 1887-?, 103–4

Kennedy, Evory, 1806-86, 16

Kenny, Méave (1936), 201

Kerr, John Martin Munro, 1868-1960, 153

Kessel, Jean (1876), 145

Killian, Gustav, 1860-1921, 146

Kirklin, John Webster, b.1917, 222

Kirschner, Martin, 1879-1942, 95, 113, 196, 213

Kirstein, Alfred, 1863-1922, 146, 190

Klein, Jacob (1849), 25

Kneeland, Samuel, 1821-88, 23

Knox, Robert, 1791-1862, 15

Koch, Robert, 1843-1910, 53–4

Kocher, Theodor, 1841-1917, 45, 91, 131, 138–40

Koeberlé, Eugène, 1828-1915, 36

Kolff, Willem Johan, b.1911, 223, 235, 236

Koller, Karl, 1857-1944, 107

Koontz, Amos Ralph, 1890-?, 114

Koster, Harry, 1893-?, 101

Kouwenhoven, William Bennett, 1886-1975, 212-3

Kraske, Paul, 1851-1930, 91

Krause, Fedor, 1857-1937, 127, 132

Krönlein, Rudolf Ulrich, 1847-1910, 39, 64

Krynauw, Rowland Anthony Harold, b.1907, 126

Küchenmeister, Gottlob Friedrich Heinrich, 1821-90, 29

Kühn, Franz, 1866-1929, 191

Kümmell, Hermann, 1852-1937, 56

Küster, Ernst Georg Ferdinand von, 1839-1930, 117, 144

Labarraque, Antoine-Germaine, 1777-1850, 22

Lam, Conrad Ramsey, 1905-?, 221-2

Landois, Leonard, 1837-1902, 182

Landsteiner, Karl, 1868-1943, 183, 184

Lane, *Sir* William Arbuthnot, 1856-1943, 161-3, 179, 184, 188, 212

Langenbeck, Bernhard Rudolf Konrad von, 1810-87, 37, 155, 162, 163, 211

Langenbuch, Carl Johann August, 1864-1901, 45

Lannelongue, Odilon Marc (1890), 233

L'Anglas (1767), 44

Larrey, *Baron* Dominique Jean, 1756-1842, 1, 9, 72-3, 111, 117, 172, 173, 211

Le Dran, Henri François, 1685-1770, 70–1

Leiter, Joseph, ?-1892, 51

Lemaire, François-Jules, 1814-?, 29

Lembert, Antoine, 1802-51, 38

Le Mesurier, Arthur Baker, 1889-?, 113–14

Lempert, Julius, 1890-?, 144

Lennander, Karl Gustav, 1857-1908, 67

Leopold I, 1790-1865, 49

Lewis, Floyd John, b.1916, 220

Lewisohn, Richard, 1875-?, 183

Lexer, Erich, 1867-1937, 227

Libavius, Andreas, 1546-1616, 182

Lilienthal, Howard, 1861-1946, 97

Lillehei, Clarence Walton, 1918-99, 216, 219, 222

Lillehei, Richard Carlton, b.1927, 233–4

Lima, Almeida (1936), 136

Lisfranc, Jacques, 1790-1847, 90

Lister, *Baron* Joseph, 1827-1912, 4, 14, 19, 20, 25, 26-32, 35, 53, 122, 162, 163, 181, 203, 243

Liston, Robert, 1794-1847, 13–15, 16

Little, Louis Stromeyer, 1840-1911, 155

Little, William John, 1810-94, 154–5

Littre, Alexis, 1658-1726, 72, 74

Lizars, John, 1787-1860, 126

Lockhart-Mummery, John Percy, 1875-1957, 94, 98

Lockwood, Charles Barrett, 1858-1914, 55

Long, Crawford Williamson, 1815-78, 10, 12, 13

Lorenz, Adolf, 1854-1946, 156–7

Lotheissen, Georg, 1868-1935, 112

Löw, Oscar (1885), 59

Lower, Richard, 1631-91, 182

Lower, Richard Rowland, b.1929, 241

Lund, Edward, 1823-98, 85

Lundy, John Silas, 1894-?, 195–6

Lyerly, James Gilbert, 1893-?, 137

McArthur, Lewis Linn, 1858-1934, 67, 113-14

McBurney, Charles, 1845-1913, 45, 65, 66-7, 88-9, 125

McClure, R.D. (1909), 135

MacCormac, William, 1836-1901, 168, 170

McDowell, Ephraim, 1771-1830, 35

Macewen, *Sir* William, 1848-1924, 33, 53, 111, 123, 130, 155, 189, 190

McIndoe, *Sir* Archibald Hector, 1900-60, 208

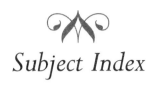

Subject Index

Plastics,
 aortic valve, 222
 arterial prosthesis, 228
 corneal graft, 143
 joints, 164
 oxygenator, disposable, 222
Plastic surgery, 178-9, 207-8
Pleural cavity, anatomy of, 187
Pneumonectomy, 189, 194, 195
 with cautery, 193
Pneumothorax, 186, 187, 188, 192, 207
 artificial, 188
Pneumoventriculography, 134
Poliomyelitis, 158-9
Polyposis, familial, 99
Prontosil, 201
Prostate cancer, 120
Psychosurgery, 136-7
Puerperal fever, 22 ff., 201
Pulmonary,
 cancer, 193, 194-5, 196
 embolism, 95, 213-14
 suppuration, 187, 193, 194, 196
 tuberculosis, 187, 188-9, 192, 196
  apicectomy, 189
  collapse therapy, 188, 192
  lobectomy, 193 ff.
  phrenic paralysis, 189
  pneumonectomy, 189
  pneumothorax, artificial, 188
  segmental resection, 196
Pulmonary valve stenosis, 214, 218, 223
Pulse charts, 118
Pyloroplasty, 40

Radiotherapy, 160-1
 breast cancer, in, 119, 120
Rectum,
 cancer, 75, 78, 79, 83, 84, 88, 90 ff.,
  93 ff., 104
 imperforate, 74, 90
Red Cross, 167
Rehabilitation, 177, 206
Relaxant drugs, 192, 196
Replantation of arm, 231
Residencies, surgical, 108
Respiration,
 artificial, 213
 paradoxical, 108
Royal Army Medical Corps, 166

Ryle's tube, 185
Saline infusion, 184, 200
Salvarsan, 201
Scribner shunt, 237
Scrubbing up, 56
Shock, 175, 176, 181, 184
Sims's position, 149
Skin grafting, 178-9, 203, 204, 208, 209
Solferino, battle of, 167
Soporific sponge, 9
Specialization, rise of, 140-1
Speculum, vaginal, 148, 149
Spencer Wells forceps, 35-6
Spinal cord, tumours of, 130
Spinal fusion, 163
Splint,
 Thomas, 175, 203
 Tobruk, 203, 209
Spontaneous generation, 22, 26
Stapes mobilization, 144-5
Statistics, 41
Sterilization, 54-5, 58 ff.
 gaseous, 59
 infra-red, 58
 irradiation, 59-60
 ultra-violet, 58
Stoma bag, Koenig-Rutzen, 99, 103
Stomach cancer, 38-9, 197
Streptomycin, 196
Subaqueous drainage, 188
Sulphonamides, 185, 201, 204, 206, 207, 208

Telemanipulation, 244
Tendon transplantation, 159, 178, 208
Tenotomy, subcutaneous, 154-5
Tetanus, 168, 172
Tetany, 139
Thalidomide, 169
Thomas splint, 175, 203
Thoraco-abdominal approach, 196-7
Thyroid gland, 107, 138 ff.
Thyrotoxicosis, 139-40
Tobruk splint, 203, 209
Tongue cancer, 138
Transplantation of organs, 230 ff.
 adrenal gland, 233
 duodenum, 233-4
 heart, 224, 230, 239 ff.
 kidney, 233, 234 ff.
 liver, 238-9